"I have known and appreciated Tina Stromsted for many years and shared the podium with her in several major conferences, bringing together my own work on trauma's defenses with her work on Authentic Movement. Here, she has collected important papers and presentations together with new material in the fine book you now hold in your hands. Her work has always been important to the field and is especially relevant now because we have finally come to understand that all trauma is an injury to the capacity to feel, and that early, unremembered trauma is encoded in the body where it remains inaccessible to rational or interpretive methods of psychotherapy. Learning how to work with the body on behalf of frozen or unconscious feelings is therefore crucial to the healing of early trauma, and Tina's enlightening book explores many such methods and provides vivid case examples of her remarkable integrative healing approach. I highly recommend this book!"

Donald Kalsched, *PhD, Jungian analyst and author of*
Trauma and the Soul

"Over the years, Tina Stromsted, a pioneer in studies of somatic psychotherapy and scholar in Jungian theory, and I, in interpersonal neurobiology, have engaged in a mutually enriching interdisciplinary dialogue. We both share a common interest in the central themes of this remarkable book—the fundamental relationships between mind and body, the critical role of emotional processes, and the development of the unconscious mind. Other areas include trauma, metaphors, spontaneous gestures, and images, all essential processes of the right brain—the neurobiological locus of Jung's anima, and the source of the feminine component of the personality. This remarkable book, the capstone of her prolific career, contains a treasure trove of fascinating case material and clinical wisdom. It is essential reading for anyone working with the deeper bodily-based strata of the human psyche."

Allan Schore, *PhD, Neuroscientist and neuropsychoanalyst, author of*
The Right Brain and the Origin of Human Nature

"Soul's *Body* is vital resource, blending Active Imagination, movement, and embodied practices with Jungian thought in ways that are profoundly applicable to our modern world. Whether you are a clinician, a health practitioner, a student, or someone seeking personal healing, you will find this book to be a wise and compassionate guide. Tina's gentle yet penetrating curiosity invites you to join her exploration as she guides us in a living dance through a process of embodied consciousness—connecting us more deeply to ourselves, one another, and the Earth itself. I know of no one better to bring you this profoundly integrative healing work."

Joan Chodorow, *PhD, Jungian analyst, author of* Dance Therapy &
Depth Psychology: The Moving Imagination

"You don't have to be a dancer to explore the emotions, memories, and dreams trapped in the cells of your body. *Soul's Body* invites the reader to tap into the story of your body through natural movement. Tina Stromsted has been a practitioner and teacher of Authentic Movement for decades, and this book charts her journey as well as the evolution of her integrative therapeutic approach. Through examples from her clinical practice with individuals and cross-cultural groups Tina demonstrates how following the imagination as it moves through the body heals the split between body and psyche. *Soul's Body* is a masterpiece—a gift to us all, extensive in its scholarship and practical in its use."

Maureen Murdock, *PhD, psychotherapist and author of* The Heroine's Journey, *and* Mythmaking: Self-Discovery and the Timeless Art of Memoir

"You are truly fortunate to have in your hands this remarkably rich, creative, engaging synthesis of psyche and soma in transformative practices that transcends the usual therapeutic categories. Tina Stromsted masterfully returns an embodied, feminine intelligence to the world in the broadest sense. Personal, clinical, and environmental forms of healing are all explored in depth. A lifetime of gathering wisdom is alchemically distilled into this enlivening elixir of a book, to be savored and enjoyed repeatedly."

Joseph Cambray, *PhD, IAAP, past-president/CEO,*
Pacifica Graduate Institute

"Tina Stromsted's long-awaited, beautifully written book is a valuable addition to the Jungian legacy that highlights the body's innate wisdom in analytic practice. Her case studies reflect her expertise and the attunement and care she provides to analysands and students on their individuation journeys. Decades of clinical experience, cross-cultural international teaching, and scholarship bear fruit in her integrative approach that combines somatic elements with the life of the psyche and the spirit. This collection offers a rich and creative perspective on embodiment, dreamwork, elements of group practice, and our essential resonance with nature."

Robert Hinshaw, *PhD, Faculty, CG Jung Institute,*
Zürich; Publisher Daimon Verlag

"This book is a precious gift to us from a woman who has courageously followed the guidance of her heart. Drawing on Jung's practice of active imagination and the experiences of mentors whose discoveries inspired her, this book is a symphony of her discoveries and the many creative practices she developed that heal both body and soul. Her approach offers a template for the teaching of moving and witnessing for adults, and in schools of the future where children could be taught the embodied wisdom our world needs."

Anne Baring, *PhD, author of* The Dream of the Cosmos:
A Quest for the Soul, Divine Wisdom, *and* Divine Wisdom
and the Holy Spirit: The Forgotten Feminine Face of God

"This beautiful book, *Soul's Body*, by expert Somatic and Movement Psychotherapist Tina Stromsted, celebrates an amazing integration of several arenas of somatic work, including active imagination, dreamwork, Authentic Movement, and embodied psychotherapy. This work, the result of decades of clinical work, international teaching, and the publication of dozens of articles, provides an excellent guide for individuals and students in this rarely integrated field. It is well-designed, incredibly well-written, and contains many illustrative case vignettes. Backed up by detailed research references, this exceptional collection conveys her unique, subtle, yet powerful contributions to the various fields of professional work. Highly recommended!"

Courtenay Young, *UK Somatic (Body) Psychotherapist,*
editor and author

"Reading this collection enriches us with the author's extensive knowledge and experience in depth-oriented embodied work. Here, Tina Stromsted explores the body as a vessel for memories and identity, drawing on renowned sources and detailed descriptions of the integrative work she has developed with individuals and groups. Her insights into conscious embodiment in the healing and growth process can benefit a range of professional disciplines!"

Sharon Chaiklin, *BC-DMT, Founding member of the American Dance*
Therapy Association, past president of the Marian Chace Foundation,
co-editor of Dance and Creativity within Dance/Movement Therapy:
International Perspectives with Hilda Wengrower

"Psychotherapy approaches limit their effectiveness when they fail to include the body, the soul, or the collective level of the psyche. In this rich book, the extremely talented, experienced, and creative Tina Stromsted makes significant theoretical and clinical contributions towards bridging the important links between the psyche, the body, the soul, and the collective and for embodying all levels of the psyche, through active imagination, Authentic Movement, and other embodiment tools. The book will be a valuable resource not only for Jungians but also for any therapist or layperson interested in ways to improve the outcomes of their work."

Dr. Raja Selvam, *PhD, senior trainer in Peter Levine's*
Somatic Experiencing (SE) professional trauma training
programs, the developer of Integral Somatic Psychology (ISP),
and author of The Practice of Embodying Emotions: A Guide
for Improving Cognitive, Emotional, and Behavioral Outcomes

"This book is a dance! It is a necessity: a multifaceted guide for those who have been wondering how to integrate movement and psyche to heal body, mind, soul, community, and Earth. Here you'll find many compelling practices and experiences explored at a depth not easily found in books. Tina is a caring and supportive mentor whose guidance in this book can be used by someone who wants to explore but doesn't easily have access to a personal teacher. This book will also be useful to more experienced practitioners, as her clinical examples reveal the potency of this body/mind integrative approach."

Judyth O. Weaver, *PhD, Teacher of Sensory Awareness,*
T'ai Chi Ch'uan, Pre/Perinatal Psychology, Body/Mind/Spirit,
and recipient of the Lifetime Achievement Award from USABP

"I am in awe of the book's depth, amazing research, and the remarkable explorations of others with whom Tina Stromsted has shared this journey. I'm likewise in awe as she ponders, with such love, the world of our dear souls and our remarkable bodies, telling the stories of our journeys of reconciliation."

Ann Skinner, *Cofounder BodySoul Rhythms® with Marion Woodman and*
Mary Hamilton. Head of Voice Emerita at Canada's Stratford Shakespeare
Festival, and former Head of Voice at the National Theatre School of Canada

"Tina Stromsted's long awaited *Soul's Body* shows us how the adversarial events of life can be turned around to bring about great healing for both ourselves and the world. Her beautifully written, deeply accessible, heartfelt book is a gift to clinicians, body-oriented healing practitioners, artists, teachers, and laypeople. A groundbreaking collection, it ties together Jungian psychology, somatic psychology, dreams, developments in neuroscience, alchemical elements, community building, and applications in the natural world. Embodied wisdom essential for our time, and all times!"

Donna Schindler, *MD, Cross-cultural psychiatrist and author of*
Flying Horse: Stories of Healing the Soul Wound

"This book is essential for anyone concerned with the interaction between mind, body, and spirit. As a Jungian analyst and master teacher, Tina Stromsted is an authority in Authentic Movement, having trained extensively with and collaborated with its early pioneers, Joan Chodorow and Janet Adler. Another vital influence is Jungian analyst Marion Woodman, a pioneer in exploring the feminine and the body. In an engaging style, Stromsted invites us to 'dance' with her through her personal journey and guides us through the facets of her unique approach— multileveled and multidisciplinary, integrating movement, neuroscience, dreams, myth, art, and voice. While Stromsted provides essential information about the field's history ('herstory'), she also offers fundamental principles and creative practices vital for its future."

Meg Wilbur, *Jungian analyst, professor emerita of UCLA's*
School of Theater, Film, and Television, cofounder
of the C. G. Jung Study Center-Southern California,
& senior faculty Marion Woodman Foundation

Soul's Body

Dr. Tina Stromsted introduces her Soul's Body® approach in this extraordinary volume, engaging the body–psyche connection in psychotherapeutic work. Through compelling case studies, the author illustrates multidisciplinary concepts, therapeutic techniques, trauma-informed practices, and essential teaching guidelines for body–psyche–spirit healing.

Stromsted's method expands Authentic Movement, rooted in Jung's Active Imagination approach, into a range of creative somatic practices within depth psychotherapy. Soul's Body® cultivates deeper self-awareness through bodily expression, dreamwork, creative imagination, empathic relationship, community engagement, and our connection with nature. This collection illuminates elements in the embodied healing process that can benefit professionals in the healing arts—Jungian analysts, clinicians, somatic psychotherapists, dancers, bodyworkers, artists, students, spiritual practitioners, and creative arts therapists. With over 45 years of clinical experience and decades of collaborations with pioneering clinicians Joan Chodorow, Marion Woodman, Janet Adler, and Stanley Keleman, Stromsted guides readers on an engaging journey toward conscious embodiment.

This book is an essential resource for anyone interested in Jungian depth work, embodied spirituality, and cultivating a vital, meaningful life.

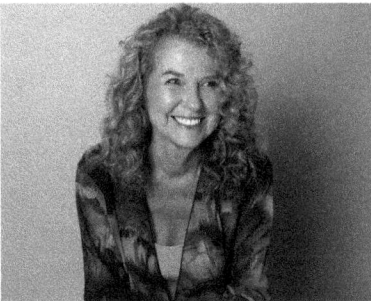

Tina Stromsted, PhD, LMFT, LPCC, BC-DMT, RSME/T, SEP, is a Jungian analyst, dance/movement and somatic psychotherapist, public speaker, and author with over 45 years of clinical experience. As the founder and director of Soul's Body® Center, she integrates Jungian depth psychology with embodied practices including Authentic Movement, BodySoul® work, DreamDancing, Embodied Alchemy, trauma integration, and Creative Arts Therapies.

Tina was cofounder and senior faculty of the Authentic Movement Institute in Berkeley, California. She was also a founding faculty of the Women's Spirituality Program at the California Institute of Integral Studies, where she served as core faculty in the Somatics Psychology graduate program and taught in the Expressive Arts Therapy Program. She has spent decades teaching in the depth-oriented Somatic Psychology doctoral programs at Pacifica Graduate Institute and the Santa Barbara Graduate Institute. Tina offers workshops and lectures at universities, conferences, and healing centers internationally. She teaches at the C. G. Jung Institute of San Francisco, Jung Platform, Inspirees Institute, and is senior faculty for the Marion Woodman Foundation, where she co-facilitated leadership training programs and served on the board.

With a background in dance and theater, Tina has a keen interest in the creative process, neuroscience, ecopsychology, attachment theory, mythology, and the development of embodied consciousness. Her extensive publications in professional journals and books delve into the intricate connections between body, psyche, and soul in relationship with community and nature. She maintains a private practice in San Francisco, and offers virtual consultation internationally. www.Authentic-Movement-BodySoul.com

Soul's Body

Active Imagination, Authentic Movement, and Embodiment in Psychotherapy

Tina Stromsted

Routledge
Taylor & Francis Group

LONDON AND NEW YORK

Designed cover image: Antelope Canyon, Navajo Nation, Arizona, USA © Shutterstock, photograph by Daniel Sockwell

First published 2026
by Routledge
4 Park Square, Milton Park, Abingdon, Oxon OX14 4RN

and by Routledge
605 Third Avenue, New York, NY 10158

Routledge is an imprint of the Taylor & Francis Group, an informa business

British Library Cataloguing-in-Publication Data
A catalogue record for this book is available from the British Library

ISBN: 978-1-032-88547-6 (hbk)
ISBN: 978-1-032-88546-9 (pbk)
ISBN: 978-1-003-53835-6 (ebk)

DOI: 10.4324/9781003538356

Typeset in Times New Roman
by KnowledgeWorks Global Ltd.

To my Mentors:

Joan Chodorow
Marion Woodman
Stanley Keleman
Janet Adler
Charles Harris

For your soulful example, profound teachings, and collaborative engagement in this work of body, soul, community, and Earth.

And to my family, friends, colleagues, students, and patients: thank you for the gifts of your presence, trust, generosity of being, and all that I continue to learn from you.

Contents

Acknowledgments

Writing a book that draws from my life experience takes not only dedication and hard work, but also the support of many others. Thank you to my editors at Routledge, Katie Randall and Manon Berset, for your patience, warmth, and guidance in bringing this book out, and to your colleagues who helped in the process. I'm incredibly grateful for my editor, LeeAnn Pickrell, for her masterful editing, help with permissions, and poetic soul. And for my dear friend Dr. Donna Schindler for her early and steady encouragement; without your suggestions and support, this book may not have come into being. Gratitude to my dear friend Dr. Teresa Doyle for your close reading and skillful editing, and to friends Amy Roberts, Paula Koepke, Maureen Kellen-Taylor, and Dave Berger for your reading and reflections on parts of this material. Special thanks to Erica Clowes and Shauna Toh for their early editing help with the book proposal, and to Tara Weaver for your valuable feedback. Warm appreciation to Sara Ellis for providing administrative support for my clinical work and teaching, as well as Jules Ough and Kathleen Maley for their help with related projects.

My sincere thanks to the artists, photographers, and poets who generously granted permission to include their beautiful, creative work in these pages.

A deep bow of gratitude to my early analysts, Neil Russack and Karlyn Ward for their authenticity, wisdom, and care. And to my analytic consultants and valued colleagues, Donald Kalsched, Suzanne Wagner, and Lou Vuksinick for your penetrating insights, guiding questions, and inspiring example of courage and contribution. My deep thanks to Weslynn Hants for your guidance and care, and to Andrew Samuels and Clara Rosemarda for your encouragement in my writing and reflections. I also want to thank teachers and colleagues Myron Sharaf, John Conger, Joseph Campbell, Arnold and Amy Mindell, and Allan Schore, and Rhiannon, for your courageous example in freeing the voice and building community.

Many individuals have accompanied me in friendship, offering inspiration and encouragement along the way, among them Anne Baring, Eleanor Criswell Hannah, Eileen Nemeth, Margaret Wilkinson, Robin van Löben Sels, Nancy Gurian, David Gerbi, Juerg Roffler, Maureen Murdock, Judyth Weaver, Renee Emunah, Rosa Maria Govoni, Toby Symington, YaYa Cantu, Machiel Klerk, and Tony Zhou. My heartfelt thanks to Meg Wilbur and Dorothy Anderson—my wonderful teaching collaborators, and Suzanne Jobling for assisting us! I also wish to thank poet Tom Centolella for his inspiring writing class!

My heartfelt gratitude to Dr. Joan Chodorow for your generous Forward to this book and for decades of soulful collaboration and treasured friendship.

To Ann Skinner and Mary Hamilton, huge appreciation for your co-leadership with Marion Woodman in BodySoul Rhythms® trainings; my learnings and our teaching collaborations have been profound.

Marion Woodman, Janet Adler, Andrea Olsen, and Irma Dosamantes-Beaudry—thank you for our interviews and for kindly allowing me to include elements from them in this book. I would like to thank Robert Hinshaw for your dedication to Diamon Press and for granting permission to republish articles that serve as the foundation for some chapters. I also appreciate the editors of the *IAAP Proceedings* for their efforts in preparing numerous publications of conference presentations, including some written by me that have been updated and published here. I wish to thank Daniela Sieff for permission to include our meaningful conversation about trauma and healing in this book. And Nancy Cater, for your inspiring work with Spring Publications and for your early invitation to publish my book.

Deep appreciation to Neala Haze for our decades of co-creation at the Authentic Movement Institute, together with the other valued faculty who joined us. I want to express my profound gratitude to Margareta Neuberger for 30 years of loving and wise professional collaboration, and to my Authentic Movement peer group—my traveling companions on inner and outer journeys over these 40 years.

A deep bow to my students and especially my patients, who have been my greatest teachers. I am truly grateful to individuals who shared their experiences as movers and allowed me to write about them.

With gratitude to my family, especially my grandmother, Astri Stromsted, my father, Erik Stromsted, and my aunt, Kate Winter, for their kind, wise, and adventurous spirits.

And finally, my very fine cat, Kachia—soft, graceful, and somewhat wild—my co-pilot at the computer and a sublime teacher of body and soul, who purred on my lap and never tired of inviting me to play!

Credits

Chapter 1

Adapted from Tina Stromsted, Authentic Movement and the evolution of Soul's Body® Work. *Journal of Dance & Somatic Practices*, 7(2), 339–357. Produced by permission of the *Journal of Dance & Somatic Practices* through PLSClear.

"The God who only knows four words" from the Penguin publication *The Gift: Poems by Hafiz* by Daniel Ladinsky © 1999 with permission. www.danielladinsky.com

Chapter 2

Adapted from Tina Stromsted (2009), Healing Soul's Body: An introduction to Authentic Movement. In P. Bennett (Ed.), *Capetown 2007: Journeys, Encounters: Clinical, Communal, Cultural. Proceedings of the 17th International IAAP Congress for Analytical Psychology* (pp. 1045–1054). Daimon.

David Whyte, "The interior angel." From *River flow: New & selected poems 1984–2007* © 2007 David Whyte. Reprinted with permission from David Whyte and Many Rivers Company, LLC, Langley, WA. www.davidwhyte.com

Chapter 3

Adapted from Tina Stromsted (2007). Embodied imagination: Form grows from emptiness. In P. Ashton (Ed.), *Evocations of absence: Interdisciplinary encounters with void states* (pp. 133–155). Spring Journal Books.

When grapes turn to wine, versions of Rumi, translated by Robert Bly, published in 1986 by Yellow Moon Press. By permission.

Chapter 4

Adapted from Tina Stromsted (2020). Shadow dances: Reclaiming "The Other." In E. Kiehl & J. Egli (Eds.), *Vienna 2019: Encountering the Other: Within us, between us, and in the world. Proceedings of the 21st International IAAP Congress for Analytical Psychology.* Daimon.

Thich Nhat Hanh, "Please call me by my true names" from *Call me by my true names: The collected poems of Thich Nhat Hanh.* Copyright © 1999 by Unified Buddhist Church. Reprinted with the permission of The Permissions Company, LLC on behalf of Parallax Press, Berkeley, California, parallax.org

Chapter 5

Used with permission of Routledge/Taylor & Francis, from Tina Stromsted, "Witnessing Practice: In the eyes of the beholder." In H. Payne, S. Koch, J. Tantia, with T. Fuchs (Eds). *The Routledge international handbook of embodied perspectives in psychotherapy: Approaches from dance movement and body psychotherapies,* 2002. Permission conveyed through Copyright Clearance Center, Inc.

LeeAnn Pickrell, "Desire." By permission of author. www.leeannpickrell.com

Chapter 6

Adapted from Tina Stromsted, Re-Inhabiting the female body. *Somatics: Journal of the Bodily Arts & Sciences, X*(1), 18–27.

"The Street Cleaner" © Corlene Van Sluizer.

Chapter 7

Reprinted from Tina Stromsted, Authentic Movement as a Gateway to Transformation, *The Arts in Psychotherapy, 28*(1), 39–55, 2001, with permission from Elsevier.

"How the Light Comes" © Jan Richardson from *Circle of Grace: A Book of Blessings for the Seasons.* Used by permission. janrichardson.com

Chapter 8

Adapted from Tina Stromsted (2007), The dancing body in psychotherapy: Reflections on somatic psychotherapy and Authentic Movement. In P. Pallaro (Ed.), *Authentic Movement: Moving the body, moving the self, being moved: A collection of essays—Volume Two* (pp. 202–220). Reproduced with permission of the Jessica Kingsley Publishers through PLSclear.

The unbroken, © 1991 Rashani Réa. By Permission.

Chapter 9

Used with permission of Rutledge/Taylor & Francis, from Tina Stromsted & Daniela Seiff, (2015), Dances of psyche and soma: Re-inhabiting the body in the wake of emotional trauma. In D. F. Sieff (Ed.), *Understanding and healing emotional trauma: Conversations with pioneering clinicians and researchers*. Permission conveyed through Copyright Clearance Center, Inc.

By permission. "The Moment that Mattered" by Rosemerry Wahtola Trommer, *A Hundred Falling Veils*, https://ahundredfallingveils.com

Chapter 10

Adapted from Tina Stromsted, Dancing body, earth body: Andrea Olsen's story. *Somatics: Journal of the Bodily Arts & Sciences*, XIII(4, 2002), 10–21.

Chapter 11

Adapted from Tina Stromsted and Neala Haze, (2007), The road in: Elements of the study and practice of Authentic Movement. In P. Pallaro (Ed.*), Authentic Movement: Moving the body, moving the self, being moved: A collection of essays— Volume Two* (pp. 56–68). Reproduced with permission of the Jessica Kingsley Publishers through PLSclear.

"Keeping Watch" from the Penguin publication *I Heard God Laughing: Poems of Hope and Joy* by Daniel Ladinsky © 1996, 2006 with permission. www. danielladinsky.com

Chapter 12

By permission. Coleman Barks (translation & commentary). Excerpt from "The Sunrise Ruby." *Rumi the Book of Love: Poems of ecstasy and longing.* HarperSanFrancisco.

Chapter 13

Tina Stromsted, (2014), The alchemy of Authentic Movement: Awakening spirit in the body. In Williamson, A., Whately, S., Batson, G., & Weber R. (Eds.), *Dance, somatics and spiritualities: Contemporary sacred narratives* (pp. 35–60). Reproduced with permission of Intellect Publishers through PLSclear.

By permission. Coleman Barks (translation & commentary). Excerpt from "Die Before You Die," *Rumi the Book of Love: Poems of ecstasy and longing.* HarperSanFrancisco.

Chapter 14

Adapted from Tina Stromsted (2000), Cellular resonance and the sacred feminine: Marion Woodman's story. *Spring: A Journal of Archetype and Culture, Body & Soul: Honoring Marion Woodman*, 72 (1–30).

Chapter 15

Adapted from Tina Stromsted (2010), DreamDancing. In P. Bennett (Ed.), *Montreal 2010: Facing Multiplicity: Psyche, Nature, Culture. Proceedings of the 18th International IAAP Congress for Analytical Psychology* (pp. 71–74). Daimon.

Chapter 16

Original poem © 1979 Nancy C. Wood, from *War Cry on a Prayer Feather*, courtesy of the Nancy Wood Literary Trust. For more poems by Nancy Wood please visit www.NancyWood.com

Chapter 17

By permission. Coleman Barks (translation & commentary). Excerpt from "The Music We Are," In *Rumi, The Book of Love: Poems of Ecstasy and Longing.* HarperSanFrancisco.

Foreword

It is a special pleasure to introduce Tina Stromsted's inspiring and beautifully written book, *Soul's Body: Active Imagination, Authentic Movement, & Embodiment in Psychotherapy*. This extraordinary work offers readers an invaluable opportunity to engage with Tina's groundbreaking integration of Active Imagination, movement, dreamwork, Embodied Alchemy, and a variety of somatic approaches—practices that illuminate and honor the profound connections between body, psyche, spirit, community, and the radiant natural beauty of the Earth we are blessed to call home.

Her work presents a rare integration of sensitive, theoretical, and experiential work grounded in her years of experience with analysands, and with students and colleagues from many cultures and parts of the world. A gifted clinician, prolific author, internationally sought-after teacher, and pioneer in movement/somatic psychotherapy and depth psychology, Tina brings a fine mind, a generous spirit, and a rare authenticity to all that she does.

I first met Tina in 1982, when she attended a course I was teaching on movement as Active Imagination. Even then, her curiosity and deep engagement with the material stood out. For more than four decades, I have had the joy of witnessing her evolution—from a student with inquisitive questions that felt Talmudic in their depth and richness, to a trusted colleague, friend, and respected leader in the field. Tina does not aim to find the "right" answers; instead, she invites inquiry and dialogue that inevitably lead to new and deeper questions, continually expanding the possibilities for exploration and growth.

Since meeting decades ago, we have collaborated closely in various settings. This includes organizing Pre-Congress Day workshops on Active Imagination in Movement for the International Association of Analytical Psychology, joined by valued colleagues from other cultures. Another setting for collaboration began in 1993 when she and her colleague, dance therapist Neala Haze, invited me and Janet Adler to join them on the faculty at their new Authentic Movement Institute (AMI). During those years my late husband, Dr. Louis Stewart, and I offered seminars on the creative healing potentials of active imagination in movement and in play. These seminars continued in my home dance studio (2004–2022), combining theory and movement practice—even meeting on Zoom during the years of the

COVID pandemic. Over the decades I've had the pleasure to engage in ongoing conversations with Tina over dinners, walks, planning sessions, and when traveling to teach; these meaningful, creative exchanges have enriched my life and work tremendously.

Tina's explorations of the roots of this work began in her formative years. Her connection with Jung's work ignited in 1972 when she read *Memories, Dreams, Reflections* as a young woman, inspired by Jung's profound respect for dreams and the psyche, a resonance reinforced by her own personal practice of journaling dreams since childhood. Descended from a family with many artists, Tina was drawn to the creative life in all its forms. Her natural attunement to the sensory-motor world of the "analytic infant" and her deep roots in dance, music, theater, and the arts gave her an intuitive ability to explore not only the personal but also the collective, cultural, and archetypal dimensions of the symbolic world and the embodied spirit.

In this book, Tina takes readers on a journey that is, at once, deeply personal, clinically engaging and empowering, and universally human. With writing that flows beautifully and accessibly, she provides a map for practitioners, students, and seekers to engage in their own embodied healing processes, as well as ways to integrate these insights into therapeutic practice.

Tina's sensitivity, informed by rigorous research and clinical expertise, is reflected in her work on trauma, particularly her recognition of how unmetabolized personal and intergenerational wounds continue to live on in the body until they can be worked with through integrative embodied approaches. Throughout this volume, Tina brings a rich, multidisciplinary perspective: weaving neuroscience, the arts, myth, fairytales, and somatic awareness into her methodology to address the suffering brought on by violence, disconnection, and our modern lifestyles. Her commitment to the healing power of Active Imagination—a cornerstone of Jungian analysis as well as Tina's embodied practice—is one of the great treasures of this text. The final chapters take this work deeper into nature, demonstrating the vital reciprocity between our bodies and that of the Earth, reminding us of the micro-macrocosmic connection so many have forgotten.

Through her decades of private practice and educational work, Tina's ability to make subtle, complex material accessible and alive is remarkable. Her insights resonate across disciplines, and her capacity to infuse material with energy and depth is complemented by her fine writing. This long-awaited book provides a lively and lovely picture of her development in and contributions to the field. It draws from her dissertation research and the treasures she has accumulated through her decades of commitment to the work she loves.

Ultimately, this book reflects Tina herself—including the depth, kindness, creativity, and transformative elements that her ways of relating exemplify. From her early love of dance and dreams to her decades of experience working with individuals, communities, and nature, Tina walks her talk with integrity and grace. Her case studies, rich with life, illustrate not only the theoretical dimensions of her work but also its universal human relevance and impact.

Through *Soul's Body*, Tina has gifted us a vital resource, blending Active Imagination, movement, and embodied practices with Jungian thought in ways that are profoundly applicable to our modern world. Whether you are a clinician, a health practitioner, a student, or someone seeking personal healing, you will find this book to be a wise and compassionate guide. Tina's gentle yet penetrating curiosity extends to you, the reader, inviting you to join her exploration as she guides us in a living dance through a process of embodied consciousness—connecting us more deeply to ourselves, one another, and the Earth itself. I know of no one better to bring you this profoundly integrative healing work!

With gratitude and admiration,
Joan Chodorow

Introduction

Authentic Movement, also known as Active Imagination in Movement, is a simple yet profound method of attending to bodily cues to facilitate healing in psychotherapy and develop embodied consciousness. A relational somatic practice, this transformative approach promotes self-discovery, emotional integrity, and creative expression by tapping into the innate intelligence of the body–psyche–spirit connection, fostering empathy and wholeness. It can also be practiced as a form of meditation or sacred dance. As a source for the creative process, Authentic Movement accesses the body's story: feelings, sensations, images, and memories within the flow of unconscious material that finds direct expression through the body.

This embodied depth approach does not require prior skill or training; instead, it calls for curiosity, respect, and courage to open to the unknown—at one's own pace and style in the presence of a compassionate witness/therapist. Authentic Movement is a transformative tool for self-discovery and creative expression with numerous applications in health, education, and the arts. Practicing with others also enhances appreciation for the diversity of human experience, promoting a greater understanding of relationships with self and the world.

This collection of essays traces the development of Authentic Movement, rooted in my long affiliation with its foremost pioneers, as well as my decades of practice and ongoing contributions as a Jungian analyst, dance/somatic psychotherapist, author, public speaker, international teacher, and cross-cultural educator. I also introduce my Soul's Body® approach, an expansion of the elements of Authentic Movement into related creative, depth-oriented somatic practices, contributing to what psychotherapists sometimes call "embodied Jung." Soul's Body work continues to extend Jung's map of the soul to include more of an embodied feminine perspective that can be lacking in some of the more cognitive, verbal psychological approaches. It also provides an alchemical lens for observing the changes that occur during this transformative work that finds expression across cultures and centuries.

I want to thank the many historical and contemporary authors who have inspired me and express my gratitude to my students and especially my patients, who have been my greatest teachers. I am deeply grateful to individuals who shared their experiences as movers and who allowed me to write about them. Some themes

DOI: 10.4324/9781003538356-1

presented here are a composite of many individuals' stories, with names and identifying details changed for confidentiality. While some material is being shared for the first time, I've also incorporated elements from my earlier publications.

Historically, writing has often used the word *he* to describe the subject. Here, I have sometimes used the word *she* to bring more accuracy and balance to the text and the term *they* to include nonbinary individuals.

This book is a dance, with each part exploring a different aspect of Soul's Body and Authentic Movement—from its beginnings to an expression of its core elements of the movement in practice and out into the world, where it fosters healing for body, soul, community, and Earth.

Part I: Spirit in the Body: Beginnings

Chapter 1, "The Evolution of Soul's Body Work," is the story of my journey with Authentic Movement, beginning with my early experiences of dancing in nature to connect with my soul during tumultuous periods in childhood. This experience of being "seen," "held," and connected to a deeper source prompted my future studies in dance, psychology, theater, spiritual practice, and later, my work as a dance/movement therapist and Jungian psychoanalyst.

Chapter 2, "Healing Soul's Body: Active Imagination in Movement," traces the history of Authentic Movement back to Jung's development of active imagination and outlines the essential elements of the process.

Part II: On the Journey: Core Elements

Chapter 3, "Embodied Imagination: From Emptiness to Form," explores how individuals can engage with absent parts of themselves through Authentic Movement. Several case vignettes provide vivid examples of the efficacy of this work, showing how natural movement arising from a deeper inner source in the presence of a safe, empathic witness can lead to a new feeling of hope and vitality.

Chapter 4, "Meeting the Shadow: Becoming More Whole," delves into the importance of working with what Jung called the "shadow." Authentic Movement provides a safe temenos for exploring previously inaccessible movements, experiencing the feelings associated with them, and verbally owning and integrating these experiences into a fuller sense of self.

Chapter 5, "Witnessing Practice: Seeing & Being Seen," explores how the deep human need to be seen, heard, and accepted for who we are can be fostered through the practice of witnessing in Authentic Movement. This chapter includes case examples and a description of the Dance of Three, a practice involving a mover and two witnesses.

Chapter 6, "Reinhabiting the Body," focuses on what it means to be "out of the body" and the reasons or processes by which women, in particular, often leave their bodies. Recovering requires a descent, which is illustrated through the myth of Demeter and Persephone and the fairytale *The Handless Maiden.*

Chapter 7, "Embodied Descent: Steps Toward Transformation," describes my research into the transformative aspects of Authentic Movement, in which I discovered themes that each reflected a facet of the embodied journey of transformation. Examples from the work of Janet Adler and Irma Dosamantes-Beaudry illustrate the potential of Authentic Movement.

Part III: Movement in Practice

Chapter 8, "The Moving Body in Psychotherapy," explores somatic psychotherapy, focusing on dance/movement therapy and Authentic Movement in clinical practice. I discuss essential elements in client assessment, readiness, and the role of the body-attuned analyst or therapist. Through two case studies, I illustrate how these methods differ in structure yet similarly facilitate transformative experiences.

Chapter 9, "Working with Trauma: Awakening Psyche and Soma," is a conversation with anthropologist and author Daniela Sieff about trauma and the body. We discuss how to heal trauma and how such healing requires working directly with our bodies to access and release what they hold.

Chapter 10, "Transforming Life: Movement as Meditation, Medicine, & Artistic Expression," takes the work outside the therapeutic context, illustrating how Authentic Movement transformed the life of dancer, choreographer, painter, educator, and ecologist Andrea Olsen.

Chapter 11, "Teaching Active Imagination in Movement," illustrates the teaching of Authentic Movement and explores how the practice has continued to evolve—using the Authentic Movement Institute, which I co-founded with Neala Haze in 1993 and was joined by Joan Chodorow and Janet Adler, as a case study.

Chapter 12, "Working with Authentic Movement in Groups," explores foundational and ethical guidelines for groups, the roles of witness and mover, and various group formats, such as Breathing Circles, Long Circles, and Naming Circles.

Part IV: Embracing the Body, Healing the Soul

Chapter 13, "Embodied Alchemy: A Pathway to the Sacred," explores the interplay between alchemy, Jung's transcendent function, and Authentic Movement, revealing the process of embodied transformation. Two case studies illustrate the alchemical journey in Authentic Movement.

Chapter 14, "BodySoul Rhythms®: Marion Woodman & the Sacred Feminine," illustrates how active imagination in movement and related conscious embodiment approaches transformed the life and work of Jungian analyst, educator, international speaker, and bestselling author Marion Woodman.

Chapter 15, "DreamDancing®: Embodied Consciousness," brings together the inner world of body sensations, feelings, dreams, and images. This chapter starts with a brief history of dreams and dreamwork and explores the neuroscience behind dreams. I share several examples of working with dreams through movement.

Chapter 16, "Earth's Body: Resonating with the Pulse of Life," highlights our connections to the Earth's body, extending Authentic Movement's holistic approach beyond the confines of the therapy room, to contribute to healing body, soul, community, and planet.

Chapter 17, "Further Reflections and Looking Forward," focuses on current developments in working with the body in analysis and various forms of healing work. It explores ways in which Authentic Movement, dreamwork, and other embodiment practices can not only assist in healing from the traumas of the world but also help heal our beautiful world itself. This chapter also reminds practitioners of the importance of retaining our embodiment, concluding with an invitation to a walking meditation.

Shall we dance?

Part I

Spirit in the Body: Beginnings

Chapter 1

The Evolution of Soul's Body Work

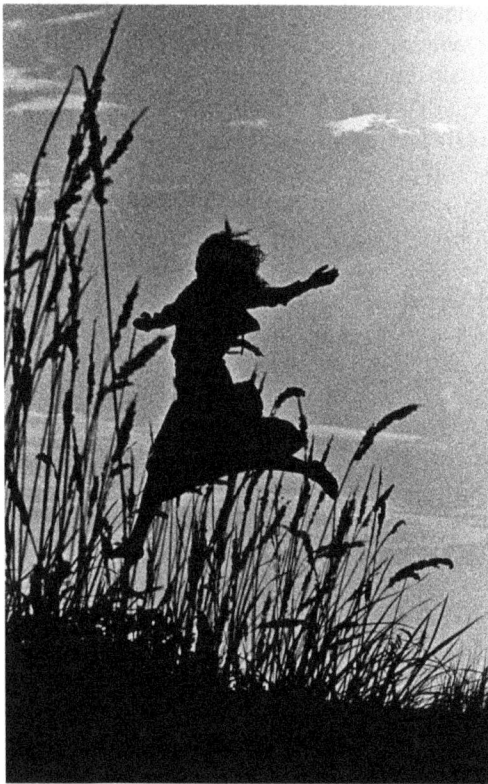

Figure 1.1 Leaping Lady, © Beverly Hall Photography.

DOI: 10.4324/9781003538356-3

Dancing in the Fields

My mother told me I danced in her belly. As a child of seven, I danced with joy and abandon to music in the large room in the back of our house, to the rhythmic hum of the winter humidifier in the living room, with the trees in the woods near the fishpond, underwater in the ocean and in the swimming pool, and in the wind that blew through the rows of corn and alfalfa before harvest. Though the adults tolerated these spontaneous expressions, their messages persisted: "Stop fidgeting," they'd say. "Can't you just stand still, like a nice girl?" (Stromsted, 2015, p. 340).

It was during this time that my parents divorced. Tension flowed through the house, and my world split apart. A year later, my father married a rational disciplinarian who struggled with feelings; she was a pendulum swing away from my childlike, reactive mother. Our household shivered with the change; we all tried to adjust. The dinner table became a stage for our divided world with my Harvard-trained engineer father sitting on one end and my stepmother, engaged in doctoral psychology studies at Radcliffe, on the other. Above the table, we engaged in intellectual conversations about books, local events, and national politics. I was more curious about what was going on *under* the table, however, where hands fidgeted, wringing napkins and soothing kneecaps, while feet pawed unspoken hieroglyphs along the floorboards.

After clearing the table, I'd head across the street into the fields. Fresh air bathed my face; swallows, chickadees, ravens, and meadowlarks sang their news as chipmunks and squirrels scurried along the dark ground and up the solid wide oaks. Tall, slim birch trees stood around the edges of the small fishpond; their arms extended toward their shadow partners reflected in the water. In the clearing at the center of the field, I began to spin, holding the horizon line steady with my eyes as my body whirled. I was free, like the blue sky, clouds, green leafy cornstalks, sweet alfalfa, and the ground under my feet. Family tension drained from my body into the soft, receptive earth.

When I danced in the fields, I could smell the moistness of the soil and feel the earth's heartbeat. I could sense the different shapes of intelligence that nature expressed and how *my* body was a part of that *larger* body. A *shimmer* ran through me—a life force that pulsed with spirit. Time stood still, and there was a sense of oneness with the natural world all around and within me. In the natural way of childhood, I had stumbled on the whirling dance practiced by the early Sufis. Feeling free and whole, my soul restored, I'd return to the house for more chores and homework. Nature was my deepest container and first witness. I'd venture there to heal my spirit, feel at one with everything, and experience myself as connected, enriched, and renewed. Then I'd take that back into my life as a child. Years later, when I was introduced to Authentic Movement, I learned that I could have a human witness. How wonderful is that?

When winter came and the roots of all things hibernated underground, I'd head to the back room of the house to sing and sway to tunes from my favorite records—Joni Mitchell, the Beatles, the Rolling Stones, the Supremes, and others. Inevitably, my two younger sisters appeared at the door, their noses and palms pressed against the panes of glass. Seeing them gave me joy; I'd wave them in, inviting them to join me in the dance. Looking back, I realize that these were my first dance therapy groups—a place to discover and express my feelings, support my sisters, and find a deeper connection to myself, my soul, and one another in the splintering household. Dance was medicine.[1]

In my twenties, while studying and performing dance and theater, I realized that my heart was not in "performing." What really interested me was *transformation* of the body, psyche, and spirit. I sought the feeling of connection I'd experienced in the fields. While guiding others' dances, I began to focus not so much on the exactness of the students' technique, but on the *shimmer* that came and went in their soul expression, the movement of light in the body. As I sought ways to support them—letting their vitality come through in the dance and reflecting those moments back to them at the end of class—many began to tell me their life stories. I realized that I wanted to better hold and understand their experiences. I began leading groups in dance, art, poetry, and nature at McLean Hospital in Belmont, Massachusetts; I trained in crisis intervention, worked the suicide hotline, and provided drop-in counseling at Project Place in Boston in the mid-1970s. These were among the seeds of my growing interest in the embodied soul.

Early Influences

Dance taught me to experience myself and others through movement, but I needed to embrace stillness as well. Moving to California in the late 1970s, I practiced zazen meditation in the Soto Zen Buddhist tradition, finding an inner quiet that brought nourishment and helped me identify unconscious sources of movement in my body. Yoga brought more fluidity, and as my investigations continued, I integrated work with the psyche through training in bioenergetics, psychodrama, and many other forms of somatic work. I enriched a quiet inner focus through weekly groups with Magda Proskauer, a wise crone and teacher of breathwork.

My study of somatics evolved, influenced by many clinical and therapeutic methods: among them Reichian, with Myron Sharaf and Charles Harris; decades of studies in Formative Psychology and body psychotherapy, with Stanley Keleman; and Gestalt therapy with Dick Price. From an integrative perspective, my work with Jungian analyst Arnold Mindell's Process Oriented Psychology expanded my knowledge of depth psychology, quantum physics, and shamanism. I discovered the wisdom of the psyche-soma connection as expressed through unconscious body cues in the present moment. Jungian analytic training and personal analysis profoundly deepened my relationship with the embodied psyche. Following that, I undertook ten years of study with Allan Schore and subsequent training in trauma work, which helped me integrate the insights of interpersonal neurobiology and regulation theory.

My concurrent involvement with the arts—dance, music, theater, and storytelling—complemented my early movement work. Dance therapist Tamara Greenberg expanded Keleman's approach through natural movement, and these explorations deepened my graduate training in dance therapy, clinical psychology, and family systems theory. Trudi Schoop, a deeply gifted mime and dancer from Switzerland and one of the grandmothers of dance/movement therapy, inspired me with movement explorations that were both uniquely personal and universal.

My early interest in myths, fairytales, and comparative religion was revitalized through studies with mythologist Joseph Campbell. I delighted in improvisation studies with the Blake Street Hawkeyes, an innovative theater troupe in Berkeley, California, and with Vocal River voice teacher Rhiannon, bringing creative spontaneity to my interpersonal work. These, and other explorations, furthered my engagement with the body-psyche-spirit community.

Discovering Authentic Movement

Then, in 1983, Joan Chodorow introduced me to Authentic Movement (Stromsted, 2025). I felt like I had come home. Here, I found the same kind of deep knowing I'd experienced in the fields as a child through a practice that allowed me to explore

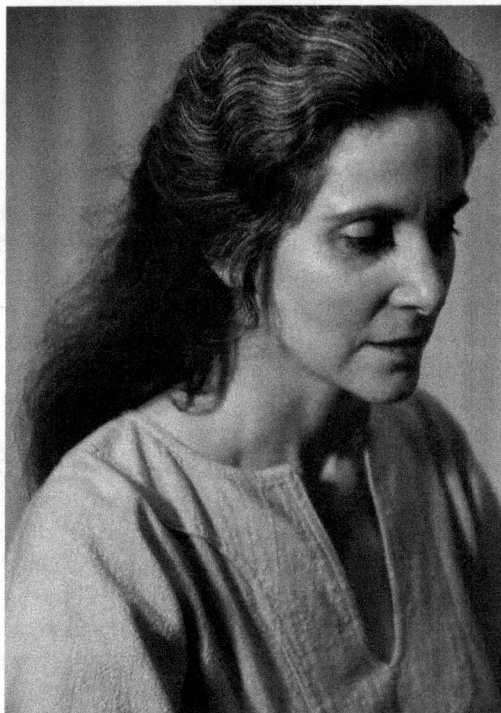

Figure 1.2 Joan Chodorow © Cara Moore 1982. Courtesy of Joan Chodorow.

inner and outer life along the spectrum from stillness to movement, this time within the context of compassionate, attuned relationship. A longtime student of pioneer dance/movement therapists Mary Whitehouse and Trudi Schoop, Joan was a senior dance therapist, Jungian analyst, and a leader in integrating the body in the Jungian world, believing as Jung did that "psyche is as much a living body as body is a living psyche" (Jung, 1998, p. 396).

Though Jung developed active imagination in 1916, and Tina Keller-Jenny and other early analysts practiced it, "*movement* as active imagination remained largely undeveloped until the 1950s, when it was taken up by Mary Whitehouse" (Chodorow, 2007, p. 33). For me, the practice of following the moving imagination in the body felt like a natural outgrowth of my early dances in the fields (Fleischer, 2024), though it was not until meeting Joan in San Francisco that I learned it was a formal practice.

Since then, Active Imagination in Movement, or Authentic Movement, has been practiced by increasing numbers of people, including therapists, artists, and spiritual practitioners as well as clients, students, parents, educators, eco-psychologists, and social activists. In my view, this is the result of a growing need to embrace the wisdom of the body and its essential role in the process of development, integrative healing, and transformation. The so-called talking cure is not enough, particularly where repressed, preverbal, or dissociated material and traumatized affects are concerned. These take up residence in the body until circumstances are safe enough to allow them to be felt, mirrored, reflected on, and healed.

Joan's warmth, depth, and wisdom enhanced my understanding of C. G. Jung's map of the soul and the active imagination process. I learned more about developmental psychology and the transformational capacities of the emotions. We also shared an interest in inclusiveness and social justice, dedicated to the advancement of tolerance and the defeat of racial and ethnic hatred. Diverse perspectives help make the world a better place (Chodorow, 1991, 1997).

In 1985 I embarked on nine years of intensive training with Janet Adler, a senior dance therapist with a background in child development, whose doctoral studies explored the relationship between Authentic Movement and mystical practice. With Janet I investigated presymbolic dimensions of the practice: experience *beneath* words (Adler, in Haze & Stromsted, 1994/1999, p. 112). Janet encouraged us to drop our narratives; movement explorations stripped us back to our most unvarnished, visceral selves, inviting preverbal experiences, new messy experiments, and moments of grace when the vibrance of the sacred came through (Adler, 1999a, 1999b, 2002).

Later, I assisted Janet with workshops in California and Italy and began teaching Authentic Movement in graduate schools and in international settings. Italy has since become a soul home where for more than 30 years I've returned to facilitate groups, often assisted by the late beloved Margareta Neuberger (2007). Throughout these years I've continued to integrate Authentic Movement in my Jungian analytic and dance therapy/somatics practice in San Francisco.

Working in embodied ways has become an intrinsic part of the fields of dance/movement, somatic, and creative arts psychotherapies for many decades. Recent developments in interpersonal neurobiology, attachment theory, and trauma work have contributed toward establishing the essential role of embodied relational processes in healing and development. As Allan Schore, a psychoanalyst and neuroscience researcher, states:

> Change does not happen when a patient is consciously reflecting on an emotion; it happens when a patient is *in* the emotion and when a resonating and actively involved therapist shows the patient a different way to be with what he is feeling. There is no room for that to happen with cognitive therapy.
>
> (Schore & Sieff, 2015, p. 134)

The attuned, containing presence of the witness/therapist in Authentic Movement allows the mover/client safe access to early, primary process-oriented parts of the self. Engaging this material establishes new neuropathways in the brain and supports the development of new behaviors, cognitions, and worldviews, leading to further integration and embodiment.

Authentic Movement and Woodman's BodySoul Rhythms®

I met Marion Woodman, a Jungian analyst, writer, and international speaker, in the late 1980s. Her work had advanced the investigation and development of embodied feminine consciousness. She was a well-known author on psyche and soma, and her intensive workshops and leadership-training programs integrated body, psyche, and spirit with creative expression and community.

Having practiced and taught Authentic Movement, I wanted to take a further step to integrate the imaginal elements of the psyche and to continue to strengthen my authentic voice and feminine standpoint. As Marion says, "Bodywork is soul work. Imagination is the bridge between body and soul" (Woodman & Mellick, 2000, p. 42). Marion helped me continue to develop a symbolic attitude in which working with metaphor was an important ingredient. Jungian analyst and neuroscience researcher Margaret Wilkinson explains that metaphor "lights up more centres of brain activity than any other form of human communication," supporting enhanced integration between the right and left brain (Wilkinson, 2013, p. 2). This became an important ingredient in my studies with Marion beginning in the 1980s, and in the BodySoul Rhythms (BSR) work she later developed with her gifted colleagues, dancer Mary Hamilton and voice and mask teacher Ann Skinner, culminating in my teaching BodySoul work for more than three decades.

Marion's work with the feminine psyche also supported the development of a more differentiated "masculine"/yang (animus) in women, further enriched through Jung's depth-psychology framework. Like Marion, I was a father's daughter who had trouble relating to and modeling my mother. Integrating dance, breath, voice

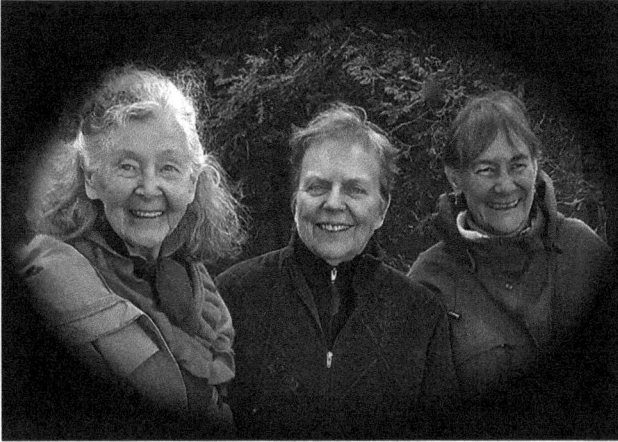

Figure 1.3 Marion Woodman, Ann Skinner, & Mary Hamilton, Grand Bend, Ontario, Canada. Photo © Meg Wilbur 2011.

work, dreams, masks, language, ritual, theater, music, art, and humor with Jungian theory, Marion, Mary, and Ann's work offered a contained, depth-oriented feminine initiation journey. Their teamwork also provided a model for collaboration among women. This brought me back to the feelings of camaraderie and joy I had experienced in my early dances with my sisters and brought hope for empowering the feminine in a patriarchal culture driven by greed, power, and competition.

Marion's discovery of Authentic Movement came about by following the active imagination process in her body to heal a kidney disorder that had resulted from her struggles with anorexia, a story I tell later in Chapter 14. Renewed, and with new insights about the body-psyche-spirit connection, Marion resumed her teaching. Then, in 1982, at Joan Chodorow's invitation, Marion participated in an Authentic Movement retreat at Jacob's Pillow in Becket, Massachusetts—a mecca for dancers and home to American's longest-running summer dance festival. Marion's experience there affirmed her sense of the potency of having a personal "witness" while moving in response to an inner prompting, elements fundamental to Authentic Movement practice. Marion's insights about the effects of the witness on the group mirrored a crucial part of my own experience. After reading her books, I was fortunate enough to take her workshop in 1989 when she visited the Jung Institute here in San Francisco, and thus began decades of studies and collaborative work together.

As BSR work continued to develop and more women requested further training, I was invited to facilitate leadership-training programs with Marion, Mary, and Ann, together with my colleagues Meg Wilbur (a talented Jungian analyst, voice teacher, and playwright and director), and Dorothy Anderson (an artist, communications specialist, and gifted teacher with an uncanny sense of humor). Our team supported the further evolution of the work by leading *Wellsprings of Feminine*

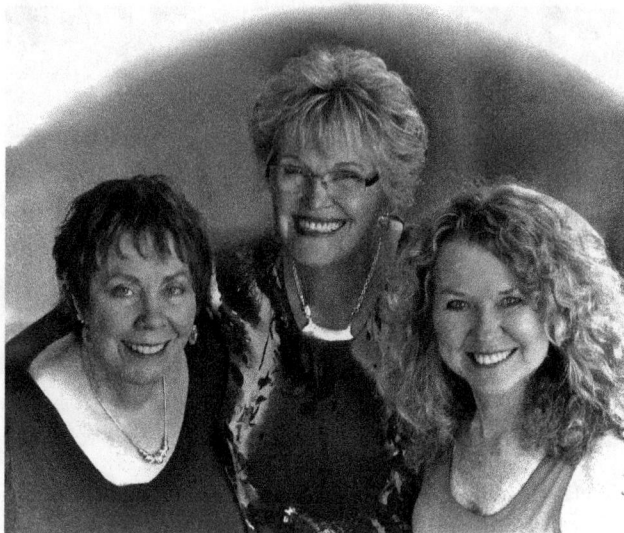

Figure 1.4 Meg Wilbur, Dorothy Anderson, & Tina Stromsted; Cambria, California 2014. Photo courtesy of Mark Winkler.

Renewal intensives, adapting myths and fairytales into plays that illuminated the feminine individuation journey integrated with other BSR elements. At Marion's recommendation, we taught an intensive course on "Jung, Woodman and the Embodied Psyche" for over a decade in the Depth Psychology/Somatics Doctoral Program at Pacifica Graduate Institute in Santa Barbara. Though Marion retired from active teaching before passing away in 2018, BodySoul Work continues to flourish through workshops sponsored by the Marion Woodman Foundation, BodySoul Europe, and in many parts of the world.

Applications of Authentic Movement

In 1993, dance therapist and somatics practitioner Neala Haze and I established the Authentic Movement Institute (AMI) in Berkeley, California, in order to further investigate this unity of psyche, body, and soul (1993–2004). We were joined by founding faculty members Joan Chodorow and Janet Adler. Joan's husband, Jungian analyst Louis Stewart, also lent his expertise in active imagination, play therapy, and embodied affect theory, a model he developed with Joan and his brother Charles Stewart, a pediatrician and child psychiatrist. All contributed their areas of expertise to teaching and curriculum development (Stromsted & Haze, 2002/2007; Stromsted & Haze, 2007), described more in-depth in Chapter 11.

Authentic Movement bridges clinical, artistic, and spiritual practice. Individual movers and witnesses also bring many facets of themselves: mind and body, personal history, persona, gender, family of origin, culture, and race. At the Institute, we invited dance/therapy and somatics colleagues to teach Authentic Movement with specific areas of application: for more challenged populations, working with women recovering from breast cancer, moving in nature, and integrating Authentic Movement with Process-Oriented Psychology and other arts and healing practices. A rich experience, the training produced graduates from a variety of professions and countries, many of whom are now teaching in different parts of the world, each steeped in their practice of the major principles of Authentic Movement.

Since then, I have been training Jungian analysts, candidates, and interns; clinicians in allied professions; health practitioners; artists; and spiritual practitioners who wish to engage the body's wisdom in healing, growth, and creative endeavors. Though I continue to resonate deeply with the transpersonal and mystical dimension of the practice, I also find myself drawn to learning more about the transformative process through relational elements, neuroscience, and the sacred dimensions of all life, including social activist and ecological concerns (Stromsted, 2009, 2014; Stromsted & Sieff, 2014).

Authentic Movement is an integral part of my own analytic, teaching, and consultation practice. It enriches empathy, helps me attend to signals and symptoms in the body, and allows me to work more deeply with dream material. Working with Jungian candidates and interns at the San Francisco Jung Institute is a joy. And I'm honored to work with analyst colleagues internationally, including decades of collaboration with Joan, Marion, and other Jungian analysts and dance therapy colleagues in congresses for the International Association of Analytical Psychology (IAAP). There, we invite analysts and candidates from many cultures to engage in embodied explorations that enrich their verbal work and support them in refining their observational skills, nonjudgmental and noninterpretive languaging, and sensitivity to their own bodies as the somatic foundation of embodied empathy and compassion in the analytic container and process.

At my Soul's Body® Center, I continue to build on Authentic Movement, Body-Soul work, and other creative, embodied healing methods. I focus on attending to natural movement and supporting the development of a conscious, embodied container. I engage the body in working with metaphors and dream images and investigating the somatic foundations of the transmission process of multigenerational family patterns. In my practice, I explore body symptoms and incorporate the use of nonjudgmental and noninterpretive language. I also offer workshops, conference presentations, webinars for the Jung Platform, and other international organizations—working with a range of integrative components to honor and engage different cultures and populations.

From the time I could read, myths, fairytales, and dreams informed my understanding of life's challenges, depicting the natural cycles of death and rebirth that illuminated the path—what Jung called the *individuation* journey. The practice of DreamDancing® draws upon this rich resource, an approach I'll discuss further in Chapter 15. During a 14-year period, I met with women in a monthly DreamDancing® group in a dance studio in San Francisco. There—sometimes joined by Rhiannon and other guest vocalists and body specialists—we explored the energies, feelings, and actions of their dreams to embody their wisdom and further integrate their guidance into daily life, supported in community.

More personally, I've continued to deepen my practice at home and in ongoing active imagination seminars with Joan Chodorow (1992–2022) here in Northern California. An intimate group of dance therapists gathered in Joan's living room each month to integrate readings from Jungian and post-Jungian theory, developmental psychology, affect theory, dance/movement therapy, neuroscience, trauma work, and the arts. Taking turns presenting personal, theoretical, and case material, we then moved from the sofas into the dance studio, where we integrated and deepened our explorations through Authentic Movement followed by drawing, writing, sandplay, and music. My Authentic Movement peer group, now in its 40th year, offers an ever-deepening and creative ground as our relationships to self, to the deeper Self, to one another, the social zeitgeist, and to the natural world continue to grow.

Moving Forward

Dissociation from unbearably traumatic experience "separates sensation, affect, and image so that an impossible meaning is obliterated" (Kalsched, 2010, p. 284). Norman O. Brown wrote in 1959 about the importance of the body: "The aim of psychoanalysis—still unfulfilled, and still only half-conscious—is to return our souls to our bodies, to return ourselves to ourselves, and thus to overcome the human state of self-alienation" (Brown, 1959). Among the many gifts of Authentic Movement, BSR practice, and trauma-informed psychotherapy is re-membering: putting the members back together (Stromsted, 1994/1995). This deeply embodied, integrative work helps restore links between body experience and the brain that became fragmented through trauma, neglect, or lack of use. As interpersonal neurobiology tells us (Schore, 2012, 2014), new nerve pathways form in the presence of a compassionate witness. The holding environment provided by the witness supports the mover's exploration of a wider range of affect tolerance, and a capacity for self-witnessing and self-regulation (Porges, 2011; Schore & Sieff, 2015; Siegel, 1999). "Eventually, the face of an attuned mother [witness] will be written into her infant's [mover's] right orbitofrontal cortex. This then acts as an emotionally containing and comforting neurobiological guidance system when she is not physically present" (Schore & Sieff, 2015, p. 117). This is the process of forming an "inner witness," a fundamental part of developing embodied consciousness.

Over the years, I have come to see Authentic Movement as *a safe-enough container*, a kind of uterus from which the client/mover may be reborn in the presence of an outer witness or *good enough mother/parenting* figure, from the *symbolic mother* of her own unconscious. This, in turn, roots the individual in the instinctual ground of all of nature, the Great Mother. My practice has made it clear to me that containment—psychic, physical, emotional, and spiritual—is necessary for deep transformation to unfold. In this cocoon, the melting of old defenses, including the body-stiffening that reflected them and held them in place, can begin to soften. At the deepest level, a dismemberment of the individual's previous sense of self can occur—through alchemical processes of *solutio* and *coagulation* (see Chapter 13)—resulting in the death of an old way of being and the reintegration of a sense of self within the context of human relatedness (Stromsted, 2014, p. 50).

An evolved awareness of self also makes possible a more sensitive and nuanced relationship with our environment—interpersonally, politically, and ecologically. The body plays a central role in this; for with a more vital, felt sense of our own embodied experience, we cannot help but resonate with the life force that animates all living beings. Instead of shutting down, dissociating, reacting with violence, or fleeing to spirit when feelings in the body are too uncomfortable to bear—thus passing them from generation to generation through unconscious trauma patterns—we can find a spiritual home in the body (Stromsted, 2015). "Shimmer" extends, and the seeds from my dances in the fields continue to grow. Fourteenth-century poet, Hafiz (Ladinsky, 1999), invites us to step in when he says:

The God Who Only Knows Four Words

Every
Child
Has known God,

Not the God of names,
Not the God of don'ts,
Not the God who ever does
Anything weird,

But the God who only knows four words
And keeps repeating them, saying:

"Come dance with Me."

Come
Dance.

Note

1 This section of Chapter 1 originally appeared as "Dancing in the Fields" in *Jung Journal: Culture & Psyche*, 18(4), pp. 156–157, DOI: 10.1080/19342039.2024.2405423.

References

Adler, J. (1999a). The collective body. In P. Pallaro (Ed.), *Authentic Movement: Essays by Mary Starks Whitehouse, Janet Adler & Joan Chodorow* (pp. 190–209). Jessica Kingsley Publishers. (Original work published in 1987.)

Adler, J. (1999b). "Who is the witness?" A description of Authentic Movement. In P. Pallaro (Ed.), *Authentic Movement: Essays by Mary Starks Whitehouse, Janet Adler & Joan Chodorow* (pp. 141–159). Jessica Kingsley Publishers. (Original work published in 1987.)

Adler, J. (2002). *Offering from the conscious body*. Inner Traditions.

Brown, N. O. (1959). *Life against death: The psychoanalytical meaning of history*. Random House.

Chodorow, J. (1991). *Dance therapy and depth psychology: The moving imagination*. Routledge.

Chodorow, J. (Ed.). (1997). *Jung on active imagination*. Routledge.

Chodorow, J. (2007). Inner-directed movement in analysis: Early beginnings. In P. Pallaro (Ed.), *Authentic Movement: Moving the body, moving the self, being moved: A collection of essays* (Vol. II) (pp. 32–34). Jessica Kingsley Publishers.

Fleischer, K. (2024). The origin and history of embodied active imagination: Authentic Movement through the life and work of its early pioneers. In C. Tozzi (Ed.), *Interdisciplinary understandings of active imagination: The special legacy of C.G. Jung*. Routledge.

Haze, N. & Stromsted, T. (1994/1999). An interview with Janet Adler. In P. Pallaro (Ed.), *Authentic Movement: Essays by Mary Starks Whitehouse, Janet Adler, & Joan Chodorow* (pp. 107–120). Jessica Kingsley Publishers.

Jung, C. G. (1998). *Nietzsche's Zarathustra: Notes on the seminar given in 1934–1939* (Vol. 1). Princeton University Press.

Kalsched, D. (2010). Working with trauma in analysis. In M. Stein (Ed.), *Jungian psychoanalysis: Working in the spirit of C. G. Jung* (pp. 281–295). Open Court.

Ladinsky, D. (Trans.). (1999). "The God Who Only Knows Four Words." In *The Gift: Poems by Hafiz*. Penguin.

Neuberger, M. (2007). Tracing the brace. In P. Pallaro (Ed.), *Authentic Movement: Moving the body, moving the self, being moved: A collection of essays* (Vol. II) (pp. 445–455). Jessica Kingsley Publishers.

Porges, S. W. (2011). *The polyvagal theory: Neurophysiological foundations of emotions, attachment, communication, and self-regulation*. Norton and Company.

Schore, A. N. (2012). *The science of the art of psychotherapy*. W. W. Norton & Company.

Schore, A. N. (2014). The right brain is dominant in psychotherapy. *Psychotherapy, 51*(3), 388–397.

Schore, A. N. & Sieff, D. (2015). On the same wave-length: How our emotional brain is shaped by human relationships. In D. Sieff, D. (Ed.), *Understanding and healing emotional trauma: conversations with pioneering clinicians and researchers* (pp. 111–136). Routledge.

Siegel, D. (1999). *The developing mind: How relationships and the brain interact to shape who we are*. Guilford Press.

Stromsted, T. (1994/1995). Re-inhabiting the female body. *Somatics: Journal of the Bodily Arts & Sciences, X*(1), 18–27.

Stromsted, T. (2009). Authentic Movement: A dance with the divine. *Body, Movement and Dance in Psychotherapy, 4*, 201–213.

Stromsted, T. (2014). The alchemy of Authentic Movement: Awakening spirit in the body. In Williamson, A., Whately, S., Batson, G., & Weber, R. (Eds.), *Dance, somatics and spiritualities: Contemporary sacred narratives, leading edge voices in the field: Sensory experiences of the divine* (pp. 35–60). Intellect Books.

Stromsted, T. (2015). Authentic Movement and the evolution of Soul's Body® Work. *Journal of Dance & Somatic Practices, 7*(2), 339–357.

Stromsted, T. (2025). Meeting Joan Chodorow: Dancing in the depths. *IAAP News Bulletin* (36), January 2025.

Stromsted, T. & Haze, N. (2002/2007). Moving psyche and soma. *Contact Quarterly, 27*(2), 55–57.

Stromsted, T. & Haze, N. (2007). The road in: Elements of the study and practice of Authentic Movement. In P. Pallaro (Ed.), *Authentic Movement: Moving the body, moving the self, being moved: A collection of essays* (Vol. II) (pp. 56–68) Jessica Kingsley Publishers.

Stromsted, T. & Sieff, D. (2014). Dances of psyche and soma: Re-inhabiting the body in the wake of emotional trauma. In D. F. Sieff (Ed.), *Understanding and healing emotional trauma: conversations with pioneering clinicians and researchers* (pp. 46–63). Routledge.

Wilkinson, M. (2013, March 16). *The embodied psyche: mind, brain, body* [Lecture]. C. G. Jung Institute of San Francisco.

Woodman, M. & Mellick, J. (2000). *Coming home to myself: Reflections on nurturing a woman's body and soul*. Conari Press.

Chapter 2

Healing Soul's Body

Active Imagination in Movement

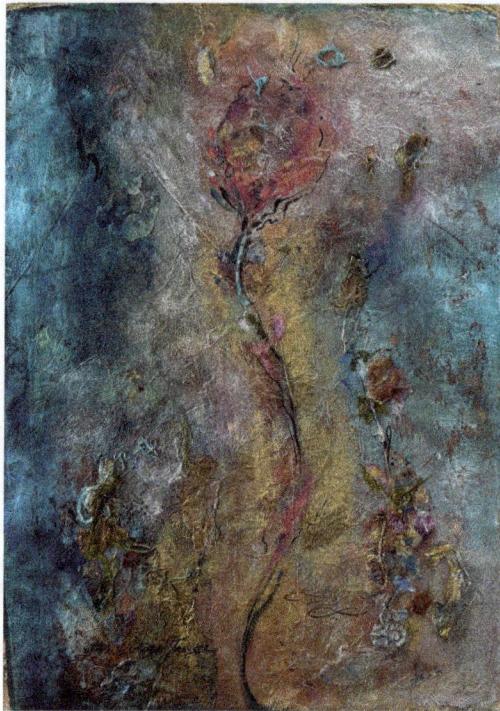

Figure 2.1 Dream Flower © 2024 by Aimee Trayser
@ https://www.aimeetrayser.net.

Healing movement has been practiced since the dawn of human history. Among traditional peoples, shamans and those seeking healing would "be moved" by an inner source, opening to a spirited flow of sensory and imaginal experiences that expressed themselves through dance (Eliade, 1964; Katz, 1982; Stromsted, 1994–1995). Communities acted as collective witnesses, forming an outer circle

DOI: 10.4324/9781003538356-4

to hold the dance, enabling the dancer to deeply follow what moved them from within. Similarly, Authentic Movement occurs within a safe container provided by witnesses. However, its focus lies not on inducing trance states but on developing individual and collective consciousness.

Authentic Movement is an inner-directed practice that utilizes nonverbal awareness in psychotherapy and in group work, with applications to daily life across cultures. The practice invites movers to attend to their embodied experience in the present moment, unfolding without agenda or plan. This process fosters emotional intelligence, as primal affects arise, are explored, brought to consciousness, and gradually integrated into a more whole personality. Genuine feelings emerge, deepening self-knowledge and connection, rather than being repressed, curated for social media or "political correctness," "acted out" in the world—or turned inward in self-destructive ways. Over time, this cultivates embodied presence and empathy—the ability to hold and receive the depths of another's experience.

This chapter explores how embodied awareness enriches analytic work, reconnecting the body with the inner world and attending to the subtleties of the intersubjective dance within the therapeutic relationship. Through the lens of Authentic Movement, I examine how the "talking cure" can be augmented by the experiences of the living body. Tracing the roots of Authentic Movement to Jung and active imagination, I outline its basic elements, which I'll expand on in later chapters. To illustrate its application, I describe an experiential session I led during the integrative Pre-Congress day at the International Association of Analytic Psychology (IAAP) Congress in Cape Town, South Africa. The event, cofacilitated by IAAP colleagues, illustrated ways to develop this approach further, engaging analysts and allied professionals in community exploration.

Active Imagination

Authentic Movement traces its origins to Jung's process of active imagination. During the period of intense soul-searching following his break with Freud, Jung discovered this "method for exploring the unknown" (Hannah, 1981, p. 4). Unlike passive fantasizing, active imagination required maintaining a conscious connection while engaging in "an active attempt to come to terms with an invisible force, … [exploring] the unknown country of the unconscious" (p. 16). Often expressed as dialogues with inner figures through various art forms, these were interactions between equals. Although Jung recognized dance as a form of active imagination, this aspect was developed more fully by others, notably Mary Starks Whitehouse.

Jung also incorporated elements from shamanism, mythology, and fairy tales—manifestations of the deeper unconscious—into his work. These elements connected patients with vital energies needed for inner transformation. Myths and fairy tales often explored dilemmas, conflicts, and resolutions, reflecting the psyche's innate healing potential (Criswell, 1997; Jung, 1968a; von Franz, 1970, 1972). Mythologist Joseph Campbell likened myths to dreams, saying, "Myths are to the culture like dreams are to the individual" (Campbell, 1978). Key myths depicting the feminine individuation journey include the stories of Demeter and Persephone (Chapter 6) and Inanna (Chapter 13).

Although Jung did not pursue embodied experience in depth, his writings made many references to the importance of the body in analytic work. He noted, for instance, that some patients danced their mandala drawings, dream elements, or feelings (Jung, 1935/1976, CW 13, p. 173). Unfortunately, he did not document these experiences in detail, leaving much of this material lost. However, the writings of his patient Tina Keller-Jenny—a physician and Jungian psychologist—vividly brought the embodiment aspect to life (Swan, 2009). Early in his career, Jung's focus on the body included experiments measuring galvanic skin responses during word association tests and observing the symbolic movements of regressed patients. He discovered gestures and repetitive actions often illuminated the patients' life histories (Jaffe, 1979, p. 39).

Over time, Jung's focus shifted from affects, which are rooted in bodily experience, to archetypes appearing as images. This transition occurred during his personal crisis following the break with Freud, when emotions threatened to overwhelm him (Chodorow, personal communication, January 2000). To manage this, Jung practiced yoga and used active imagination to connect affects with their corresponding images, introducing form and reflection to his emotions. Although this shift influenced his later work, Jung maintained that affect (and its bodily enervations) *and* image—both integral to archetypes—were inseparable.

Jung also acknowledged the value of art, sandplay, dreams, and movement in facilitating personal growth and wholeness. Post-Jungian analysts like Joan Chodorow, Marion Woodman, Arnold Mindell, Anita Greene, and others have expanded on Jung's early considerations of the body's role in analytic work. Their contributions, alongside contemporary object relations theory and interdisciplinary research, have profoundly enriched my understanding. As Jung wrote:

> If we can reconcile ourselves to the mysterious truth that the spirit is the life of the body seen from within, and the body the outward manifestation of the life of the spirit—the two being really one—then we can understand why the striving to transcend the present level of consciousness through acceptance of the unconscious must give the body its due.
>
> (Jung, 1928/1970, CW 10, p. 195)

Authentic Movement

Authentic Movement was pioneered by Mary Starks Whitehouse, who integrated her studies at the Zurich Jung Institute with her training under German modern dancer Mary Wigman and dancer/choreographer Martha Graham (Stromsted, 2025). However, the seeds of this practice had been sown decades earlier. Around 1924, Tina Keller-Jenny, a patient of Jung and later a Jungian-oriented psychologist

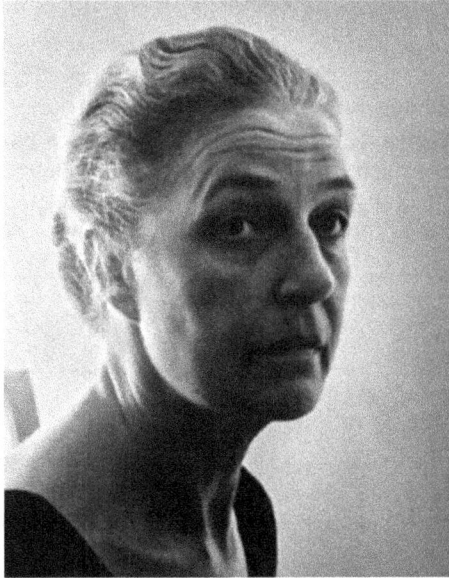

Figure 2.2 Mary Starks Whitehouse, Santa Monica, California, 1967, with kind permission from Berti Klein and Paula Sager on behalf of the Authentic Movement Community.

and physician herself, described an experience of moving during an analytic session with Jung's associate Toni Wolff:

> When I was in analysis with Miss Toni Wolff, I often had the feeling that something in me hidden deep inside wanted to express itself; but I also knew that this "something" had no words. As we were looking for another means of expression, I suddenly had the idea: "I could dance it." Miss Wolff encouraged me to try. The body sensation I felt was oppression; the image came that I was inside a stone and had to release myself from it to emerge as a separate, self-standing individual. The movements that grew out of the body sensations had the goal of my liberation from the stone just as the image had. It took a good deal of the hour. After a painful effort I stood there, liberated. This very freeing event was much more potent than the hours in which we only talked. This was a "psychodrama" of an inner happening, or that which Jung had named "active imagination." Only here it was the body that took the active part.
>
> (Keller, 1972, p. 22, translated by R. Oppikofer)

Mary Starks Whitehouse, a modern dancer and pioneer in dance/movement therapy, returned to California to explore a form of active imagination through movement. From the 1950s until her death in 1979, she worked with dancers and those seeking personal growth. During this time (1958–1971), Keller-Jenny, who had moved to Los Angeles, occasionally joined Whitehouse's studio classes. Also known as *Movement in Depth* or *Active Imagination in Movement*, Authentic Movement facilitates contact with and response to unconscious material as it finds bodily expression (Whitehouse, 1999).

Active Imagination, as defined by Jung, involves two phases: letting unconscious material emerge and coming to terms with it. Building on Jung's framework, Marie-Louise von Franz described five subdivisions, which analyst Janet Dallett later condensed into four:

1 Opening to the unconscious,
2 Giving it form,
3 Ego's reaction, and
4 Living it (Chodorow, 1997, p. 11).

Jung himself emphasized that it was not enough to gain some understanding of the images that arose during the process, but that once these insights had arisen into consciousness, we had an "'ethical' obligation" to live them (Jung, 1961, pp. 192–193).

Authentic Movement has broad applications as psychotherapy, meditation, sacred dance, creative exploration, ecopsychology, social activism, and community development. It can amplify dreams, offering clarity, depth, and meaning as images are consciously embodied (DreamDancing is explored in Chapter 15). Incorporating expressive movement with other creative media like drawing, painting, sculpture, writing, music, and theater, Authentic Movement facilitates the integration of unconscious material into conscious awareness (Chodorow, 1997, p. 7).

An essential aspect of the practice is discerning whether a mover's experiences, images, or dreams reflect unresolved personal material or broader transpersonal implications. The object relations approach explores how early developmental experiences with significant figures—parents, siblings, and others—shape the client's sense of self and influence current relationships (Scharff & Scharff, 1991; St. Clair, 1986). These insights, drawn from Gestalt, Family Constellations, and Internal Family Systems, build on Jung's work with inner figures and complexes. They shed light on the role of early life experiences and their effect on character development and relationship dynamics, helping to understand the fantasies and projections in the transference–countertransference dynamics that inevitably arise between the mover and the witness in Authentic Movement during the course of the analytic work.

Moving and Witnessing

Authentic Movement involves a mover (or group of movers) and a witness (or multiple witnesses, as in some forms of group work detailed in Chapter 12). The mover closes their eyes to focus inwardly, listening to and following their inner experience without choreography or plan. Eyes may open slightly for safety when necessary. This process of internal attention—known in neuroscience as *interocep-tion* (Schore, 2001)—is performed in the presence of a witness.

The mover's role is to engage with their experience attentively and respectfully, allowing the body to be moved from within, exploring their inner world at a pace and depth that feels appropriate. The witness, seated to the side, holds the space, ensures its privacy, and tracks the agreed-upon session length. Like an analyst in psychotherapy, the witness provides a containing function, observing the mover while also attending to their own feelings and somatic and imaginative responses evoked by the mover's experience. This dual awareness is critical for creating the safety required for embodied descent.

After the movement, the mover reflects on their experience and may seek feed-back from the witness. The witness's role is to respond nonjudgmentally to what they observed and what they experienced without interpretation, containing and owning any projections that may have been stirred within them. This process allows the mover to revisit and integrate deeper layers of experience. Repressed *shadow* el-ements—suppressed or underdeveloped aspects—often shaped by family, cultural, or religious influences—can emerge, be acknowledged, and transformed, fostering a sense of physical, psychological, and spiritual wholeness. The practice nurtures presence within oneself and in relationship, offering a framework for profound complexity and depth with applications that extend beyond the consulting room.

The mover's willingness to explore and integrate this material is essential for transformation. By attending to kinesthetic imagery (movement-related images [Dosamantes-Alperson, 1987]), dreams, body symptoms, and relationship patterns, themes emerge within the mover–witness dynamic, and meaningful synchronici-ties often play a role.

Witnessing Language

Witness feedback is nonjudgmental, noninterpretive, and free of aesthetic evalua-tions like "beautiful" or "awkward," minimizing any inclination the mover might feel to control or perform. Instead, the witness reflects literal movements and expres-sions, sharing how these affected their own sensations, emotions, images, memories, and stories—while explicitly owning these reactions. This approach helps the mover recall and deepen their experience, builds embodied consciousness, and affirms the relational healing power for both mover and witness (Stromsted & Haze, 2007).

Creating a Safe Container

Establishing a safe and trustworthy container—a *temenos*—is foundational in this practice. A "good enough" witness-figure (Winnicott, 1971) is essential to hold the mover's experience and facilitate transformation. Without a witness who main-tains open eyes, a nonjudgmental presence, and ego consciousness, the mover may struggle to relax their vigilance—the internalized self-protective system shaped by early negative experiences (Kalsched, 1996). A safe container enables the mover to engage with unconscious material freely, providing the "sheltered space" described by Dora Kalff (1980) or Winnicott's "transitional space" (1971). As shadow material surfaces for both mover and witness, the container supports its exploration and integration, fostering greater consciousness—a process further elaborated in Chapter 4.

Embracing Sacred Energy

As individuals engage in Authentic Movement, their "inner witness"—self-reflective consciousness—evolves, becoming more compassionate and better able to accept and integrate the full spectrum of human emotions. The practice also fosters an inner evolution that helps movers reconnect with their inherent divine nature—the God or Goddess within and in the world. The feminine aspect of the divine, often represented as *Sophia* in matter or the *Shekinah*, descended into the Abyss with the rise of patriarchal religions. Engaging in this work awakens deep knowing rooted in the body and embodied feelings, enabling a conscious feminine principle to emerge. Here, *feminine* refers to yin energy—an essence present in all people regardless of gender or sexual orientation. Qualities like *process, presence, being here now, paradox, resonating, receiving, surrendering,* and *listening* are at the heart of this aspect of being, as we seek wholeness in our ongoing dance with the opposites (Woodman, 1993).

Through Authentic Movement, individuals awaken their embodied awareness, accessing intuitive, nonverbal, and relational ways of knowing and resonating. This practice deepens the connection to self and others, affirming the sacredness of the body as a vessel for wisdom and transformation.

Community, Culture, and the Collective Body

While traditional analytic work often centers on individual journeys, Authentic Movement integrates the individual into the context of their broader networks—family, kinship groups, communities, nation, and planetary life. In group settings, experiencing a sense of belonging and purpose in a larger community or "collective body" often emerges as a powerful theme (Adler, 1999; Jung, 1968b).

The process invites awareness of the collective myth or story arising from the group's shared movements. For example, one participant may express grief while another embodies joy, highlighting the interplay of life's opposites. Projections are acknowledged and explored, multiple perspectives expressed and heard, fostering a dynamic balance between individual authenticity and communal relationships, key elements in individuation.

As analysts and somatic psychotherapists, we have much to learn from earlier shamanic traditions, where the larger group or tribe actively participated in an individual's rite of passage, creating transformation not just for the person but for the collective as a whole (Eliade, 1964; Henderson, 1967; van Löben Sels, 2020; Vuksinick, 1997). These ceremonies were deeply intertwined with myths—narratives that illuminated the web of relationships binding individuals to themselves, one another, the natural world, and the gods.

Jung highlighted how the symbolic imagery in myths serves as a guide, revealing the stages of life, the obstacles encountered along the way—the complexes, impasses, or "storms" where energy becomes stuck—and the steps necessary for more conscious development. Authentic Movement often evokes elements of these shamanic traditions, offering participants an opportunity to engage with embodied energies. These energies may manifest as figures, animals, or natural elements, becoming allies that help individuals navigate conflicts, traverse forests, scale mountains, or cross seas—each symbolizing the unique challenges of their life path. Practiced individually and in groups, Authentic Movement bridges the unconscious and conscious, personal and communal, daily experience and the sacred dimension, fostering transformative change that resonates beyond the therapy room (explored further in Chapters 16 and 17).

Embodied Depth and Neuroscience

Historically, therapeutic practices often disregarded the body's role, yet ancient traditions understood its significance. From shamanic dances to South African Sangomas' rituals, movement has long been a pathway to healing the individual and their community (Henderson, 1967).

Authentic Movement revitalizes this understanding, integrating body, psyche, and spirit. Contemporary neuroscience underscores its relevance, emphasizing early right-brain dominance where nonverbal communication forms the foundation of human connection. Within the therapeutic context, the body continually "speaks its mind," revealing the unconscious through subtle, embodied interactions between patient and therapist.

In honoring the body as a pathway to the soul and a medium for unconscious expression, Authentic Movement reinforces Jung's reminder to "give the body its due," cultivating a profound synthesis of ancient wisdom and modern insight.

Experiential Session

At a Pre-Congress experiential session in Cape Town in 2007, Joan Chodorow guided participants in exploring the principles of Authentic Movement through inner-sourced exploration. Beginning in a large circle, participants learned the practice of moving and witnessing, engaging in movement with an inner focus, followed by shared reflections with a partner. Jackie Gerson (2007), an analyst from Mexico, then presented on "Body Sensing as Emotional Communication," highlighting how unconscious "walls" manifest in stiffened musculature and sensing membranes, reflecting a lack of receptivity in relationships. These dynamics parallel the rigidity individuals, and even nations, often show toward one another. Gerson connected these insights to dyadic therapeutic work, where such walls can obscure relational depth.

Building on these themes, Antonella Adorisio (2007) shared her video exploring the union of nature and spirit, while Margarita Mendez (Chodorow et al., 2007) discussed Venezuela's historical complexes. Mendez illustrated how Jungian psychology, combined with dance and psychodrama, helped community leaders navigate colonialism's lingering effects, fostering greater tolerance and conflict resolution.

The earlier presentations led to a concluding experiential session in which I led a warm-up that deepened awareness of the body and breath, exploring movements like pressing against the floor and walls. These gestures amplified Gerson's distinction between rigid walls and healthy boundaries.

I invited the group to ground their bodies while opening to imagery from nature. We began by embodying a tree, feeling its roots sinking deep into the earth, and then transitioned to its opposite: exploring the sensations of a bird pressing off the ground to soar. In this way, we traversed the continuum between earth and sky, matter and spirit. Participants then moved to music blending African drumming with Australian didgeridoo, moving through space in ways that deepened their exploration of both inner and outer landscapes. Each person discovered the unique essence of their tree and bird before releasing these images to follow their own inner-directed active imagination.

With eyes closed, the group continued moving for twenty minutes, observed by five cofacilitators who held a quiet, grounded presence in the corners of the room. Afterward, participants stayed in the space with their eyes still closed, reflecting on their movement experience "like recalling a dream." They were then invited to revisit a shape or gesture that had felt particularly significant, repeating it a few times to deepen their clarity before concluding their movement.

To give form to the energy, participants expressed their experience through colors on paper. They then partnered to share their reflections, starting with the movement that stood out and the emotions it evoked. Each partner mirrored the other's gesture and offered a word or phrase describing how it resonated in their own body. The mover then shared additional aspects of their journey that felt ready to be voiced. The witness held a receptive, attuned presence, later reflecting back words or themes that carried particular resonance.

After switching roles and completing the process, participants returned to the larger group to share their drawings, insights, and discoveries. Through this layered and reciprocal practice, a profound sense of connection and understanding emerged.

Our day-long workshop integrated film, lecture, movement, and dialogue, culminating in reflections on the integrative power of Authentic Movement. Participants described a sense of wholeness and universality, affirming the approach's relevance across cultures and how many of the elements could be effective for working with children, teenagers, and others less responsive to verbal methods. In the context of Africa, many posed a pivotal question: "How can we continue to bring the body into analysis and training programs?" a question I hear in many parts of the world.

Jung's wisdom resonated throughout the session:

When the great swing has taken the individual into the world of symbolic mysteries, nothing comes of it ... unless it has been associated with the earth, unless it has happened when that individual was in the body ... And so individuation can only take place if you first return to the body, to your earth; only then does it become true.

(1976, CW 18, para. 473)

This grounding in the body roots symbolic mysteries in lived reality, supporting the ego in its engagement with the unconscious. By reclaiming a cellular intelligence that connects psyche and spirit, participants left with a renewed understanding of Authentic Movement's potential to bridge individual and collective transformation.

> One day the hero
> sits down,
> afraid to take
> another step,
> and the old interior angel
> limps slowly in
> with her no-nonsense
> compassion
> and her old secret
> and goes ahead.
>
> "Namaste"
> you say
> and follow.
>
> David Whyte (2007), from "The Old Interior Angel"

References

Adler, J. (1999). The collective body. In P. Pallaro (Ed.), *Authentic Movement: Essays by Mary Starks Whitehouse, Janet Adler, and Joan Chodorow* (pp. 190–204). Jessica Kingsley Publishers.

Adorisio, A. (2007, August 12). Mysterium – Body/spirit coniunctio in analytical psychology: Testimonials [Paper and DVD]. XVIIth International Congress for Analytical Psychology, Cape Town, South Africa.

Campbell, J. (1978). The hero's journey: Mythological and somatic perspectives [Lectures and workshop]. Co-taught with Stanley Keleman, Carmel, California. Sponsored by the Center for Energetic Studies, Berkeley, CA.

Chodorow, J. (Ed.). (1997). Introduction. *Jung on active imagination* (pp. 1–20). Princeton University Press.

Chodorow, J., Fay, C. G., Adorisio, A., Gerson, J., Mendez, M., & Stromsted, T. (2007, August 12). Moving journeys-embodied encounters: The living body in analysis [Presentation]. Pre-congress Day, XVIIth International Congress for Analytical Psychology, Capetown, South Africa.

Criswell, H. E. (1997, Spring/summer). Reflections of the editor. *Somatics: Magazine-Journal of the Mind/Body Arts and Sciences, XI*(2), inside cover.

Dosamantes-Alperson, I. (1987). Transference and counter-transference issues in movement psychotherapy. *The Arts in Psychotherapy, 4,* 209–214.

Eliade, M. (1964). *Shamanism: Archaic techniques of ecstasy.* Princeton University Press.

Gerson, J. (2007, August 12). *Bodily sensing as emotional communication* [Presentation]. XVIIth International Congress for Analytical Psychology, Cape Town, South Africa.

Hannah, B. (1981). *Encounters with the soul: Active imagination as developed by C. G. Jung.* Sigo Press.

Henderson, J. L. (1967). *Thresholds of initiation.* Wesleyan University Press.

Jaffe, A. (Ed.). (1979). *C. G. Jung: Word and image.* Princeton University Press.

Jung, C. G. (1961). *Memories, dreams, reflections.* Vintage Books, Random House.

Jung, C. G. (1968a). *Analytical psychology: Its theory and practice.* Vintage Books.

Jung, C. G. (1968b). The psychology of the child archetype. In *The archetypes and the collective unconscious* (Vol. 9i). Princeton University Press. (Original work published 1940.)

Jung, C. G. (1970). The spiritual problems of modern man. In *The collected works of C. G. Jung: Vol. 10. Civilization in transition.* Princeton University Press. (Original work published 1928.)

Jung, C. G. (1976). The Tavistock lectures: On the theory and practice of analytical psychology. In *The collected works of C. G. Jung: Vol. 18. The symbolic life.* Princeton University Press. (Original work published 1935.)

Kalff, D. (1980). *Sandplay: A psychotherapeutic approach to the psyche.* Sigo Press.

Kalsched, D. (1996). *The inner world of trauma: Archetypal defenses of the personal spirit.* Routledge.

Katz, E. (1982). *Boiling energy.* Harvard University Press.

Keller, T. (1972). IV. Körperempfindung und bewegung in der psychotherapie (Chapter IV. Body awareness and movement in psychotherapy). *Wege inneren Wachstums: Aus meinen erinnerungen an C.G. Jung (Pathways to inner growth from my memories of C. G. Jung)* (pp. 22–27). Bircher-Benner Verlag.

Scharff, D. & Scharff, J. (1991). *Object relations family therapy.* Jason Aronson, Inc.

Schore, A. (2001). The effects of early relational trauma on right brain development, affect regulation, and infant mental health. *Infant Mental Health Journal, 22,* 201–269.

St. Clair, M. (1986). *Object relations and self psychology: An introduction.* Wadsworth, Inc.

Swan, W. (2009). *Memoir of Tina Keller-Jenny: A lifelong confrontation with the psychology of C. G. Jung.* Spring Journal Books.

Stromsted, T. (1994/1995). Re-Inhabiting the female body. *Somatics: Journal of the Bodily Arts & Sciences, X*(1), 18–27.

Stromsted, T. (2025). Psyche's body: A brief history of engaging the body in analysis and psychotherapy. *IAAP News Bulletin* (36), January 2025.

Stromsted, T. & Haze, N. (2007). The road in: Elements of the study and practice of Authentic Movement. In P. Pallaro (Ed.), *Authentic Movement: Moving the body, moving the self, being moved: A collection of essays* (Vol. II) (pp. 56–68). Jessica Kingsley Publishers.

van Löben Sels, R. (2020). *Shamanic dimensions of psychotherapy: Healing through the symbolic process.* Routledge.

von Franz, M.-L. (1970). *Apuleius's golden ass.* Spring Publications.

von Franz, M.-L. (1972). *The feminine in fairy tales.* Spring Publications.

Vuksinick, L. (1997). Serpent fire arousal: Its clinical relevance. In D. F. Sandner & S. H. Wong (Eds.), *The Sacred heritage: The influence of shamanism on analytical psychology* (pp. 101–110). Routledge.

Whitehouse, M. S. (1999). Essays. In P. Pallaro (Ed.), *Authentic Movement: Essays by Mary Starks Whitehouse, Janet Adler, and Joan Chodorow* (pp. 14–101). Jessica Kingsley.

Winnicott, D. W. (1971). *Playing and reality.* Tavistock Publications.

Woodman, M. (1993). The conscious feminine. In *Conscious femininity: Interviews with Marion Woodman* (pp. 81–90). Inner City Books.

Whyte, D. (2007). The interior angel. In *River flow: New & selected poems 1984–2007.* Many Rivers Company.

Part II

On the Journey:
Core Elements

Chapter 3

Embodied Imagination

From Emptiness to Form

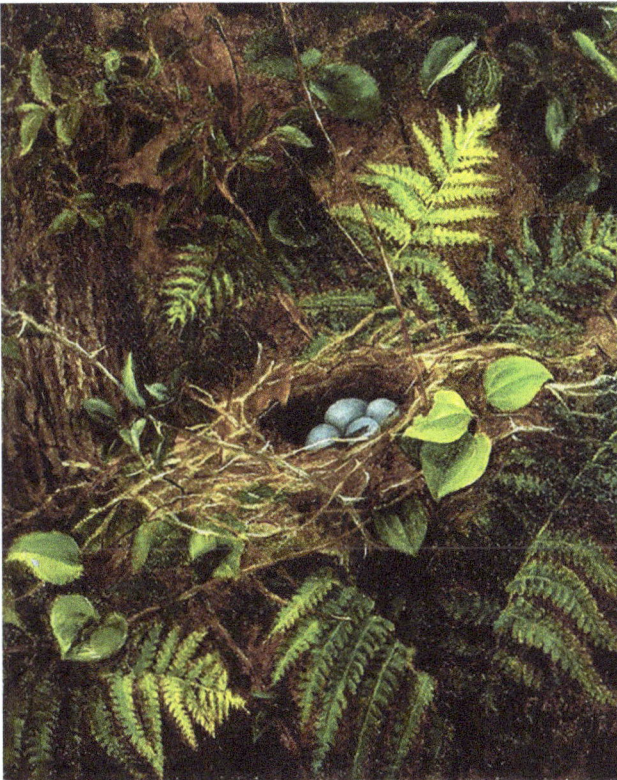

Figure 3.1 Still Life with Robin's Nest by Fidelia Bridges (1834–1923).

The Upanishads ask, "If you cannot find it in your own body, where will you go in search of it?" (Prabhavananda & Manchester, 2002, p. 21). How can we live a meaningful, embodied life in today's fast-paced, mechanized, and materialistic world? How do we reconnect with the sacredness of our bodies and everyday Eros

DOI: 10.4324/9781003538356-6

amid the polarizing tensions of the cultural–political landscape, the ravages of oppression and war, the sensual detachment of the internet, and the exploitation of our planet's resources for consumerist gain? How do we address the emptiness that consumption cannot fill? And how do we find the courage to embrace the unknown—the fertile void—and uncover the creativity, healing, and mystery it holds? These reflections arise from my experiences with individuals and groups exploring these questions through Authentic Movement.

Authentic Movement is a process of being guided into movement from within while being witnessed in that unfolding. The mover closes their eyes, waits, and responds to sensations, impulses, emotions, and images arising in the body. With curiosity and open attention, they "listen" to what emerges, allowing themselves to be guided spontaneously. As the witness, I sensitively track and hold the mover's experience, creating a container that supports their descent into the depths their psyche draws them toward. Together, we slow down to listen inwardly and reflect on what we discover—essential for attuning to our deeper nature.

In this process, we encounter challenging feelings, unmet needs, and moments of sweet surrender. It often mirrors the night sea journey that challenges who we thought we were, musters unexpected strength, and heightens our ability to navigate darkness. Ultimately, this practice deepens our capacity to help others see in the dark in uncertain times. It fosters resilience and well-being in the embodied psyche, guiding us as we encounter the devastating losses, rapid shifts, and inspiring innovations of contemporary life. Previously unrealized images and energies can surface, renewing our faith that "some-thing" can emerge from "no-thing."

The Evolving Self

The roots of this work trace back to our earliest beginnings. From the moment an infant enters the world, the foundation of human existence is laid: they experience and are experienced. In infancy, sensations dominate, shaping how the infant encounters life. As they grow, their perceptual world deepens and becomes more complex, integrating physical, cognitive, psychological, relational, moral, spiritual, and ecological dimensions into a unified whole. They begin to *see* and *be seen* by the world around them (Stromsted & Haze, 2007, p. 56). Within this first primary relationship, usually with the mother, *being seen* is, ideally, deeply present.

In this first relationship, the mother or primary caregiver provides an empathic, nonintrusive, and holding environment that allows the child to discover their sense of self. The caregiver's ability to hold and reflect the full spectrum of the child's emotions, as well as their experiences of health and illness, fosters a deeper awareness of inner states. "If the mother [or primary parenting figure] is not able to reflect accurately the child's affective states, the child will not be able to develop a reliable sense of self," notes psychoanalytic dance therapist Arlene Avstreih (1981, p. 22). Authentic Movement supports the transformation of unsatisfactory experiences within this early dyad by enabling the mover (child/client) and witness (parent/therapist) relationship. This interaction can establish a "holding environment" and a "potential space," offering new pathways for healing and self-discovery.

The Role of the Witness

In the practice of witnessing, therapists refine their skills in observation and empathic listening. They learn to recognize interpersonal themes and group dynamics from an embodied perspective while deepening their understanding of the creative process and the multimodal approach of active imagination. As Janet Adler observes, "Inherent in being a person in the cultures of the West, is a longing for a witness. We seem to want, deeply want, to be seen as we are by another" (Alder, 1999, p. 158).

T. S. Eliot's *Four Quartets* illuminates the paradox of holding opposites—will and surrender, concentration and open attention—central to Authentic Movement for both mover and witness:

I said to my soul, be still, and wait without hope

For hope would be hope for the wrong thing; wait without love,

For love would be love of the wrong thing; there is yet faith

But the faith and the love and the hope are all in the waiting.

Wait without thought, for you are not ready for thought:

So the darkness shall be the light, and the stillness the dancing.

(Eliot, 1943)

At the conclusion of their movement session, the mover recounts the physical, emotional, and imaginal elements of their journey. The witness, who has been holding space and presence for the mover, responds without judgment or interpretation, sharing sensations, images, and feelings experienced while observing. Maintaining receptive, curious attention, the witness refrains from directing or shaping the mover's process. Through this engagement, somatic countertransference can arise as the witness holds and metabolizes the unmentalized, presymbolic material the mover is exploring. Each encounters emptiness before form, embracing the unknown through direct, embodied experience.

Empathic mirroring by the witness helps address void states—feelings of invisibility, emptiness, or even nonexistence, stemming from inadequate early mirroring. The witness's attentive presence, along with verbal exchange, supports the mover in accessing and integrating cellular memories. The mover's potential will unfold in its own time.

Through this work, preverbal memories, unresolved developmental material, and transpersonal experiences may surface, enriching both participants' interpersonal, creative, and spiritual capacities. Movers gain access to unconscious energies, feelings, and primal or numinous imagery. Witnesses are often deeply moved by the authenticity of the mover's process, evoking potent insights and emotions. Listening inwardly with conscious attention supports healing early wounds and recovering unlived life; it helps both mover and witness build stronger, more flexible, embodied vessels for navigating challenging feelings and channeling sacred energy—an essential element for living a meaningful, soulful life.

Within the safe, intentional container provided, the process begins to soften coping mechanisms and outdated self-images through the direct experience of suffering and beauty, making way for compassion. Movers often become more graceful as they surrender conscious control, experiencing a sense of being moved by something greater than the ego. Mover and witness alike often experience transformative shifts, as the boundaries of time and space begin to soften. They may also experience a union of self and other, a profound participation in the larger resonant field or life force.

After moving, creative exploration through drawing, sculpting, or writing can further integrate the mover's experience. These expressions often anchor insights and energies, deepening their impact. Dialogues between mover and witness allow these discoveries to ripple into the mover's broader life, enriching relationships and deepening self-awareness. Dreams, too, can be explored through this method, with formative images becoming consciously embodied.

The following examples illustrate the healing and transformation made possible through Authentic Movement. (I use present tense to preserve their vitality and reflect the language of the work.)

Mandala Body

In 1977, during a workshop in San Francisco, I was witnessed by the late Magda Proskauer (1980), a physical therapist and wise teacher of breathwork. It was there that I had the following experience:

As I lie on my back, I bring my awareness to the inner spaces and bony support structures of my skeleton. I particularly focus on the major ball-and-socket joints in my body. I lift my shoulders and hips before lowering them to the floor. Later, I feel the connection between my upper and lower body by twisting along the long diagonal axis in my body, letting my knees drop toward the floor to the left as my head rolls to the right. I make these movements consciously and with feeling, supported by the natural rhythm of my breath. After moving this way for several minutes, I feel a warm glow wash through me. My mouth fills with a sweet taste, and I hear a kind of buzz within me that reminds me of the sound that bees make around a hive. It's as though they are circulating throughout my body in my bloodstream ... or is it my nervous system ... or perhaps my energetic body? Though the specific "location" is unclear, since it is an overall body sensation, what is undeniable is how full and peaceful, yet vibrantly alive I feel. In the next moment, I have an image of a mandala, the sacred circle that plays an important role in many Eastern meditative practices. What is unusual about this one is that it is not two-dimensional like the ones I have seen in books. Instead, it is a sphere, three- or perhaps four-dimensional. It feels timeless, eternal. Seeing it, I realize that my body too is a mandala—my dearest, most intimate mandala. With this resonating awareness, I begin to weep sweet tears of gratitude, which gives me a felt connection to my Self, to everyone in the room, and, simultaneously, to all of life.

Upon reflection, I realized this moment followed months of painful separation from a long-term partner—a chaotic time that had distanced me from my body. Held safely in the witness's presence, I could breathe deeply, descend into my depths, and rediscover a sense of wholeness. Years later, I occasionally revisit that sweet humming sensation in Authentic Movement practice. While mysterious, it often emerges after a disconnection—from myself, others, or the Self—prompting movement that arises from the void. The atmosphere feels paradoxically light yet textured, like honey with an electrical buzz to it, and charged with healing energy that is bright and spirited. Sometimes, tears and a taste of sweetness accompany it.

Working in Groups

In nonanalytic group settings, the process shifts slightly while maintaining core principles (discussed further in Chapter 12). Witnesses form a circle, creating a contained space for movers. Often, the empty center symbolizes the void—a source of new life and eventual return. Movers enter the circle only when an inner stirring or "call" arises. Like meditation, the presence of an engaged community deepens awareness. Within the witness-circle's safety, movers explore the unknown, responding to their inner rhythms and the group's co-creation.

At such times, I often feel in tune with a shared frequency, resonating along a harmonic continuum. I envision bees in a hive, each moving instinctively, without forethought, guided by a deeper source. This evokes a sense of participation in a dance that builds the hive and keeps the community alive with living music, transforming pollen into honey. A palpable hum vibrates through my body. When discussing these experiences within the circle, others often echo similar sensations—a spirited energy, a shared story, or the sweetness of connection.

Years later, I discovered the ancient Bee Goddess of Regeneration, depicted in Minoan Crete's art and rituals. She signified the indestructible life that comes out of the carcass of death;she inspired rites echoed in the Eleusinian Mysteries connected with the myth of Demeter and Persephone and the Dionysian rite. Devotees of these cults heard "the 'voice' of the goddess, the 'sound' of creation" in the humming of the bees (Baring & Cashford, 1991, pp. 118–119). Such divine energies, I believe, remain encoded within us, reconnecting us to the larger life force. They also remind us of the crucial role that honeybees, now endangered by pesticides and dwindling landscapes, play in the interdependent web of life.

Healing the Vessel

One student I worked with used Authentic Movement for inner discovery and self-knowledge. "Sabeth's" loss occurred so early in life that she had no conscious memory of it.

Earlier in the day, "Sabeth" had felt drawn to witness "Anna," who was wearing a red smock and cradling her six-month-old fetus in her belly. Now Sabeth enters the movement, closes her eyes, and stands in the center of the circle of witnesses, her feet planted shoulder-width apart and her arms raised over her head, appearing solid and fully grounded. Gradually her arms lower to a horizontal position, remaining outstretched and still for ten to fifteen minutes; her expression is intensely focused. Others enter the circle, following an inner prompting to become movers. As I witness the group of movers, I feel drawn to Sabeth's powerful inward-gathering of energy. My gaze returns to her again and again, and I note that I feel increasingly present as it does so. I feel firm, full, and aware of my contact with the ground. Very soon, I sense a stream of energy moving up from the floor, through Sabeth's legs, womb, and heart, and out through her arms and hands. As I watch, I feel my heart opening, and my spine begins to tingle with electricity and warm with heat. There is a buildup of pressure behind my eyes. I close them for a moment, catching a vision of a ball of radiant, bright light. Just as the tension reaches its peak, something in Sabeth is released, and the energy appears to drain from her, leaving her limp, as if lifeless. I notice a draining of my energy as this happens. Moments later, another mover comes up from behind her and presses the front of her body into Sabeth's back. At first, Sabeth's body stiffens, pulling forward and away from the contact. Soon, however, she releases her weight, allowing this new companion to support her. When the movement round comes to an end, Sabeth opens her eyes and returns to the circle to speak about her experience.

While moving, she says she felt drawn to replicate the gestures of the pregnant woman from earlier. To Sabeth, Anna represented the Healing Mother or Divine Feminine. When Sabeth extended her arms, an image of an angel appeared, her arms becoming wings, and her womb felt "full of red." She experienced herself as both the angel delivering the annunciation and the Virgin Mother receiving it. In this process, she felt healed.

Sabeth then felt "full of tears," though she couldn't grasp their meaning. This was followed by a sense of being cut off from her pelvis and legs as she "hung there," arms outstretched. Initially resistant to contact, an "inner shift" allowed her to accept the support and presence of the other mover at her back, which became a source of comfort. As Sabeth shared her experience, she realized how the support had helped, giving her the backbone that allowed her to move beyond her "stuck" place.

In response, I told her that, for me, her outstretched arms evoked the image of the crucified Christ—first in ecstasy, filled with light, then in despair, limp and bleeding. Although I felt despair, there was a sense of a "rightness in the sequence," an inevitability, as if the sacrifice "*had* to be." Later, her body resembled a vessel, filling with light and energy before draining out. The image of the Sumerian Goddess Inanna came to mind, hanging in the underworld after receiving the death gaze of her dark sister, Erishkigal (described more in detail in Chapter 13), whom she had come to comfort. At first, I, too, felt ambivalent when the other mover arrived, not wanting anything to "interfere" with Sabeth's experience. However, when Sabeth's body softened into the support, I felt my weight shift, a grounding peace settling in.

Sabeth nodded upon hearing my reflection and described how the contact helped her "bring spirit into [my] legs, light into dense matter. It was excruciatingly painful in the beginning," she says. "I felt as though I would be torn in two opposing directions, but there was nothing I could do but stay there. When the other mover came, I realized that I could embrace her from that part of myself that needs support and that I can love and accept the love of another. It was not at all what I had expected to happen, and by the end, I felt more fully myself." Placing her hands on her pelvis and belly, she adds, "This is where I have always felt most uncertain and wounded." She then recalled how her mother had spoken of the terror she felt during violent contractions while bombs dropped around them in her rural European village during World War II (WWII). Quietly, Sabeth acknowledged that the movement had offered profound healing she couldn't yet fully articulate (Stromsted, 1996, pp. 26–28).

In Sabeth's work, I saw the personal, cultural (Henderson, 1984), and archetypal layers of the unconscious—the embodiment of some of Western culture's earliest mythic forms. C. G. Jung described a "collective unconscious" that allows individuals to access the experiences of all previous life forms (Jung, 1966, CW 7). As Sabeth's witness, I sensed the presence of a larger energy. Something deep within me recognized archetypal images of suffering and redemption, death and resurrection. As a fetus in the womb of a mother in war-torn Europe, a mother who lacked adequate support, Sabeth had been wounded. But now, Sabeth could open to an energy beyond her personal mother, finding support through her connection with another mover and through her link to the Great Mother, a deep, sacred source.

The annihilatory anxiety between mother and fetus during the bombing had terrorized them both, an original trauma that constricted Sabeth's ability to sense herself as an empowered woman. Sabeth's ability to linger in the unknown and to hold the opposites, expressed through the tension in her outstretched arms, evoked the emergence of the *transcendent function*—the capacity to hold the tension between opposites until a new, third energy emerges, often unexpected and more than the sum of its parts, a new birth. Warm light moved through her, healing energy that brought with it a fuller sense of her vital, womanly self.

A critical challenge in our time is the reintegration of mind, body, and spirit—a special issue for women, who have been more closely associated with the body than men in a culture alienated from it (Stromsted, 2001). Women's menstrual cycles, experiences of giving birth, and nursing bring them closer to the cycles of nature within their bodies. Yet, they are also imprinted by their mothers' uncertain connection to feminine wisdom or seduced by media images of the "perfect" female body. As in Sabeth's case, world events and cultural constraints can create a sense of the void. Growing up within this context, girls often suffer an inherent sense of loss, a "homelessness" hard to name, and Authentic Movement can offer a pathway home. As Marion Woodman writes, "When there has been a radical split, I believe a somatic container must be prepared to receive the psychic labor. There must be a greeting of the spirit, a chalice to receive the wine" (Woodman, 1982, p. 69).

Moving Men: Re-membering the Emotional Body

Men, too, face challenges in re-inhabiting their bodies. Often, they report a deep sense of alienation due to societal pressures to perform and the denial of their feelings. Through movement practice, many rediscover their body's emotional wisdom, sense of worth, and genuine longing for connection.

Some time ago, I taught an Authentic Movement course to a group of men and women in their midtwenties to midforties. They were all in their first quarter of graduate training in Somatic Psychology at the California Institute of Integral Studies in San Francisco. The course focused on developing embodied presence and exploring the somatic nuances of the transference–countertransference relationship. Authentic Movement provided a means to explore personal movement patterns, body image issues, and relationship dynamics unconsciously embodied in their family of origin and ethnic background.

As we began moving and witnessing, I observed the entire group while modeling nonjudgmental witnessing language. Over the weeks, they shifted from outwardly focused, dynamic movement to a more receptive, meditative, inner focus, allowing them to access deeper feelings and states of being. In "Keith's" experience, fragments of psyche, body sensation, feeling, memory, and relationship dynamics gradually integrated into a more cohesive sense of self.

> Closing my eyes, I feel unsteady, like an infant. Then I sense myself moving into young adulthood and feel angry, restricted, and inhibited. When Tina asks us to imagine ourselves in the context of our "family's dance," I feel my family moving in tight dance steps in small circles, reflecting our strict Irish Catholic heritage, which inhibited freedom of expression. My movements are wild Dionysian lunges away from them. "Is how I feel inside being perceived on the outside?" I wonder. As I begin to move I feel the mystery of expectation in an experience that is completely unknown to me. "Will anything happen?" I wonder, "And how deep will it go?" Beginning with controlled Tai-Chi movements, I immediately feel chills in my body. This makes me close up and drop to my knees—a

closing up that seems to happen when I stop controlling my actions. As I give up control, I don't know how to act; my natural instincts feel as if they have died of inactivity. On my knees, anger rises up in me. I get up and begin to walk across the room and then pace back and forth. I feel very agitated and want to explode and let whatever is holding me so tight come pouring out.

Then something happens so naturally that I am not even aware of the change. The anger and agitation give way to a sadness that feels as far away as it is present. I sit down and lean against the wall, feeling small and innocent, and begin rubbing my right leg. I am lost in this moment for a few minutes when all at once I realize what I am doing. Tears come to my eyes. Was I not being seen? Was my pain not valid? It was months of this pain before my parents took me to the doctor. I remember looking at my mother in front of the doctor's office and saying, "I hope something's wrong with me so Dad won't be mad." There was something wrong, but it took the doctors two years to find the cancerous tumor in my right hip. When we gather together after the movement I share what I experienced, feeling deeply touched, vulnerable, and astounded that so much memory and feeling could be recovered in that simple gesture of rubbing my leg. It feels good to be heard and important to have my feelings and pain acknowledged. I feel a lost piece of myself return.

(CIIS student, personal communication, 1999)

Keith, an attractive, powerfully built man in his early thirties, exuded easy self-confidence. But inside, he felt empty and inadequate, as though his life were not his own. Through surrendering to his inner experience, contained by supportive, non-judgmental witnesses, Keith reconnected with his feelings, reintegrating forgotten parts of himself. This experience ignited a renewed faith in his inner knowing and a fresh interest in life.

Giving Birth to Myself: Embodied Voice

Authentic Movement supports the integration of sensation, emotion, and imagery within the mover. Often, the next step involves finding an authentic voice to express embodied truth. This practice may tap into the roots of sound, helping movers discover and own their voice to express their emerging sense of *be-ing* in the world. For many women, vocal expression can be challenging. Voices often become muted, squeaky, cut off, or distorted as they attempt to conform to a largely patriarchal, disembodied, and mechanistic culture. Group work explores ways to support and expand each person's authentic voice.

After a workshop in London, one participant, "Christina," described how revitalization began for her after reading an article I provided. Here are her words:

Before reaching the end of your article I feel the urge to do some Authentic Movement on my own. I decide to move for ten minutes and simply ask that I be shown all I need to be shown at this point in time. I am standing and start to jiggle my knees in an upward/downward motion. The movement becomes faster and faster, and as I breathe I begin to vocalize, pushing sound out on the out-breath. My abdomen suddenly contracts, and I create a louder, sharper sound. It sounds animal to me. The sounds continue, and my mouth begins to stretch wider and wider till it feels enormous. I have an image of a wide-open vagina, and then I begin to feel a baby's head emerging from my mouth. I am both baby emerging into the world and mother giving birth. I have a sense of something profound happening and quite spontaneously I imagine you witnessing, [and this] encourages me to continue with the movement. I certainly don't feel so alone.

In my original birth, I was born with the cord around my neck, and when I begin to feel the baby's head emerge from my mouth, the baby becomes stuck once the head has emerged. This experience of birthing brings feelings of wonder, amazement, and relief all at the same time. I then become the present me, the mother, giving birth, and I move to the floor on hands and knees, pelvis wide open, and begin to pant as though resting between contractions. In my movement I alternate between being the baby being born and myself giving birth to my baby. My hands reach toward my head and I gently rotate it. I sense a vast silence surrounding me. My head begins to move forward slightly and my throat feels clearer. I take some breaths and imagine that any restriction around my throat is gone. I continue to move forward and slide onto my stomach on the floor. I am sad because no one has witnessed my birth, but then I think of you witnessing me, God witnessing me, and witnessing myself, and I feel OK. I open my eyes and look at the world.

Christina wrote: "My sense is that I am finally giving birth to myself and can move forward after weeks, months, and years of feeling stuck" (Personal communication, 2002). Despite years of study, Christina's well-developed intellect couldn't quell the deep sense of not belonging, of being stranded between worlds. Embodied active imagination allowed her to return to the "stuck place" encountered at her birth and follow the wisdom of the Self to deliver her anew. As Mary Stark Whitehouse wrote, "Movement, to be experienced, has to be found in the body, not put on like a dress or a coat. There is that in us which has moved from the very beginning; it is that which can liberate us" (Whitehouse, 1999, p. 51). Christina's growing capacity to experience vitality in her body, find her standpoint, and express herself in her natural voice allowed her to feel present, empowered, and more fully engaged in her life's journey.

Science and Mystery

Though the energies, openings, and healings I've described may seem idiosyncratic, they stem from what is universal within us. Brian Swimme, a mathematical cosmologist, writes about this universe within and around us:

The universe emerges out of an all-nourishing abyss, not just fifteen billion years ago but in every moment. Each instant, protons and antiprotons flash out of, and are suddenly absorbed back into, this abyss. It is not a thing or a collection of things, but a power that births and absorbs existence at its annihilation. The foundational reality of the universe is this unseen ocean of potentiality.

(Swimme 1996, p. 100)

In a contained space, the mover surrenders ego control, becoming receptive to energetic currents and images from the Self beneath the adaptations of the personality. This often fosters a profound connection—with themselves, others, and the natural world. Muscular armoring, overdetermined boundaries, and dichotomous thinking soften as mover and witness experience their individual standpoints, along with a sense of union. This can bring a sense of belonging to the human community across time and culture, and to the natural world.

It also becomes clear that the "talking cure," initiated by Freud, is insufficient. Contemporary neuroscience research points to the right brain's receptivity to nonverbal elements—facial expressions, tone of voice, movement, affect, music, imagery, and the play of symbols in dreams and poetry (Bazhenova et al., 2007; Schore, 2003; Siegel, 1999). From our earliest moments, empathic relating is crucial for self-formation. Affective mirroring and embodied presence build the foundation for consciousness in the cells, as well as a sense of well-being and belonging in the world. By being sensitive to the body, analysts can attend to this language, hear the soul's call, and address the obstacles that prevent a response.

Through the practice of accessing bodily sensation and allowing movements rooted in a deeper source, movers give embodied form to myths that have shaped humankind since creation. "Transcendental power," says dancer and scholar Maria-Gabriele Wosien, "articulates myth and ritual as it articulates the shapes of plants and trees, the structure of the nervous system, or any other processes beyond men's deliberate control" (Wosien, 1974, p. 30). Authentic Movement reconnects movers and witnesses with the instinctual resources and spiritual intelligence embedded in their cells. Through waiting without knowing, they embrace mysteries and may recover unlived parts of their nature, on intra-, inter-, and transpersonal levels.

Listening Forward

As we bring consciousness to our most genuine resource—the life energy expressed through the movement of our bodies—profound healing and change unfold. Emptiness may give rise to fullness, and the void may become nourishing darkness. From the experience of loss to the vital "hum" of bees, from a woman giving birth to herself to a man becoming internally integrated, all of this may be facilitated by the consciousness gained through Authentic Movement. As modern people, our bodies still have the capacity to engage us in meaningful experiences that are deeply personal and universal, spanning continents and centuries. Now, more than ever, we need the pathway toward a paradigm shift that embodied active imagination offers.

In this work, rather than adopting outer images or gods, I stay close to what holds the most truth for me—the direct, embodied experiences of the sacred.

The practice invites me to linger in emptiness, listen to my body's deeper callings, and give shape to the feelings and images that surface from underground wellsprings toward consciousness. The presence of an outer witness fosters the development of a compassionate "inner witness," responding to the self's longing for the Self. Beneath the infant-mother dyad, and the analytic dyad, lies a deeper one—the nascent ego's yearning for the beloved, the divine, the Self. What was once the "void" now has the potential to transform into a fertile darkness, a tolerable emptiness that gives rise to deeper experiences of the Self. This work's power lies in its holistic approach, touching physical, psychological, spiritual, social, aesthetic, and ecological dimensions. As movers, we are supported in exploring what is necessary for our healing, while witnesses are enriched by what has been transformed. Together, we take our place in an ever-widening circle, embracing the larger community and the planet (Stromsted, 2001, pp. 54–55).

> The body developed out of us, not we from it. We are bees,
> and our body is a honeycomb.
> We made
> the body, cell by cell we made it.
>
> Rumi (Bly, 1986)

References

Adler, J. (1999). Who is the witness? In P. Pallero (Ed.), *Authentic Movement: Essays by Mary Stark Whitehouse, Janet Adler, and Joan Chodorow* (2nd ed.). Jessica Kingsley Publishers.

Avstreih, A. K. (1981). The emerging self: Psychoanalytic concepts of self-development and their implications for dance therapy. *American Journal of Dance Therapy, 4*(2), 21–32.

Bazhenova, O. V., Stoganova, T. A., Doussard-Roosevelt, J. A., Posikera, I. A., & Porges, S. W. (2007). Physiological responses of 5-month-old infants to smiling and blank faces. *International Journal of Psychophysiology, 63*(1), 64–76. doi: 10.1016/j.ijpsycho.2006.08.008.

Baring, A. & Cashford, J. (1991). *The myth of the Goddess: Evolution of an image*. Penguin Books.

Bly, R. (Trans.) (1986). The body developed out of us, not we from it. In Rumi (Ed.), *When grapes turn to wine*. Yellow Moon Press.

Eliot, T. S. (1943). East coker. In *Four quartets*. Harcourt, Brace, & Co.

Henderson, J. L. (1984). *Cultural attitudes in psychological perspective*. Inner City Books.

Jung, C. G. (1966). On the psychology of the unconscious. In *Two essays on analytical psychology* (Vol. 7). (R. F. C. Hull, trans.) Princeton University Press. (Original work published 1917.)

Prabhavananda, S., & Manchester, F. (Trans.) (2002). *The Upanishads: Breath from the eternal: The wisdom of the Hindu mystics*. Signet Classics/Penguin Random House.

Proskauer, M. (1980). The relationship between body & psyche as it manifests itself in my work. *Journal of Biological Experience, 2*(2), 56–62.

Schore, S. (2003). *Affect regulation and the origin of the self* and *Affect dysregulation and disorders of the self* (2 vols.). W. W. Norton & Company.

Siegel, D. (1999). *The developing mind: Toward a neurobiology of interpersonal experience*. The Guilford Press.

Stromsted, T. (1996). Authentic Movement as embodied transformative practice: A study of the experience of the witness from psychological and mystical perspectives [Unpublished PhD paper]. California Institute of Integral Studies.

Stromsted, T. (2001, January). Re-inhabiting the female body: Authentic Movement as a gateway to transformation. *The Arts in Psychotherapy*, *28*(1), 39–55.

Stromsted, T. & Haze, N. (2007). The road in: Elements of the study and practice of Authentic Movement. In P. Pallaro (Ed.), *Authentic Movement: Moving the body, moving the self, being moved: A collection of essays* (Vol. II) (pp. 56–68). Jessica Kingsley Publishers.

Swimme, B. (1996). *The hidden heart of the cosmos: Humanity and the new story*. Orbis Books.

Whitehouse, M. S. (1999). Physical movement and personality. In P. Pallero (Ed.), *Authentic Movement: Essays by Mary Stark Whitehouse, Janet Adler, and Joan Chodorow* (2nd ed.). Jessica Kingsley Publishers.

Wosien, M.-G. (1974). *Sacred dance: Encounter with the gods*. Thames & Hudson.

Woodman, M. (1982). *Addiction to perfection: The still unravished bride*. Inner City Books.

Chapter 4

Meeting the Shadow

Becoming More Whole

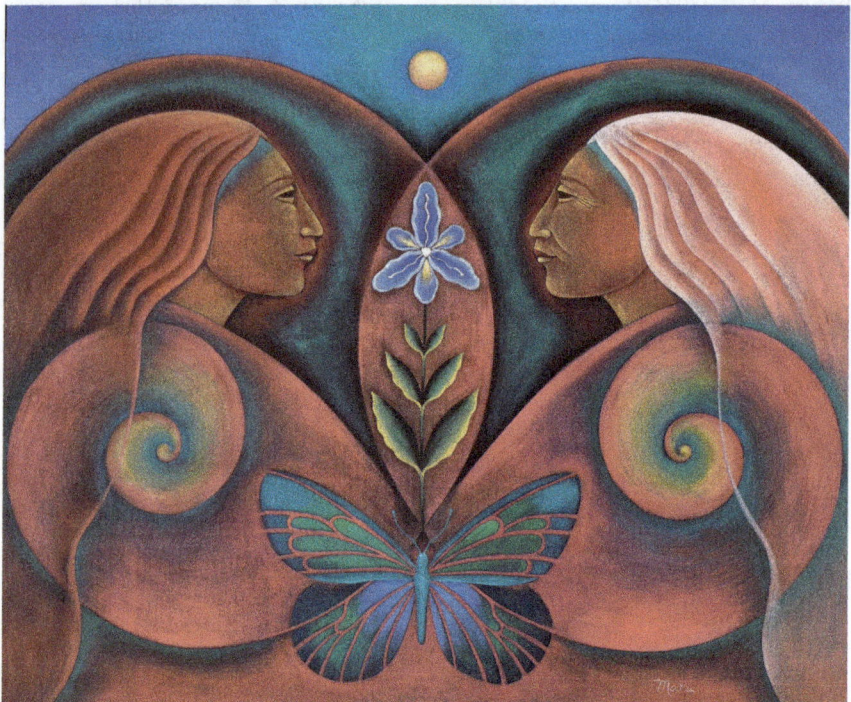

Figure 4.1 Mirror of My Future, Reflection of My Past © 1995, by Mara Berendt Friedman @ www.newmoonvisions.com.

Transformation is an embodied, cellular process involving the reclamation of re-jected parts of the self necessary for wholeness. Re-integrating shadow material projected onto others is crucial. As Jung says, "One does not become enlightened by imagining figures of light, but by making the darkness conscious" (Jung, 1967, CW 13, para. 335). What might emerge if we reclaim this "Other?"

DOI: 10.4324/9781003538356-7

"It is often extremely difficult to recognize in ourselves the tendency to project unwanted emotions onto others" (Chodorow, 1991, p. 55). Guilt and anxiety frequently accompany contact with these split-off, rejected parts of the self. Yet many of these aspects, unwanted in childhood (like aggression and sexuality), are necessary for healthy adult functioning when we are better equipped to handle them. Extreme projections lead to denying, demeaning, and annihilating the other—fueling sexism, racism, xenophobia, and warfare.

By bringing these qualities to consciousness and re-integrating them rather than "acting out," individuals increase their capacity for self-regulation and healthy emotional expression. They expand their sense of self and improve their decision-making. This process—exploring forbidden movement behaviors, experiencing related feelings, and verbally owning the experience—releases energy previously tied up in dissociation and repression. Engaging with shadow aspects in the psyche's natural timing within a safe *temenos* frees parts of the self unconsciously held in the tissue—energies vital for growth and wholeness. Authentic Movement bridges body and psyche, enabling a descent within a secure environment.

The Shadow in Psychotherapy

Therapy, particularly body-oriented psychotherapy, addresses these lesser-known, often frightening feelings, qualities, and viewpoints—what C. G. Jung called "the shadow" (Jung, 1959, CW 9i, para. 291). Jung described the shadow as "the thing a person has no wish to be" (Jung, 1966, CW 16, para. 470). These are the parts of ourselves that we may deny, devalue, shun, or project onto others. This occurs when one attitude dominates and another falls into the unconscious. For example, a child shamed for acting "silly" or "too needy," expressing anger, sensuality, or differing views, may feel their affection and safety are at risk, leading to the creation of a "pleasing" persona. In extreme cases, the child suffers a sense of annihilation, developing accommodating behavior, intellectualizing, or numbing out through addictions, violent reactions, or projection, instead of authentic expression in vulnerable circumstances.

Exploring hidden material is essential. As poet Robert Bly, paraphrasing Jung, observes, "When sunlight hits the body, the body turns bright, but it throws a shadow, which is dark. The brighter the light, the darker the shadow" (Bly, 1988, p. 7). Repressing the shadow requires immense energy. When experienced, differentiated, and integrated, this energy becomes available for transformation. The shadow also holds positive elements—"everything that is yet unborn or not yet conscious within us" (Bolen, 1989, p. 289).

Shadow elements often surface through unconscious gestures, tone of voice, breathing patterns, and moods. This work requires readiness, as clients must confront shadow aspects without further distancing from feelings. Active imagination in all its forms is effective in fostering a conscious relationship with shadow energies, promoting their integration into the personality and fostering balance. By accessing what has been stored in the body, we bridge the unconscious, help regulate the nervous system, and free life energy vital for growth, creativity, and deeper self-knowledge (Stromsted, 1998).

Compassionate witnessing is key to experiencing goodness and wholeness. Trauma often leaves individuals feeling they must do everything alone (Kalsched, 2013). Early neglect or endangerment can lead to a profound distrust of others and the environment. Authentic Movement, described as "an active, relational approach," helps repair attachment wounds, rebuilding trust in bodily responses, others, and our connection to the natural world and the cosmos. (Stromsted, 2019, p. 11). This practice invites us to "see" with the heart and senses, transforming both the "seer" and what is seen, contributing to a better world.

Relationships are essential for healing and transformation. Alienation and isolation—shadows of relationship—are products of a modern world that connects us through the internet while maintaining sensual distance. Embracing the shadow through embodied practices like Authentic Movement enables us to practice intimacy and facilitates deep relational work. Such practices equip analysts and other healing professionals with tools to support transitions between the unconscious and conscious, individual and community (Stromsted, 2009).

The following case studies illustrate how the shadow manifests in the body and some of the ways I work with it.

Embodying the Positive Shadow: Anya's Story

A tall, dark-skinned, successful professional woman, Anya grew up feeling she was "too much." Her body size, feelings, and needs were "too big." When I asked her about her feelings, she described keeping them "shoved in her body," holding on tightly. This manifested in stooping to reduce her height, hunching her shoulders, and collapsing her chest.

Her body posture reflected invisibility, self-doubt, and defeat. She often felt angry and suffered from anxiety and depression. Relaxing amplified her inner critic, so she avoided unstructured time by being constantly busy, which quieted the critical voice.

In Malaysia, Anya's mother, a successful businesswoman, left childcare to others. Anya felt abandoned and wondered what was wrong with her. Moving to the US intensified her sense of being "too big," as her features didn't match Western body ideals. Cultural body ideals compounded her personal struggles, a crisis many women, and increasingly men, face in our consumerist society. Rather than addressing the deeper roots of inadequacy, many seek to "fix" themselves through costly products, surgery, or implants—choices that often fail to resolve underlying issues.

To help Anya ease into movement, I suggested starting with a structured approach, rather than an inner-sourced method such as active imagination, I asked, "Are there any female role models you admire, who feel genuine, have height, and embrace it?"

She immediately thought of Michelle Obama and Beyoncé! Regarding Michelle, she said, "Grace, articulateness, and integrity. A professional woman and a mother who cares about people, about health care, education, children's nutrition, exercise, and equal rights for everyone. She's powerful, yet warm and approachable."

I invited her to become aware of what she felt in her body as she imagined Michelle, first seated, then standing. As she stood, her posture became relaxed and solid; she lifted her chest, squared her shoulders, and made direct eye contact. Her breath deepened, and she appeared fuller, tall, and powerful, but not intimidating.

Anya described Beyoncé as "sexy, powerful, creative, wealthy, and successful. A hardworking professional woman, married with a child." While imagining Beyoncé, she lifted her chin and walked with strength and fluidity, swinging her hips. Though initially self-conscious, she grew playful and potent in her movements. Drawing from these positive shadow figures allowed her to explore qualities within herself that had been undeveloped.

By naming and embodying these strengths, and addressing early family and cultural biases, Anya grew more self-confident and embraced her fullness professionally. She became more relaxed in her marriage and began discussing the possibility of motherhood. When I think of Anya, one of Ranier Marie Rilke's quotes from *Letters to a Young Poet* comes to mind: "Perhaps all the dragons in our lives are princesses who are only waiting to see us act, just once, with beauty and courage. Perhaps everything that frightens us is, in its deepest essence, something helpless that wants our love" (Rilke, 1993, p. 43).

Experiential Session

Engaging the unconscious is essential to therapy and can be deepened and further integrated through embodied exploration. To illustrate, my colleagues and I co-facilitated a day-long active imagination in movement workshop with analysts and allied professionals at the beginning of the International Association for Analytical Psychology Congress (IAAP) in Vienna. Later, at the Congress's conclusion, I led another workshop focused on shadow work blending lecture, discussion, movement, and creative arts (Stromsted, 2020). Participants explored rediscovering light in darkness, burnishing the gold we've shunned.

After a short warm-up to heighten body and breath awareness, participants were invited to explore "the other" within. First, they embodied a positive figure in their lives, developing a movement phrase representing this person and reflecting on their feelings and worldview in that posture. Next, they embodied a person they disliked, crafting a movement phrase for this figure with similar reflections.

Transitioning between these two figures, participants discovered a movement pathway bridging these opposites, creating a new "dance" that held their tension. This dance became the starting point for each participant's Authentic Movement practice. I encouraged participants to follow their movements, trusting how they evolved into a new "third" position. Jung described this transcendent function as, "a movement out of the suspension between two opposites, a living birth that leads to a new level of being" (Jung, 1975, CW 8, para. 189). Joan Chodorow described this process as polar energies converging into a "symbolic position which contains both perspectives. 'Either/or' choices become 'both/and,' but on a new and unforeseeable level" (Chodorow, 1999, pp. 236–237).

Next, I invited participants to stay quietly with their experience and bring the energy from their movement onto paper through color and line in a brief essence drawing. In this way, they gave further form to their experiences before transitioning from the emotional, image-based right brain engagement to left-brain-oriented verbal language. In pairs, they practiced reflective witnessing. The mover then expanded on their journey, while the witness echoed words that carried a particular resonance for them—a listening practice I term "re-call." Roles were reversed, and afterward, participants shared their drawings and insights with the larger group.

At day's end, coinciding with the Congress's conclusion, participants shared reflections. Many described the work as deeply integrative, leaving them "more centered and substantial," with a profound sense of "vitality and wholeness." Several were surprised by the depth they accessed so quickly, while others marveled at the connections they felt with their partners.

Listening to Self

Says Marion Woodman, "If you can listen to the wisdom of your body, love this flesh and bone, dedicate yourself to its mystery, you may one day find yourself smiling from your mirror" (Woodman & Mellick, 2000, p. 44). Here, in this large room at the IAAP conference, it was heartwarming to see 85 colleagues from 30 to 40 different countries moving and witnessing together. Beginning and concluding the IAAP Congress with embodied explorations felt important and promising, especially at this time in our world. Together, we worked to hold the tension between the opposites within us, between us, and in the world to discover a new third potential with increasing consciousness and care. Buddhist monk and peace activist Thich Nhat Hanh speaks to this in his poem, "Please Call Me By My True Names" (Nhat Hanh, 1999).

> Don't say that I will depart tomorrow—
> even today I am still arriving.
>
> Look deeply: every second I am arriving
> to be a bud on a Spring branch,
> to be a tiny bird, with still-fragile wings,
> learning to sing in my new nest,
> to be a caterpillar in the heart of a flower,
> to be a jewel hiding itself in a stone.
>
> I still arrive, in order to laugh and to cry,
> to fear and to hope.
> The rhythm of my heart is the birth and death
> of all that is alive.

I am a mayfly metamorphosing
on the surface of the river.
And I am the bird
that swoops down to swallow the mayfly.

I am a frog swimming happily
in the clear water of a pond.
And I am the grass-snake
that silently feeds itself on the frog.

I am the child in Uganda, all skin and bones,
my legs as thin as bamboo sticks.
And I am the arms merchant,
selling deadly weapons to Uganda.

I am the twelve-year-old girl,
refugee on a small boat,
who throws herself into the ocean
after being raped by a sea pirate.

And I am also the pirate,
my heart not yet capable
of seeing and loving.

I am a member of the politburo,
with plenty of power in my hands.
And I am the man who has to pay
his "debt of blood" to my people
dying slowly in a forced-labor camp.

My joy is like Spring, so warm
it makes flowers bloom all over the Earth.
My pain is like a river of tears,
so vast it fills the four oceans.

Please call me by my true names,
so I can hear all my cries and laughter at once,
so I can see that my joy and pain are one.

Please call me by my true names,
so I can wake up
and the door of my heart
could be left open,
the door of compassion.

References

Bly, R. (1988). *A little book on the human shadow*. Harper & Row Publishers.

Bolen, J. S. (1989). *Gods in everyman: Archetypes that shape men's lives*. Harper & Row.

Chodorow, J. (1991). *Dance therapy and depth psychology: The moving imagination*. Routledge.

Chodorow, J. (1999). Dance therapy and the transcendent function. In P. Pallaro (Ed.), *Authentic Movement: Essays by Mary Starks Whitehouse, Janet Adler, & Joan Chodorow* (pp. 236–252). Jessica Kingsley Publishers. (Original work published 1977.)

Jung, C.G. (1959). The psychology of the child archetype. In *The archetypes and the collective unconscious* (Vol. 9i). Princeton University Press. (Original work published 1940.)

Jung, C.G. (1966). The psychology of the transference. In *The practice of psychotherapy* (Vol. 16). Princeton University Press. (Original work published 1954.)

Jung, C.G. (1967). The philosophical tree. In *Alchemical studies* (Vol. 13). Princeton University Press.

Jung, C. G. (1975). The transcendent function. In *The structure and dynamics of the psyche* (Vol. 8). Princeton University Press. (Original work published 1916.)

Kalsched, D. (2013). *Trauma and the soul: A psycho-spiritual approach to human development and its interruption*. Routledge.

Nhat Hanh, T. (1999). Please call me by my true names. In *Call me by my true names: The collected poems of Thich Nhat Hanh*. Parallax Press.

Rilke, R. M. (1993). *Letters to a young poet* (M. D. Herter Norton, Trans.). W. W. Norton & Company.

Stromsted, T. (1998). The dance and the body in psychotherapy: Reflections and clinical examples. In D. H. Johnson & I. J. Grand (Eds.), *The body in psychotherapy* (pp. 147–169). North Atlantic Books.

Stromsted, T. (2009). Healing soul's body: An introduction to Authentic Movement. In P. Bennett (Ed.), *Journeys & encounters: Clinical, communal, cultural, Proceedings of the 17th International IAAP Congress for Analytical Psychology*. Daimon Verlag.

Stromsted, T. (2019). Witnessing practice: In the eyes of the beholder. In *The Routledge international handbook: Embodied perspectives in psychotherapy: Approaches from dance movement and body psychotherapies*. Routledge.

Stromsted, T. (2020). Shadow dances: Reclaiming "The Other." In E. Kiehl & J. Egli (Eds.), *Vienna 2019: Encountering the other: Within us, between us, and in the world. Proceedings of the 21st International IAAP Congress for Analytical Psychology*. Daimon.

Woodman, M. & Mellick, J. (2000). *Coming home to myself: Reflections for nurturing a woman's body and soul*. Conari Press.

Chapter 5

Witnessing Practice

Seeing and Being Seen

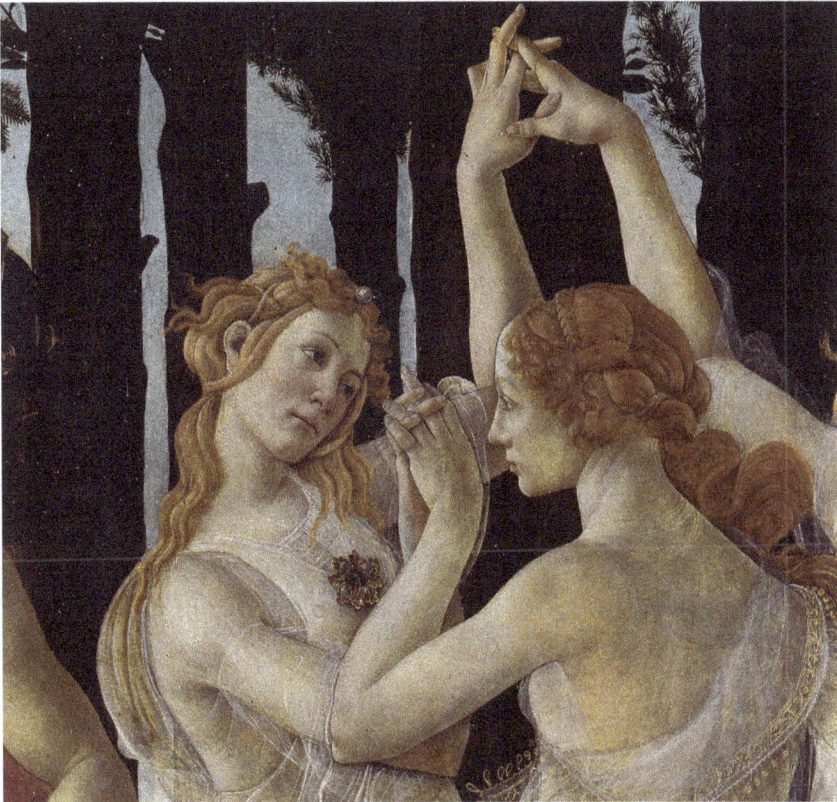

Figure 5.1 Sandro Botticelli, *Allegoria Della Primavera (Allegory to Spring)*.
Detail: Two of the Graces. Tempora on wood.
© Gabinetto Fotografico delle Gallerie degli Uffizi.

DOI: 10.4324/9781003538356-8

What does it mean to be *seen*, to be *heard*, and to be received for who we are? To experience ourselves as real people and to belong? Witnessing practice, at its core, promotes these experiences. When such deeply human needs have not been met in a person's early development, or have been thwarted or injured through subsequent life experiences, they can be fostered through the practice of moving and witnessing in Authentic Movement.

In Authentic Movement practice, the mover/client closes their eyes, waits, and then, in the presence of their witness/therapist, moves in response to body-felt sensations, movement impulses, emotions, memories, dreams, or internal images. The opportunity to be *seen* by a witness who is not *watching* or *observing* the mover, but rather *holding* her in a receptive, compassionate gaze—without interpretation or judgment—allows the mover to experience and to follow the immediacy of her own authentic experience safely. While teaching, I often say to my students, "In this practice, my body is my teacher, and I am the student who follows." In this way, the mover can reconnect with her instinctual ground of being, discovering and transforming emotions and undeveloped capacities held in the body beneath the level of consciousness. During the mover's explorations, the witness sits to the side with her eyes open, bringing a sense of quiet warmth, receptive focus, and presence to the space. She also monitors the time allowed for the session while maintaining an awareness of her own embodied experience.

Following the movement session, the mover often shares significant moments from her movement journey and receives verbal reflection from the witness if she wishes. Witnessing language is rooted in describing movement literally, using the present tense to stay with the immediacy of the experience (Stromsted & Haze, 2007, p. 65). For example, "I see your head bow down and a tear stream down your cheek; as I see this, I feel a release in my jaw and softening and warmth in my chest." Witnesses use the language of neutral observation instead of interpretation, such as "I see you crying and bowing your head, so I imagine that you are ashamed." Sometimes witnesses share images that come to them as well, although they are careful to own them as their own. This leaves the mover free to be curious about them, without needing to take them on. As such, witnessing represents a departure from the interpretive language that is often a part of psychotherapy. In this way, the mover remains the expert of her own experience, a democratic format that allows each to *be* in the other's presence.

Over the years, I have found that witnesses who are psychotherapists often make interpretations, as they have been trained to do in verbal psychotherapy, thinking it was helpful to the mover. However, in some of these instances, the mover experiences a sense of being hurt, judged, or simply unseen at a time when she is deeply vulnerable, having just emerged from movement explorations that were sourced in her unconscious. I have often heard witnesses, with the best of intentions, unconsciously using evaluative language like "You looked a little stiff," "I wish you'd kept going with that," or even, "You were absolutely beautiful!" This last sounds affirming, but it may leave the mover with the take-away message that she needs to be beautiful for her witnesses (Stromsted, 2015, p. 348). Thus, the witness needs to strip language down to its essential ingredients, stay true to the mover's personal metaphors, and acknowledge her own embodied experience as a witness, when asked. To this end, Janet Adler introduced the concept of *percept language* adapted from her studies with psychologist John Weir (Haze & Stromsted, 1994/1999, p. 114). Using "I" statements to own my experience, this nonjudgmental, noninterpretive way of speaking provides additional clarity, safety, and depth for movers and witnesses alike.

I've also introduced a practice I term *re-call*, where the witness reflects the mover's words and describes their own embodied resonance. For example, if a mover says, "After standing for some time, I surrender to the floor, and my hair falls over my face like a waterfall," the witness might respond, "Standing, surrender, floor, waterfall: As I hear you speak, I feel a deepening in my breath, a release in my spine, and a softening sensation in my face" (Stromsted, 2015, pp. 348–349).

The Gaze

The mover–witness process has parallels to the process of child development. D. W. Winnicott, a child psychoanalyst and pediatrician, spoke of the importance of the mother's gaze for an integrated sense of self, a sense of "being real." Self-psychologist Heinz Kohut described this responsiveness as the "gleam in the mother's eye" that gives the child a sense of being safe, secure, and loved (Kohut, 1966, p. 251). The mother's face is the "precursor of the mirror" (Winnicott, 1971, p. 111), reflecting her pleasure in her baby. When the baby sees his mother's loving expression, he feels lovable and good. Over time, as the baby sees himself in her "mirror," he comes to see himself. As Winnicott says, "When I look, I am seen, so I exist" (p. 114).

But how does healing occur when the gaze has been distorted, or less than loving? Parents may not have received enough emotional containment and empathic mirroring themselves. When this is the case, they—mother, father, or other primary caretaking figures—are thwarted in being able to embody their own genuineness, their own sense of goodness and enoughness, to mirror and pass down this sense of wholeness to their children. Kohut asserted that parents' failure to empathize with their children—and their children's responses to these failures—were "at the root of almost all psychopathology" (Nersessian & Kopff, 1996, p. 661).

Witnessing addresses this by providing a relational environment that can reflect the "real self." Crucial to the process of witnessing is the quality of the witness's gaze. Having a "good enough" witness/therapist/mother-figure (Winnicott, 1971, p. 81), one who is capable of containing the mover's experience, makes it possible to explore unconscious material safely. This allows for regression, which is necessary in order to access earlier developmental experiences. It also gives space for exploration, expression, and reintegration, leading to transformation. New experiences can arise as the mover feels safe enough to leave the familiar shore and embark on a deeper journey. Over time, the experience of being held and mirrored by an attuned witness allows the mover to develop an "inner witness" (Adler, 2003/2007, p. 25;

Sager, 2015; Stromsted, 2009b, p. 207). This inner witness offers the mover the capacity to pause, contain, and reflect on their own experience. This brings about a deeper sense of embodied awareness, emotional literacy, and discernment—an embodied wisdom that becomes a potent guide in the person's life.

The following example illustrates how the witness helps the mover explore painful emotions generated by childhood and adult relationships, integrating them into a more fully embodied sense of self.

Elia, the mover, has just gone through a wrenching breakup with her partner when she meets with her Authentic Movement peer group. *At first, she walks aimlessly, meandering around the circle with her eyes closed. Sensing the warmth of a pool of light she comes to a standstill and begins to play with the material of the baggy white blouse she is wearing, swooping her arms up and away from her body in wide, vigorous arcs and figure eights. Gradually she comes to a pause, wraps her arms around her chest, and begins to sway.*

Following Elia's sharing of her experience in the circle, a witness says that at first she feels distraught as Elia walks in different directions throughout the space. Then, as Elia pauses and swings her arms, the witness feels strength in her spine and torso, with a growing sense of warmth and comfort as Elia begins to sway. "Throughout your movement I find myself very drawn to your feet," her witness re-calls. Elia responds that it is affirming to hear the witness's experience, and that the attention to her feet helps bring her own awareness from her upper body down to her feet, allowing her to feel more grounded during a time of disorientation.

A second witness shares that as Elia makes figure eights with her billowing blouse that an image of "a sailboat with gusts of wind filling its big white sail" comes to her, "moving as if lost at sea before finding its home harbor. I feel really sad and unmoored at first, then revitalized as you play with your shirt, and at peace when you come to a resting place at the end."

Elia nods and responds, "Hearing your feelings and the image of the sailboat coming into harbor helps me find meaning in my movement. I feel seen at a really painful time in my journey. Now I can begin to find my way home."

Following the movement session, Elia journals about her experience and re-members the anguish she felt when her mother left her father when she was five years old. Her breath releases and tears come, softening her jaw and her heart as a new sense of spaciousness and belonging emerge. Here, sensation, movement, emotion, image, and memory come together, generating an embodied experience in the safety of a contained space of conscious, compassionate witnesses.

Witnessing also helps mitigate the rise of narcissism, the "me-first-and-most" character traits that a growing percentage of the population seems to suffer from. The rampant use of "selfies" may be a symptom of insufficient, inaccurate mirroring. Witnessing provides a safe container (*temenos*) from which the authentic self can emerge from beneath the "adapted" or socialized "false self" (Winnicott, 1965, p. 140). This is increasingly important in advantaged communities in today's world, where a person's outer image must be manicured, managed, and "branded," converting personhood into a commodity valued in terms of beauty, fame, or net worth, threatening to overshadow genuine feelings, experiences, and meaningful relationships.

In an Authentic Movement group I facilitated in East Asia, a participant I'll call Jade reported the following dream:

> *I am alone on the top floor of a tall skyscraper; when I look out the window I tumble down toward the sidewalk below. Though I am terrified that I will die from the impact, I wake up before I land.*

Afterward, I ask her if it would be okay for me to slowly mirror the movements I saw her do as she shared her dream. We could have interpreted the dream verbally, though her body told the story. Her shoulders had been pulled in and raised up around her ears, her breath shallow, her eyes wide, and her mouth turned down.

My mirroring gave her a sudden insight. "It's as if I'm coming down from the tower of my head where I have been living, finding my way to earth. I didn't even know how much I lived there, until I was afraid of falling … But you are catching me now." Ultimately, as the witness I was doing what the mover's own mother had not done: provide a safe container, mirror her feelings, and accept her body, so that she could inhabit it. Jade continued, her voice at first sad and then vibrant, "When I was born, [my mother] was profoundly disappointed; while she was pregnant she went to a doctor and a shaman to get medicines, herbs, and prayers to be sure I'd be a boy, and has always been angry with me for being a girl … I could feel my curves on the floor yesterday, and felt safe and accepted for who I am. Today is the first day that I can feel that I have a woman's body."

In this movement exploration and integrative dream sequence, I see a young woman "descend" into her softening body. The process brought consciousness to her cellular experience. Her emotions opened; she began to grieve and was joined by many other women in the workshop who resonated with her experience of being a woman in a culture in which women are to be accommodating and men tend to be more prized. Sometimes, men, too, have the experience of being a disappointment to their mother or father at their birth, an early imprint that can influence their subsequent sense of self.

Witnessing practice can also be deeply moving and healing for the witnesses themselves. As a witness maintains an open, receptive presence, they may be deeply touched by what they see and sense, as their mover engages experiences that go to the deepest levels of human experience. Some years ago, a participant in a cancer recovery group I was leading asked me whether, in my own psychotherapy practice, *I* was the mover and my *client* the witness. When I looked surprised, she explained, "I felt so deeply touched by witnessing my mover that it brought tears, and such warmth in my heart." This sense of being profoundly moved by another's humanity is a feeling that I, too, have experienced on many occasions. "When two strings of an instrument resonate … each is changed by the impact of the other" (Siegel, 2010, p. 54).

Contributions from Neuroscience

What about the science behind the gaze? Advances in interpersonal neuroscience indicate that witnessing is supported by the mirror neuron system, among others. This system is thought to be the root of empathy, contributing to our capacity to "resonate" with another (Cozolino, 2006, p. 187; Gallese, 2003). Mirror neurons "fire" in the brain of a witness when she observes her mover performing an action that is familiar to her (Berrol, 2006; Damasio, 2010, p. 104). In this way, "we pick up not only another person's movement but her emotional state and intentions as well" (van der Kolk, 2014, p. 59).

Though the witness may resonate with her mover's experience, she maintains a quality of stillness, containing the mover's response, instead of enacting it in the moment. As she "holds space" for her mover's experience and for her own, information from her body—particularly from the primitive, survival-oriented areas in the brainstem and limbic system—forges links and deeper levels of connectivity and integration with the higher cortical centers in the brain (the prefrontal cortex). This provides an opportunity to reflect on and bring language to what she is sensing and feeling. The process of pausing, breathing, and bringing sustained attention to the witness's own responses and knee-jerk reactions quiets the limbic system, invokes the parasympathetic (rest/digest) nervous system, and supports insight, self-knowledge, and self-regulation.

The presence of an empathic witness also supports the mover in widening what psychiatrist and neuroscience author Daniel Siegel calls the "affect window of tolerance" (Ogden & Fisher, 2015; Siegel, 2010, p. 252). Intolerable emotions can arise in the presence of others, as old relational issues surface. These are often accompanied by emotions that weren't acceptable to the mover's parents or caretakers, which resulted in shaming, abandonment, or abuse. Working with a safe witness can make it possible for the client to begin to tolerate a wider range of feelings—such as hate, rage, shame, contempt, disgust, grief, joy, hope, and love. Then they can experience them safely in the body, become curious about them, and explore them in a relational context. This, in turn, helps to create trust, repair early wounding, and foster the development of healthy attachment and a capacity for more flexible, reciprocal relating. This is essential for self-care, for relating to others, and for preserving and fostering community (Homann, 2017; Keleman, 1985; Schore, 2012; Schore & Sieff, 2015; Siegel, 2010, p. 55; Wilkinson, 2010, p. 46).

The Dance of Three

One of the first embodied exercises I learned from Marion Woodman was the Dance of Three. Initially developed by Mary Hamilton, a former Royal Canadian Ballet trainee and modern dance teacher at the University of Western Ontario, it was later refined in collaboration with Marion Woodman and Ann Skinner, a highly attuned voice coach and mask-maker formerly with the Ontario Stratford Shakespeare Company (Hamilton, 2009, pp. 93–94). The *Dance of Three* uses embodied active imagination to explore psychotherapy's nonverbal foundations through bodily sensations, emotions, imagination, voice, and empathic witnessing in a safe and relational setting. This practice involves three roles: a primary mover, a responder, and a reflective witness. Participants alternate between moving, witnessing, and containing, deepening their presence with themselves and others. The triad framework fosters regeneration through natural movement and empathic responses, inviting respect and empathy in relationships (Stromsted, 2009a).

The mover follows inner impulses with closed eyes, while the "mirroring witness" synchronizes with her gestures and sounds, reflecting without leading. The "containing witness" provides a safe boundary for the dyad, holding space with unconditional acceptance and ensuring the group remains psychically and physically secure. After each round, the mover shares her experience and receives feedback before roles rotate.

Participants frequently extend the process by drawing, writing, or using clay to give form to emerging material—often childhood experiences or feelings stored in the body. This process brings dormant emotional seeds into language and consciousness. Reflecting on such work, body-psychotherapist Pat Ogden notes that change occurs through empathic, psychobiologically attuned interactions that allow clients to safely contact and regulate inner experiences (Ogden et al., 2005, p. 22).

Empathic relational experiences are foundational to self-formation, as shown by advances in interpersonal neurobiology, which highlight the right brain's receptivity to nonverbal cues like voice, tone, facial expression, movement, music, and symbolism in dreams and poetry. Practices like Authentic Movement allow developmental experiences stored in the body and brain to surface, be explored, and integrated into conscious awareness (Stromsted & Sieff, 2015).

Unlike Authentic Movement, which is silent as movers listen for an inner prompting, the Dance of Three incorporates music. While teaching internationally, I began diversifying beyond Marion Woodman's preference for Chopin's Nocturnes, selecting music that resonates with different cultural backgrounds. This inclusion of the "cultural unconscious" (Henderson, 1984) enriches the practice, allowing participants to explore individual and cultural differences while affirming shared human experiences. The Dance of Three provides a framework for reflection and communication essential to therapeutic settings, relationships, and the broader social world.

I have since shared the Dance of Three with diverse groups, including analytic candidates, international therapists, nuns and priests, and participants at the US Body Psychotherapy Conference (Stromsted, 2020). In these settings, participants alternated between roles of mover/client, engaged witness/therapist, and container/supervisor. Before beginning, witnesses asked movers if they wished for supportive touch—standing side by side, back-to-back, or engaging respectful contact at areas like the forehead, neck, heart, or low back. Witnesses were encouraged to offer presence rather than intervention, while movers were guided to adjust or decline support as needed.

This process highlights a profound paradox: at times, we yearn for support that is unavailable, while at others, we may struggle to receive the support that is already present. After a few moments of this connection, witnesses gently removed their hands, leaving a residual sense of support as movers stepped into their dance. Variations of the Dance of Three include roles like the "Witness of the Heart," who holds a space of compassionate presence, and the "Dynamic Witness," who accompanies movers by naming body parts to invite awareness or movement into potentially blocked areas.

Culture's Body

Witnessing is not only important in the therapeutic process, but crucial for our development as human beings. It prepares us to become family members, friends, parents, workers, and world citizens. *Being seen* with all of our contradictions in the wholeness of our experience enables us to see others, including others who are not like us: children at school, colleagues at work, partners or spouses, our own children, people on the street, citizens of other countries, those who have emigrated from other parts of the world, and those who were born in our own country but look different from us.

Authentic Movement practice is deeply shaped by different cultures and yet opens to profoundly universal, archetypal experiences as well. For example, while teaching in Japan, I learned that direct eye contact is sometimes experienced as intrusive and that bowing is a more accustomed way to greet someone. I invited movers and witnesses to explore a soft gaze that included the face and shoulders of their partner rather than focusing on the eyes. In groups in Argentina with a history of dictators, military juntas, and "disappeared" people, movements expressing protective containment and discipline oscillated with those of smoldering wildness and the elegant intimacy of tango! Also notable was a deep capacity for reflectiveness, resilience, and passion in connection. Moving and witnessing in post-apartheid South Africa affirmed the importance of reconnecting with their deeper cultural heritage, integrating more nontraditional embodied approaches into contemporary verbal psychotherapy. My experience in these and other cultural settings has helped me gain a deeper appreciation for the diversity both in the mover, and in the projections, biases, and new learnings possible in the "eyes of the beholder."

Witnessing and Community

The body is the bedrock of who we are. Being in touch with one's self is the root of empathy; without it, other people's feelings don't register in us, nor do they matter. This creates an environment where we must live from "image," a condition promulgated by consumerist culture. Being split off from our bodies also means being disconnected from others and from the world around us. This not only leads to a sense of alienation, both from ourselves and from others, but also ultimately creates the conditions for unrestrained aggression. Boundaries between "us" and "them" are rigidly maintained. This is like an autoimmune disease in the cultural body, which seeks to reject what could help it grow.

Today, children and adults in industrialized cultures are learning to occupy themselves in isolation, and to work without time boundaries via the ever-available email, text, or tweet. In industrialized countries, children do much of their work on personal computers, iPads, or cellphones rather than engaging in games that involve safe touch or physical proximity to others. In this setting, children now are learning to self-regulate through machines rather than learning to *co-regulate* in a healthy, reciprocal way with others.

Adults are also profoundly impacted by their use of technology. Astonishingly, even the number of adults who are on their smartphones while having sex is on the rise (Porges, 2016). Though it's beyond the scope of this chapter, the implications of this "selfie culture" deserve more attention. We want to be seen, known, and accepted for who we are. It's a profoundly human need, as is contact and co-regulation through the intersubjective dance of relationship with others. These are among the reasons that witnessing practice is so relevant for psychotherapy, education, and daily life.

Authentic Movement is an active, relational approach that helps repair attachment wounds, allowing us to rebuild trust in our own bodily responses, in others, and in our vital connection to the natural world and the cosmos. Shakespeare said the eyes are the windows to the soul. Witnessing practice invites us to "see" with the heart and with all of our senses, a practice that transforms both the "seer" and what is seen, and helps create a better world.

Desire

Desire causes suffering—the second noble truth,
which builds on the first noble truth, there is suffering.

If I didn't desire I wouldn't suffer.
But to be human is to dig in the mulch of despair,
dirt under my fingernails. Without sorrow
can I learn to dance?

Or dance, not learn to, to just move my body,
spin through the living room
drawing shapes through the air
in my pink "Hello Gorgeous" pajamas.

Desire is why I've left and why I've stayed.
Why as we both stand in the kitchen
waiting for the coffee to brew,

you take my hand to twirl me around—
the cat looking on from the doorway—
as we dance to a song we make up as we go.

LeeAnn Pickrell

References

Adler, J. (2003/2007). From autism to the discipline of Authentic Movement. In P. Pallaro (Ed.), *Authentic Movement: Moving the body, moving the self, being moved: A collection of essays* (Vol. II) (pp. 24–31). Jessica Kingsley.

Berrol, C. (2006). Neuroscience meets dance/movement therapy: Mirror neurons, the therapeutic process and empathy. *The Arts in Psychotherapy, 33*, 302–315.

Cozolino, L. (2006). *The neuroscience of human relationships: Attachment and the developing brain.* Norton & Company.

Damasio, A. (2010). *Self comes to mind: Constructing the conscious brain.* Pantheon Books.

Gallese, V. (2003). The roots of empathy: The shared manifold hypothesis and the neural basis of intersubjectivity. *Psychopathology, 36*, 171–180.

Hamilton, M. (2009). *The dragonfly principle: An exploration of the body's experience in unfolding spirituality.* Colenso Island Press.

Haze, N. & Stromsted, T. (1994/1999). An interview with Janet Adler. In P. Pallaro (Ed.), *Authentic Movement: Essays by Mary Starks Whitehouse, Janet Adler, & Joan Chodorow* (pp. 107–120). Jessica Kingsley Publishers.

Henderson, J. (1984). *Cultural attitudes in psychological perspectives.* Inner City Books.

Homann, K. (2017). Dynamic equilibrium: Engaging neurophysiological intelligences through Dance/Movement Therapy. In H. Payne (Ed.), *Essentials of dance movement psychotherapy: International perspectives on theory, research, and practice* (pp. 37–52). Routledge.

Keleman, S. (1985). *Emotional anatomy: The structure of experience.* Center Press.

Kohut, H. (1966). Forms and transformations of narcissism. *Journal of the American Psychoanalytic Association, 14*, 243–272.

Nersessian, E. & Kopff, R. (1996). *Textbook of psychoanalysis.* American Psychiatric Press.

Ogden, P. & Fisher, J. (2015). *Sensorimotor psychotherapy: Interventions for trauma and attachment.* W. W. Norton & Company, Inc.

Ogden, P, Pain, C., Minton, K., & Fisher, J. (2005). Including the body in mainstream psychotherapy for traumatized individuals. *Psychologist-psychoanalyst, XXV*(4), 19–24.

Porges, S. W. (2016, April 22). Connectedness as a biological imperative: Understanding the consequences of trauma, abuse, and chronic stress through the lens of the Polyvagal Theory [Keynote lecture]. ADTA 51st National Dance Therapy Conference, Bethesda, Maryland.

Sager, P. (2015). Journey of the inner witness: A path of development. *Journal of Dance and Somatic Practices: Authentic Movement: Defining the Field, 7*(2), 365–376.

Schore, A. N. (2012). *The science of the art of psychotherapy.* W.W. Norton & Company.

Schore, A. N. & Sieff, D. (2015). On the same wave-length: How our emotional brain is shaped by human relationships. In D. Sieff (Ed.), *Understanding and healing emotional trauma: Conversations with pioneering clinicians and researchers* (pp. 111–136). Routledge.

Siegel, D. (2010). *The mindful therapist: A clinician's guide to mindsight, and neural integration.* W. W. Norton & Company.

Stromsted, T. (2009a) Healing soul's body: An introduction to Authentic Movement. In P. Bennett (Ed.), *Proceedings of the 17th international IAAP congress for analytical psychology: Journeys & encounters: Clinical, communal, cultural.* Daimon Verlag.

Stromsted, T. (Summer, 2009b). Authentic Movement: A dance with the divine. *Body Movement and Dance in Psychotherapy Journal, 4*(3), 201–213.

Stromsted, T. (2015). Authentic Movement & the evolution of Soul's Body® Work. *Journal of Dance and Somatic Practices: Authentic Movement: Defining the Field, 7*(2), 339–357.

Stromsted, T. (Spring/Summer, 2020). Embodied wisdom: The dance of three. *International Body Psychotherapy Journal: The Art & Science of Somatic Praxis, 19*(1), 50–54.

Stromsted, T. & Haze, N. (2007). The road in: Elements of the study and practice of Authentic Movement. In P. Pallaro (Ed.), *Authentic Movement: Moving the body, moving the self, being moved: A collection of essays* (Vol. II) (pp. 56–68). Jessica Kingsley Publishers.

Stromsted, T. & Sieff, D. (2015). Dances of psyche and soma: Re-Inhabiting the body in the wake of emotional trauma. In D. Sieff (Ed.), *Understanding and healing emotional trauma: Conversations with pioneering clinicians and researchers*. Routledge.

Van der Kolk, B. (2014). *The body keeps the score: Brain, mind, and body in the healing of trauma*. Viking.

Wilkinson, M. (2010). *Changing minds in therapy: Emotion, attachment, trauma, and neurobiology*. W. W. Norton.

Winnicott, D. W. (1965). Ego distortion in terms of true and false self. In *The maturational process and the facilitating environment: Studies in the theory of emotional development* (pp. 140–157). The Hogarth Press and the Institute of Psycho-Analysis.

Winnicott, D. W. (1971). *Playing and reality*. Routledge.

Chapter 6

Reinhabiting the Body

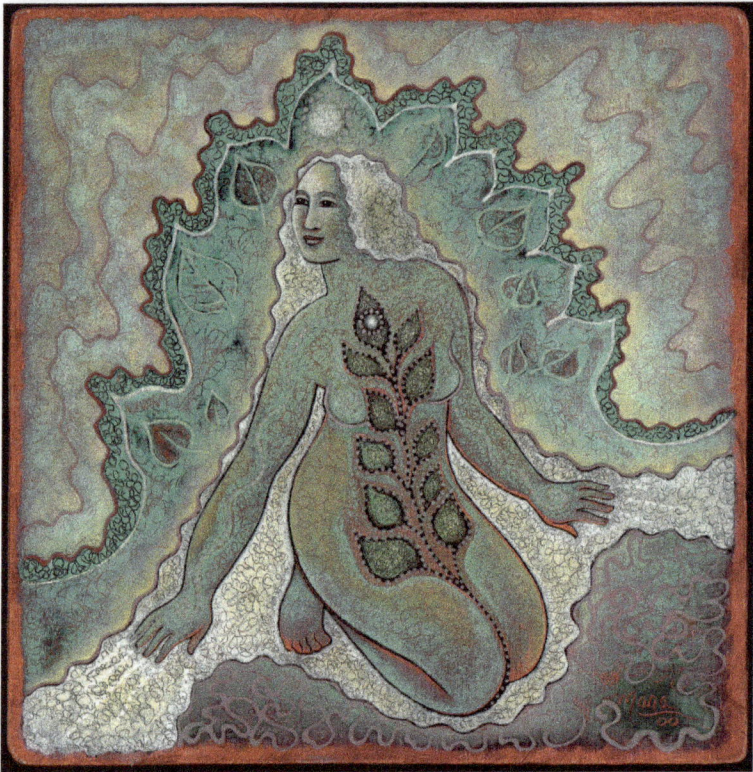

Figure 6.1 Blossoming Spirit © 2001, by Mara Berendt Friedman @ www.newmoonvisions.com.

Some years ago, while rushing too fast on a dimly lit path to teach a class at Esalen Institute on the California coast, I fell and pulled both hamstrings so badly that I had difficulty walking and sitting for months. This time would have been difficult for anyone, and for me, a dancer who could no longer move freely, it was a time of

DOI: 10.4324/9781003538356-9

coming to terms with how I had literally "overextended" myself. It showed me how concretely my body was able to provide limits that my psyche was not yet able to acknowledge. Injury, stillness, or paralysis is the shadow side of the dancer. This experience offered an important vehicle for me to sit with the sensations, feelings, images, and truths that arose as my body slowly took me through a process of introspection, grieving, and healing, resulting in what gradually felt like new, more feeling-full feminine legs.

Spirit and Matter: How We Leave Ourselves

Before we can "reinhabit the female body," we must first consciously understand how we leave ourselves, how the split between body and psyche, spirit and matter, has trickled down to the body level. Although I include some elements that can be helpful to men and nonbinary individuals as well, here I will focus primarily on women's experience. First, I will examine what it means to be "out of the body," that is, how we experience it in our culture in the present moment. Next, I will discuss some of the reasons or processes by which we leave our bodies. Upcoming chapters are then devoted to how we—across genders—can reinhabit our bodies, or "find our way home."

How We Leave the Body

There are many ways to "leave the body." Although clearly there can be no hard divisions between the mind, the body, and the spirit, these categories can offer helpful frameworks for organizing the variety of responses.

In the area of the mind, people may use a range of intellectual defenses such as denial, intellectualization, or rationalization that move them "upstairs," away from conflicts, needs, and pain. Through the mechanism of projection, they can then attribute these to someone or something else.

In more severe cases, a person may abandon their "reality" altogether through psychosis, losing ground in the personal realm to founder in the waters of the unconscious. Social scientist Gregory Bateson (1985) once said that "the schizophrenic drowns in the same waters that the mystic swims in." Whatever the case, the body as the reservoir of powerful unbidden impulses, memories, and feelings is no longer experienced as a friendly place to live and becomes distorted. As therapists, we may encounter this in a client's reluctance to engage in expressive movement or through their body-image drawings revealing overly elongated necks, no hands or feet, and even machine parts in specific areas of the body.

Severe trauma often gives rise to dissociation to survive what feels unbearable; its amplified disturbance in dissociative identity disorder (DID) offers another, albeit often fragmenting, psychological attempt at a solution to the problem. Struggling with this disorder the individual may split off from and have amnesia regarding specific experiences, qualities, emotions, and memories that cannot be tolerated or integrated into the "host" personality or sense of self. This disorder is often associated with a history of severe physical, sexual, and emotional abuse. Research (Van der Hart et al., 2006) has found that the body may play a specific role within the same person. A splinter personality or state of being may have a particular food allergy, rash, or any other presenting symptom; in contrast, another part of the personality may be free of these ailments and virtually unaware of them. (It is noteworthy that integrating the different sets of movements characteristic of each personality aspect or "inner part" may facilitate recollection, re-embodiment, and some integration of these aspects of the self.)

Posttraumatic stress disorder (PTSD), which often follows trauma, is another way a person can leave their body as a means of seeking protection against otherwise terrifying experiences at the moment. However, they may later re-experience them through nightmares, flashbacks, panic attacks, sweats, and other somatic symptoms when triggers reminding them of the earlier trauma present themselves. Multigenerational trauma patterns can also be readily triggered and reenacted in cycles of violation and abuse if there hasn't been a healing process. Engaging with the emotions, thwarted actions stored in the body, and the relational dynamics that trigger them is essential to bring these issues to consciousness for healing and repair.

Politicizing can be disembodying, too, functioning as a way to externalize our drives, needs, anger, fear, cravings, and what we find intolerable in ourselves. When not used to manipulate truth for gain, conspiracy theories may reflect an attempt to provide certainty in an uncertain world. Political action is an essential social force, though unexamined traumatic emotions and a desire for power can sometimes drive it. When this is the case, action substitutes for feeling—a defense against experiencing vulnerability or the loss of privilege as others strive for greater autonomy, access to resources, and equitable human rights. If enacted unconsciously, politicizing can make the mistake of turning the tables by identifying with the aggressor—for example, supporting the "strong man," no matter how damaged or punitive—rather than reflecting the organic development of an individual standpoint.

An unbalanced approach to spirituality is another method for leaving the body. As distinct from a deep connection to one's faith, here the individual may engage in a kind of "spiritual bypass" of the body's experience. A misinterpretation of most teachings, the goal here may be to "transcend," instead of experiencing feelings and the limitations, suffering, and needs that accompany human life in the body. Through this route there may be denial, minimization, ego inflation, or a glossing over of personal complexes. When this is the case, the individual is encouraged to remain at the level of positive affirmations and an unexamined transference onto the often remote or ingratiatingly rewarding love object or guru.

In this way, someone can linger in the light instead of dropping down into the darker resources of the body and the shadow material that may be "housed" there and is most certainly evoked within human relationships. Spiritual bypass can keep them floating above the troubles below, which out of awareness, can then be readily projected onto others. Finding a haven in religiosity may mean claiming a higher ground and, in more extreme cases, even a "righteous" wish to control or punish others. Or giving up their own experience, sensations, values, and authority in favor of outer forms and structures, exchanging mystery, chaos, and uncertainty for stability and predictability.

There are, however, more readily recognizable bodily signals that often arise when we leave our bodies, which provide a foundation of our sense of self: freezing parts of the body through a marked withdrawal of energy away from the extremities and toward the core is a form of distancing from the body. In this state, a client may dream of ice or snowy landscapes, followed by greener springtime scenes once thawing has begun, perhaps through analysis and sensitive bodywork.

Numbing is a related experience in which breath, blood flow, or energy may be constricted or withdrawn enough into a particular area so that the woman is often unaware of or "out of touch" with that part of herself. This can manifest to the point where that body part may even be omitted, as in the case of the body-image drawings of anorexic women that lack breasts, hips, and genitals, or in the portraits of disempowered women who can be seen without hands, needed for enacting a life in the world, or feet to stand on.

Other ways the body can become compromised as a result of challenging life experiences includes *body armoring* of all kinds, a concept introduced by Wilhelm Reich (1933/1980), a medical doctor, psychoanalyst, and younger protégé of Sigmund Freud. *Muscular armoring* is another way to "leave the body," or perhaps selectively inhabit it in a way that cordons off sensations in particular areas.

Addictions provide another way to "leave the body" through overstimulation or understimulation by "self-medicating." Through a variety of means, addictions represent an escape from the reality of how a person experiences themself in the present moment, coupled with a longing for a particular "altered state," which is often the opposite of how they really feel. Addictions may also, paradoxically, represent a misdirected urge toward wholeness.

Compulsive internet scrolling and social media use can distance us from genuine feelings and deeper interpersonal needs. Although social media can offer positive social contact and support, algorithms are designed to keep users engaged, which can contribute to increasing loneliness and mental health issues (Orben et al., 2024). "Binge watching" movies, game shows, or "reality TV" can provide other ways to "leave the troubles" of daily life behind. Compulsive news intake without pacing oneself may amplify vigilance or flood the brain, mind, and body.

Workaholism is another addiction, especially in fast-paced American culture. People often rush around, overwhelming themselves to fill an emotional void or escape anxiety and depression. Perfectionism or an unbalanced drive for achievement can also pressure them, a drive that is often rewarded in today's culture. Physical overactivity can also take the form of an addiction, whether a person is addicted to running, aerobics, or working out. These are generally considered positive ways to get the "feel good" endorphins to soar to high levels. Still, they may also, if overdone, serve as defenses against feeling or as ways to fortify preexisting body armor. These defenses can resemble a "fight response" in the fight, flight, freeze survival model, protecting vulnerability through overperforming in mechanical, disembodied movements (based on a view of the body as a machine, which must be brought in for regular tune-ups).

Years ago, when I stopped going to mime school and dancing several hours a day, I lost a significant amount of body tone. As my tissues softened, I began to feel my sadness and to touch deeper memories of loss, simultaneously experiencing myself as a feminine person in ways I hadn't been able to access or embody before.

Some people "leave the body" by attempting to circumvent the aging process, insisting on maintaining a shape that mirrors the culture's icons and stereotypes of what a man or woman "should" look like. Together with such shape-contorting images, there is often a personal image that each person may "hold" of themselves. This image might be held consciously, but more often it's unconscious, corresponding to an age and shape for which they received validation. For instance, a woman might have been "daddy's little girl" at one point. Alternatively, she may have endured trauma or abuse that left her imprinted or "stuck" at a certain developmental phase—reflected in her startled eyes, sunken chest, held pelvis, or a childlike voice.

Some people take such beliefs to an extreme and are convinced that they will only be lovable if they get rid of parts of their body. I read about a man who, hating his perfectly healthy legs, tried to find a surgeon who would amputate them (Orbach, 2009, pp. 24, 28–29). None would agree; however, his hatred ran so deep that he packed dry ice around his legs and caused himself such severe damage that both limbs had to be amputated. This man had grown up when polio was common, and as a child he noticed how kind and empathetic people were to those who had lost limbs. Having never been treated with kindness, he developed the unconscious belief that he would only become lovable if he did not have legs. Thus, he grew to hate his legs because he believed that they stood between him and love.

Facelifts and Botox can bring different problems. During conversations, we depend on nonverbal cues from the "social engagement system" to help us understand what is happening in somebody's internal world. After cosmetic surgery, those cues are less available, so it may be challenging for us to engage with a person who has undergone such work (Porges, 2011). However, our lack of engagement may leave the person feeling they are still not attractive enough and that may drive them toward more cosmetic procedures. But more procedures may make their predicament worse; the way through is to address the emotional issues that lie beneath the surface of the skin.

Throughout history, men have also had to achieve body ideals, including standards of physical prowess through workouts, competition, and heroic deeds, though less often with cosmetic adjustments. Now they, too, are increasingly going under the knife, injecting facial Botox, often referred to as *Brotox*, and having eyeliner tattooed around their eyes. Then there is the dangerous habit of pumping up on anabolic steroids to enhance muscle bulk and strength during workouts—sometimes beginning in the early teens. Men may also seek to achieve the "perfect manly" bodies they see on social media, without necessarily addressing the vulnerability that lies beneath the skin. That said, how we look is not the same as how we truly feel (Flinders University, 2024).

Rejecting her body's genetic heritage is another way that a woman can leave herself, particularly if her genetic makeup does not match the cultural ideal. Clarissa Pinkola Estes (1992), who was adopted and raised by Hungarian parents, speaks about her stout, square body and how startling it was when she visited the Mexican village of her biological parents, where she met women broader than she who insisted that she was too lean and tried to fatten her up. What's remarkable is how "at home" she felt in her own body when she found herself in the midst of women of her heritage whom she could embrace and who could embrace her for being herself.

Why We Leave Our Bodies

After decades of clinical experience, I believe many women flee their bodies due to a history of abuse. Studies show that one in four women in this country has experienced molestation or sexual abuse as a child. These experiences are often underreported because of fear of reprisal, disbelief, shame, or other inhibiting factors. As I think about this issue, both as a clinician and as a woman, a broader context comes to mind. Why has sexual abuse taken the foreground in our awareness and work over the past several decades? (I would like to say here, again, that although there are men who have been abused, I think it's safe to say that the cases involving women as victims of sexual abuse significantly outnumber those involving men, and it is the woman's experience that I will focus on here.)

Sexual abuse has persisted for millennia, with rapes in domestic news and wartorn nations serving as cruel reminders of this fact. However, a new development has emerged following the women's movement: the "conscious feminine." This awareness asserts that a woman's body is her own and that it is sacred. It recognizes that *matter* has consciousness and that matter and spirit are not separate. The body is alive, possessing its own wisdom. Intuition and "gut feeling" are important, and the body has a remarkable ability to continuously repair and regenerate new tissue, healing itself in ways that the medical profession still struggles to fully understand.

Painfully, even in modern times, patriarchal governments and radical religious movements continue to seek to remove these hard-won human rights, such as the harsh restrictions on women's education, work, freedom to affiliate, drive cars, and even choose how they wish to dress in some cultures. Here in the United States, we experienced the shock of the overturning of *Roe v. Wade*, which protected a women's reproductive freedom—a perilous pendulum swing many of us hope will be reversed as bias and corruption at the highest levels in the executive and judiciary systems become better regulated through ethical standards.

Men, nonbinary, and transgender individuals also suffer in environments that discourage access to feelings, capacity for intimacy, and tolerance for vulnerability. Society often discourages them from honoring their *anima*, or inner feminine, as Jung described. Many do not receive the modeling and support needed to develop this wholeness, including a genuine masculinity that emerges as they grow. Men are not born that way: studies show that male babies are very emotionally responsive to their mothers (Tronick & Cohn, 1989). However, society often discourages emotional expression beyond toughness by the age of 15 or younger.

Many other factors can impact "leaving our bodies." Some of these include:

- Early childhood illness, difficult births, birth impairments, challenges with physical functioning, or traumas to the body over which we had no control as children.
- Other traumas to the body, including accidents and invasive surgery.
- Attachment failures and poor early object relations in which the mirroring and support by parental figures necessary for the child to develop a healthy sense of self may have been inadequate.
- Inadequate or disturbed boundaries regulating interpersonal relations between family members, caretakers, or in educational, work, religious, political, military, or other community settings.
- A sense of shame or criticism projected onto a daughter by a mother who did not love or feel at home in her own body or by a rejecting or invasive father. Feeling inadequate or unwanted for being a female or male infant or identifying as gay or nonbinary.
- Early abandonment or neglect, or a sense that the girl's or boy's body or quality of aliveness did not conform to the cultural ideal or to the family's pattern or style.
- Judgment, rejection, shame, or punishment related to a person's race, ethnicity, religious beliefs, gender identity, sexual preference, women's reproductive freedom, and other elements of personal choice, including who one loves.
- Religious devaluation of the body's sensuality, needs, and role as the crucial foundation of our own perception, standpoint, and access to the sensed world.
- Survival of accidents and natural disasters, Generalized anxiety related to the increasing ecological crisis and sociopolitical tensions, and domestic or community violence. These include human-made disasters, such as the eradication of indigenous populations, the Holocaust, other genocides or wars, and the lasting effects of colonization, slavery, and other traumas affecting human life and dignity.

This, then, is the political, social, and developmental context within which the therapy or healing process takes place. Embedded in this thinking is the materialistic way in which the body—particularly the female body—has been viewed: as an object to be dieted, exercised, dressed up, disguised, fattened, surgically altered, controlled, or repressed. The body has been in shadow, but women are now awakening in our awareness, both personally and at a planetary level in the body of the earth; this often arrives, however, with a great deal of accumulated pain. The hope in this work is in contacting the soulfulness that enlivens the body. The challenge lies in the journey of recovering our bodies, which the remainder of this book addresses.

Descent as a Feminine Path to Individuation

During the past decades, my work has taken me into a deeper investigation of this question: once we have experienced wounding by trauma, or loss that has resulted in a subjective experience of having left the body, how do we get back? For those with early developmental trauma, this may involve finding a home in their body for the first time—as some analytic patients and participants in my classes have attested. My long-term work as a Jungian analyst and dance therapist who integrates somatic process, dreamwork, and creative arts therapies has taught me that there are many roads to healing.

From a broader perspective, dance therapist and Jungian analyst Joan Chodorow speaks of what she calls the "Unholy Trinity": the Body, the Shadow, and the Feminine (Chodorow, 1983), describing the chthonic underworld triad Jung pointed to in his reflections on some of the consequences of the reification of the Christian story (Jung, 1959, CW 9ii, p. 63). Having been repressed for millennia, this trinity is now unmistakably making its way toward the surface, toward consciousness, toward re-embodiment, upsetting the patriarchal culture with its emphasis on solar consciousness, linear or digital time, rugged individualism, competition, and the elevation of logos above all other ways of knowing.

My concern is that having been raised for so many generations according to patriarchal images of spiritual "ascent," together with the quest for personal and individualistic power, we have forgotten its vital counterpart: the feminine path to individuation through "descent." It is as though we must engage in an archeological dig that is at once psychological, spiritual, and physical to recover what is lost. This descent is not just at the level of metaphor, but requires a woman to release and surrender into the depths of her body—reclaiming memories, feelings, and capacities for pleasure and new, life-enhancing and empowering energies that are critical to the healing and transformative process.

To discover a larger framework for their growth process and evolutionary development, women are beginning to remember some of the earliest recorded stories, such as the ancient Sumerian myth of the goddess Inanna (see Chapter 13), or the Greek myth of the mother–daughter relationship shared by Demeter and Persephone. In this story, Persephone is abducted by Hades, god of the underworld. Held captive in his dark kingdom, she refuses to eat until one day she succumbs and eats six seeds from the pomegranate he offers her.

Once returned to her mother's care in the upper world, Demeter carefully questions her as to whether she has eaten anything in Hades. Because she has, Persephone must return to the underworld for six months each year. The story provides a Western example of a myth that underlies the cycles of death and rebirth in our seasonal and psychological changes. Demeter, goddess of nourishment and nature, grieves each year when she has to relinquish her daughter, bringing cold and snow, or in other parts of the world, drought and famine. In springtime, when her daughter is returned to her, she rejoices, causing the rain to fall, to which the earth responds with flowers and the growth of life-giving crops.

In Persephone's case, we see abduction by the dark masculine, implying a death to the innocence and sense of security of the maiden who, assuming immortality, feels impervious to human suffering. Psychologically, we might think of this as the necessary deflation that follows an inflated identification with the archetypal energies of the goddess. Through her ordeal, Persephone integrates shadow and light, reaching a new level of conscious development and maturity.

From a somatic perspective, the psychological terms *inflation* and *deflation* are bodily energetic states. They accompany particular states of consciousness. We get puffed up seeking the expansive, inflated, underbounded, high-energy state of the light goddess through drugs, alcohol, anorexia, or addictive sexual enactments. Then we "crash" in the narrowed, densely weighted, depressive phases that follow on the heels of these airborne surges if we identify too personally with the goddess. Our chest collapses, our head hangs or pulls, turtle-like, into the body, our eyes are dull, and our movement slows. Alternately, we may unconsciously reach for these deflated states through binge eating, overworking to the point of exhaustion, partnering with possessive and demanding mates, and a myriad of other ways. What's essential is to build a conscious, embodied container that is strong enough and flexible enough to withstand the tides of archetypal energy and big feelings.

What we have forgotten and need to relearn is how to surrender to this descent process, trusting that something rich and good can come from it. That we have forgotten is no wonder—we live in an age where feminine qualities, such as feeling, intuition, interpersonal relating, and direct embodied knowing, are undervalued.

This was true, for the most part, in our mothers' and grandmothers' time as well, when the female body was not cherished for what she was. How can a woman expect to love her own body if her mother, her earliest model of what it means to be a woman, has not valued her own? How can you surrender to the depths of your own body if you have not experienced being held as an infant in a way that offers support for your weight, your skin, your breath, your inner organs, your goodness reflected in a loving gaze? Such a gaze assures you can let go to "something larger" without fear of being dropped or abandoned. Over mothering can also be a risk, where you might feel swallowed up or psychologically sucked back into the womb and the mother's identity.

Jungian analyst Marie Louise von Franz has this to say about the process of descent:

Every dark thing one falls into can be called an initiation. To be initiated into a thing means to go into it. The first step is generally falling into the dark place and usually appears in a dubious or negative form—falling into something or being possessed by something. The shamans say that being a medicine man begins by falling into the power of the demons; the one who pulls out of the dark place becomes the medicine man, and the one who stays in, the sick person. You can take every psychological illness as an initiation. Even the worst things you fall into are an effort at initiation, for you are in something which belongs to you, and now you must get out of it.

(1993, p. 74)

What we need to relearn is how to navigate through the lower worlds without fear that we'll be gobbled up there, encountering an abusive parent or going crazy, or dying, never being released to the upper worlds again. What we need are the skills, the courage, and the compassionate support to face the shadow.

Authentic Movement is one avenue for inviting a descent into the body and psyche within a safe environment. Here, a woman may go at her own pace, finding a style and rhythm that is uniquely her own. In this way, she will find her own challenges, which often involve literal reenactments of the embodied movement patterns surrounding the trauma, wound, or stuck place, the places where the resources ran out or she had to cower, freeze, or puff herself up just to survive. What I have learned through my years of practicing embodied depth analysis and of moving and witnessing people move is that *transformation is the other side of the wound*. It is as if they are two sides of the same coin. If we can return to the site of the wound, the "scene of the crime" as it were—the feelings, bodily states, and the meanings we have made of them—with the additional resources of adulthood, we can heal ourselves. This process mirrors the shaman's journey, who, after suffering from a psychotic break or near-death experience, develops a knowledge of the descent and the way through again.

The Handless Maiden: A Story of Healing and Transformation

The Grimms' fairytale "The Handless Maiden"—a poignant yet ultimately empowering tale for our time—tells the story of a miller's daughter whose hands are cut off by her father who has been tricked by the devil into promising her in exchange for wealth. Duped by desperation and greed, the father thinks he is only handing over "what stands behind his house"—the "old Apple Tree." In fact, his daughter was sweeping the yard at that moment. However, when the devil comes to claim his prize, he cannot take the girl while her hands are pure, so he forces her father to sever them or risk losing his own life.

The father is distraught, and the mother is helpless to intercede. The miller—representing something outworn in the collective that wants to continue in the old way—together with the missing feminine, represented by the mother, are swept into a horrific act. The father begs his daughter's forgiveness, asking, "What else can I do?" As a naive "good girl," the maiden at first consents, telling him, "Dear Father, do with me what you will; I am your child" (Grimm & Grimm, 1944, p. 161), illustrating her willingness to give herself away to appease patriarchal demands, at the risk of losing her literal hands and her soul. Says von Franz, "From the miller's standpoint, his daughter would represent his anima figure—that is, a part of his feeling and emotional life which is now sold to evil and falls into the devil's hands." If taken from the feminine standpoint, "one could say that this represents the case of a woman who through a negative constellation of her father complex has fallen into the greatest danger" (von Franz, 1993, p. 87).

Despite her parents' pleas to stay, the Handless Maiden leaves, seeking compassion elsewhere. In the forest, an angel aids her, and she finds refuge in a king's garden.

The King, captivated by her purity, marries her and has silver hands fashioned for her. Outwardly, the King is "the personification of a dominant content of the collective consciousness of the culture"; inwardly, he symbolizes a carrier of wholeness, sovereignty, solar brilliance, and spiritual insight (Woodman, 1992a, p. 11).

When the King goes to war, the devil intervenes again, altering messages to have the Queen and her newborn son killed. The King's mother, refusing to shed innocent blood, sends them away to the woods, where an angel again guides them. Although the Brothers Grimm Christianize the tale, in an earlier version, while on her way through the woods to a cabin, the Queen becomes thirsty and seeing a spring leans over to take a drink (von Franz, 1972/1993, p. 99). Suddenly, her baby slips from her body and falls into the water. In anguish, the Queen thrusts her silver hands into the water to prevent him from drowning, and her flesh and blood hands grow back! It is through the act of reaching out with love for what she values most that her hands grow back; her love for her child restores her real hands. After seven years, the King finds them, and they return to the castle, celebrating a second wedding; there is great joy throughout the community, and they live happily until the end of their days.

Here, we see the alchemical "sacred marriage"—the *coniunctio*—the union of the more developed masculine/yang and feminine/yin elements. Two aspects of the self that have come together at a deeper level of integration having grown through travails, each through their own individuation journeys. This results in the "divine child," the new life that flowers from this union. The Handless Maiden illustrates a journey through wounding, suffering, and the development of a sense of agency, personal identity, and empowerment. Having first identified as an obedient "father's daughter"—a girl or woman who identifies more with the father's psychology than with the mother's—she comes into her own as a woman, a soul, a mother, and a Queen. Through the process she achieves a higher level of conscious development and fulfills her destiny.

The tale illustrates both healing from trauma and the development of genuine feeling, courage, agency, and capacity in the world—a connection with a healthy *animus*. Tracing the movement from cultural repression to perseverance, from wounded child to whole healed woman, and from impoverishment to the mistress of her destiny, the heroine demonstrates a pathway for creativity and manifestation in life—from oppression to transformation. She can now "take her life into her own hands."

Descent & Ascent: Reintegration

Though this conscious embodiment process is something dance/movement and body-oriented practitioners have understood for some time, more recently the neurosciences have begun to track brain function related to traumatic injuries. Neuroscientist Ruth Lanius works with functional magnetic resonance imaging (FMRI) scans and other modalities to study the effects of traumatic experience on the brain, mind, and body, examining ways in which "the consciousness of embodiment, or people's sense of having, 'consciously being in,' owning, and belonging to a body can be altered by the experience of psychological trauma" (Frewen & Lanius, 2015, pp. 188–189). Lanius, Judith Herman (1997), Bessel van der Kolk (2014), Allan Schore (2012), Stephen Porges (2011), and other prominent clinicians, neuroscience researchers, and dance/movement and somatic psychotherapists underscore the vital role of embodied methods for healing from trauma, oppression, and other potentially debilitating conditions.

Furthermore, trauma doesn't happen in isolation; it's a symptom of a far broader systemic problem. Herman uses her research on domestic violence and studies combat veterans and political terror victims to highlight similarities between private traumas like domestic violence and public ones like terrorism. She emphasizes that understanding psychological trauma requires considering the social context in which it occurs.

In this chapter, I have described some of the major ways we leave our bodies and why we leave. Recovering begins with descent. Marion Woodman reflects on the process in her work as an analyst.

> So often at the psychic level the process is moving in a very healing direction. But then I may reach out to touch my analysand and the body pulls back. It doesn't feel worthy. It says, "I am unlovable." (This reaction comes regardless of what they might be consciously thinking or wanting.) As I go deeper into their dreams, I realize that the voice [of the complex] that says, "I am unlovable" is in the cells [where it may have been for generations]. Therefore it's at that cellular level that the transformation has to take place.
>
> (Woodman, 1992b)

As my women clients and students make the necessary descent into themselves and their bodies, I often see their struggles between "the nun"/ascetic and "the prostitute"/sexual woman, the Virgin Mary/maternal figure and Mary Magdalene/ the lover, the all-sacrificing mother and the innocent daughter, the witch and the country maid, mirroring the feminine split in many primarily patriarchal cultures. Working with these courageous women has allowed me to witness them bridge their way back to their bodies and instincts. I see them reclaiming what has been taken from them and finding hope as they heal the split within themselves. In the process, they step into a more authentic, mature female sexuality—a sense of self-worth, soulfulness, and the ability to finally "come home" to themselves, take their place in the world, and make meaningful contributions.

It is my hope that whether you are a clinician choosing to use or develop more active movement or body-based interventions in your work, a man nurturing your inner feminine, a woman listening for your own deeper instinctual callings, or an individual with more fluidity in your sense of "ascribed" gender that you will allow your body to tell its story, receiving it with love as you find ways to take the feminine by the hand, welcoming her back from the shadows and into the light.

The Street Cleaner

She had a purpose
Cleaning the streets
Some days it was dirt
Some days it was trash
And some days it was
Rose petals
From funeral marches
Strewn on the road
By insane mothers and fathers
Who lost their sons and daughters
Infants and grandchildren
To war

She heard the voices
Which arose from the dead
Bodies never buried

With her broom in hand
She dutifully
Made circles of rose petals
In the quiet places
To honor them
A touch of beauty
She thought
In this time of darkness
She then moved on
Her palm frond broom in hand

Cleaning
          Corlene Van Sluizer

References

Bateson, G. (1985, May). *From metaphors and butterflies* [Guest lecture]. Stanislav Grof's seminar, Esalen Institute, Big Sur, California.

Chodorow, J. (1983). *Dance therapy and the unholy trinity: Feminine, body, shadow* [Lecture]. General session of the Eighteenth Annual American Dance Therapy Conference, October 21–24, 1983, at the Asilomar Conference Center, Pacific Grove, California.

Estes, C. P. (1992). *Women who run with the wolves: Myths and stories of the wild woman archetype*. Ballantine Books.

Flinders University. (2024, October 30). The dangerous pursuit of muscularity in men and adolescent boys. *Science Daily*. Retrieved November 25, 2024, from https://www.sciencedaily.com/releases/2024/10/241030150853.htm

Frewen, P. & Lanius, R. (2015). *Healing the traumatized self: Consciousness, neuroscience, treatment*. W. W. Norton & Company.

Grimm, J. & Grimm, W. (1944). *The complete Grimm's fairy tales, introduced by Padraic Colum with commentary by Joseph Campbell*. Pantheon Books.

Herman, J. (1997). *Trauma and recovery: The aftermath of violence—from domestic abuse to political terror*. Basic Books.

Jung, C. G. (1959). *The collected works of C. G. Jung: Vol. 9ii. Aion* (R. F. C. Hull, trans.). Bollingen Foundation, Inc.

Orbach, S. (2009). *Bodies*. Picador Press.

Orben, A., Meier, A., Dalgleish, T., et al. (2024). Mechanisms linking social media use to adolescent mental health vulnerability. *Nature Reviews Psychology, 3*, 407–423. https://doi.org/10.1038/s44159-024-00307-y

Porges, S. (2011). *The polyvagal theory: Neurophysiological foundations of emotions, attachment, communication, and self-regulation*. W. W. Norton & Co.

Reich, W. (1980). *Character analysis*. Farrar, Straus & Giroux. (Original work published 1933.)

Schore, A. (2012). *The science of the art of psychotherapy*. W. W. Norton & Company.

Tronick E. Z. & Cohn J. F. (1989). Infant-mother face-to-face interaction: Age and gender differences in coordination and the occurrence of miscoordination. *Child Development, 60*(1), 85–92.

Van der Hart, O., Nijenhuis, E. R. S., & Steele, K. (2006). *The haunted self: Structural dissociation and the treatment of chronic traumatization*. W. W. Norton & Co.

Van der Kolk, B. (2014). *The body keeps the score: Brain, mind, and body in the healing of trauma*. Viking Press.

von Franz, M. L. (1993). *The feminine in fairytales*. Shambhala. (Original publication 1972.)

Woodman, M. (1992a). *Leaving my father's house: A journey to conscious femininity*. Shambhala Publications.

Woodman, M. (1992b). A meeting with Marion Woodman. In *Conscious femininity: Interviews with Marion Woodman*. Inner City Books.

Chapter 7

Embodied Descent
Steps Toward Transformation

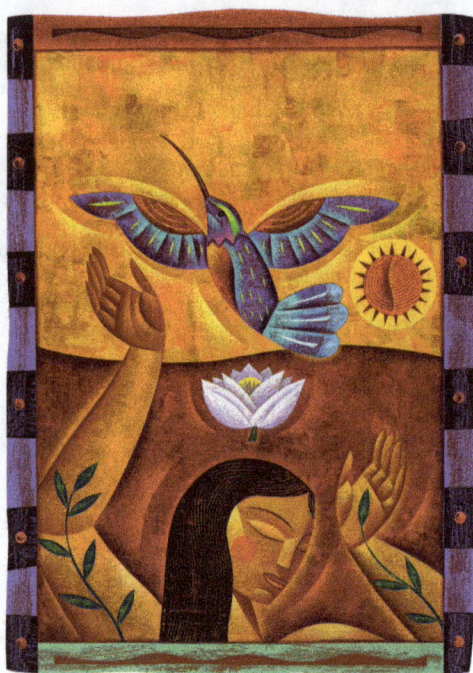

Figure 7.1 Colibri © 2008, by Rafael Lopez @ https://rafaellopez.com/.

Our bodies may be our closest link to the unconscious, expressing the soul's longing through breath, gesture, the rhythm of our steps, and the music of our speech. This chapter expands on my dissertation research, which explores the transformative potential of Authentic Movement for women, emphasizing the body's central role in healing, spiritual growth, and creative expression. This practice has been a pivotal part of my life for more than forty years, informing my work as a dance/somatic psychotherapist, teacher, and Jungian analyst.

DOI: 10.4324/9781003538356-10

Dance has been a vital and healing force for me since childhood, laying the foundation for my journey as a dance therapist, Authentic Movement practitioner, and psychoanalyst. Over the years, I have had the privilege of working with thousands of women and men in various settings: clinical environments, graduate training programs, professional organizations, and international workshops. These experiences inspired a desire to articulate the deep, nonverbal, embodied wisdom I have witnessed and practiced. My study involved reflecting on my own learnings and engaging in dialogue with women whose lives have been deeply shaped by Authentic Movement, exploring how their stories intersected with and enriched my own.

Challenging memories, a sense of distance from one's deeper vitality, and trauma, both physical and emotional, often reside in the body, held in stasis until they can be consciously integrated. The practice facilitates transformative experiences by allowing genuine expression to emerge and become part of lived reality. Despite its power, these embodied experiences remain underrepresented in the professional literature, making it crucial to share and articulate them. My dissertation was a way to explore this further, combining my story, the history of Authentic Movement, and the narratives of key practitioners. This chapter focuses on Janet Adler and Irma Dosamantes-Beaudry, with later chapters delving into Andrea Olsen's and Marion Woodman's contributions. As Dr. Joan Chodorow, a pioneering innovator and teacher of this work, was the cochair of my dissertation research committee, I've not profiled her specifically here. However, her profound contributions are reflected throughout this book and in her publications, which have been translated into dozens of languages (Stromsted, 2025).

During my research, I conducted in-depth, audio-recorded interviews, visiting each co-researcher in their own setting. I recognized the impact of my own subjectivity, acknowledging how my experiences shaped my interpretations while remaining open to the insights my co-researchers shared. Their wisdom, often overlooked in a culture that disregards the body's intelligence, illuminated the significance of embodied knowledge in healing and personal growth.

Embodied Descent

Authentic Movement helps women reconnect with instinctual knowing. As noted in previous chapters, they often describe it as a process of "descent" into themselves—one that they emerge from with new insights. This theme of descent and return is mirrored in ancient myths, such as those of *Inanna, Demeter and Persephone, Psyche* and *Eros*, and many of non-Western origin. Though these stories are ancient, the process itself, buried for so long in our culture, is as potentially meaningful for women today as it was then. Says Jungian analyst Marion Woodman, "Though a modern woman cannot go back to the Dionysian Mysteries, she must nevertheless make the journey into the dark regions below and back again" if she is to experience and integrate the less conscious "shadow" aspects of herself and become more whole (Woodman, 1980, p. 111). Woodman writes about the necessity for modern women to rediscover the sacred within their bodies, describing dance as a way to reconnect with this inner mystery and facilitate transformation. "Dance is one practical way of listening to her body" she explains, allowing women to experience themselves as vessels of divine energy (p. 111).

Psychoanalyst and dance therapist Irma Dosamantes-Beaudry emphasizes the importance of having a trusted companion during this journey. She notes that transformative work can evoke periods of instability, likening it to a "mini break-down" where old patterns dissolve and a woman's sense of self is radically altered. Authentic Movement, as a form of "active imagination in movement," provides a structure for this process, enabling women to heal and transform in their own unique way and at their own pace.

Methodology

In recent decades, qualitative research methodologies have evolved, moving be-yond the positivist view that reality exists objectively, independent of perception. Constructivist paradigms acknowledge the role of the researcher in shaping and interpreting data, emphasizing holistic and relational approaches. Instead of seek-ing a linear, causal analysis, qualitative methods offer a "holistic perspective that describes the interdependence and relatedness of complex phenomena" (Patton, 1990, p. 424). An approach that can embrace more feminine ways of knowing, it emphasizes "illumination, understanding, and extrapolation rather than [only] causal determination, prediction, and generalization" (Creswell, 1994, p. 6). My re-search embraced the Organic Research Method, integrating feminist and heuristic principles that respected the evolving, embodied nature of the inquiry. This method allowed for a deep exploration of experience rooted in sensory and intuitive know-ing, reflecting the practice of Authentic Movement itself.

Conducting the research also allowed me to develop my own consciousness, thereby enhancing my ability to affect change. In addition, accessing women's voices—their descriptions of their direct experience before they had been further abstracted or rein-terpreted through the lens of the still-dominant patriarchal cultural paradigm—was an essential aspect of this process, mirroring the practice of Authentic Movement.

The Organic Research Method (Clements et al., 1998), influenced by the work of Clark Moustakas (1990), provided a research paradigm that could do justice to the intuitive and sensory-grounded dimensions of the work. Likened to the process of a seed growing into a tree—the same image that Jung uses to describe the individu-ation process (Jung, 1961, p. 4)—this approach guided my research through five stages: Sacred (preparing the ground), Personal (planting the seed), Chthonic (the roots emerging), Relational (growing the tree), and Transformative (harvesting the fruit). This approach honored the unfolding nature of the work, recognizing that intuitive insights, dreams, and embodied experiences played a crucial role in the research process. The methodology allowed for an authentic representation of how movement facilitates transformation.

The research itself was transformative, in that it brought about changes in me, my co-researchers, and our readers, who reported a deep sense of recognition and inspiration as they moved through the text.

Co-Researchers: Selection Criteria and Role

My co-researchers were carefully selected based on their maturity and depth of experience in the field: Andrea Olsen, whom I discuss in Chapter 10, because of her engagement in the artistic and physiological arenas of the creative process, performance, experiential anatomy, and the relationship between body and place; Marion Woodman, whose story I explore in Chapter 14, for her work in the analytical psychology of C. G. Jung, bodily expression in women's individuation process, dreams, working through addictions, and the development of the conscious feminine principle. In this chapter, I focus on Irma Dosamantes-Beaudry, who has developed the work further in the psychoanalytic, object relations, and cross-cultural arenas; and Janet Adler for her exploration of the area of mysticism and in the further development of the Discipline of Authentic Movement.

Irma Dosamantes-Beaudry, PhD, BC-DMT, trained as a psychologist, psychoanalyst, dance therapist, and dancer. She served as director of the Graduate Dance/Movement Therapy Program in the World Arts and Culture Department at University of California Los Angeles (UCLA) (1977–1990), where she taught generations of Dance/Movement therapists and supervised Fulbright and Visiting Scholars. Past president of the American Dance Therapy Association and the American Association for the Study of Mental Imagery, she was the recipient of the Chace Memorial Foundation Award for her lifetime contribution to the field of Dance/Movement Therapy and served as editor-in-chief of *The Arts in Psychotherapy Journal* (1990–2003). Her research and writing have centered around contemporary psychoanalysis; sacred female healing traditions; the arts as healing and therapy; cultural, developmental, and subjective aspects of self-construction; and the role of the body as an instrument of consciousness (Dosamantes-Alperson,

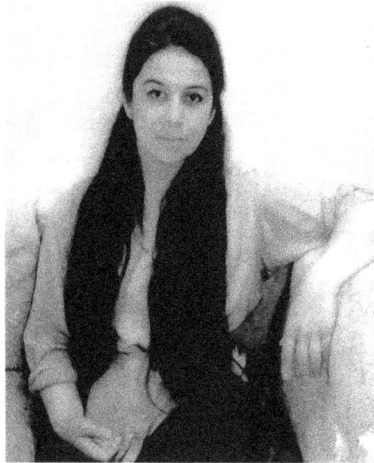

Figure 7.2 Irma Dosamantes-Beaudry. Reproduced courtesy of Irma Dosamantes-Beaudry.

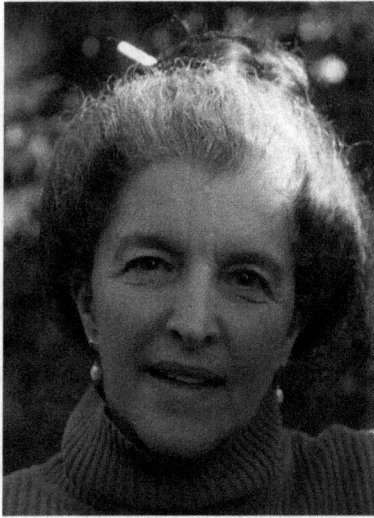

Figure 7.3 Janet Adler, Sebastopol, California © D.A. Sonneborn 1997.
All Rights Reserved.

1974, 1983, 1986, 1987; Dosamantes, 1992a, 1992b, 1993; Dosamantes-Beaudry, 1997a, 1997b, 1998; Fairweather, 1994). Her book, *The Arts in Contemporary Healing* (Dosamantes-Beaudry, 2003), was selected for inclusion in Greenwood Publisher's Significant Contribution to Psychology Series (Dosamantes-Beaudry, 2024).

Janet Ader (1941–2023) studied with pioneering Dance/Movement therapists Mary Starks Whitehouse and Marian Chace. Janet made substantial contributions to the development of the practice, particularly in the role of the witness, and as an avenue to mystical experience, calling it the Discipline of Authentic Movement, which she taught for fifty years. She founded Circles of Four (2013) and was the author of three books: *Arching Backward: The Mystical Initiation of a Contemporary Woman* (Alder, 1995), *Offering from the Conscious Body: The Discipline of Authentic Movement* (Alder, 2002), and *Intimacy in Emptiness: An Evolution of Embodied Consciousness* (previously published papers, edited with commentary by Bonnie Morrissey and Paula Sager, Alder, 2022). She also made two films: *Looking for Me* (1968), a reflection of her early work with autistic children, and *Still Looking* (1998), a film about her work at that time in the Discipline of Authentic Movement. Her archives, The Janet Adler Collection, are housed at the New York Public Library for the Performing Arts.

The stories of Janet Adler and Irma Dosamantes-Beaudry, along with those of Andrea Olsen and Marion Woodman, form a rich tapestry of wisdom, illustrating the profound impact of Authentic Movement on women's individuation journeys. This depth-oriented practice continues to deepen and evolve, underscoring the essential role of embodied experience in our quest for wholeness.

Initial Interview Questions

The study aimed to uncover and articulate the core elements of Authentic Movement that facilitate transformative experiences for women. To guide this exploration, I posed the following open-ended questions to my co-researchers:

1 How have Authentic Movement and related practices transformed your life and contributed to your development as a woman? What matters to you now, and what advice would you offer to other women?
2 In your work, how does Authentic Movement transform women? What themes emerge around transformational experiences? What key elements or processes are crucial for healing and transformation? Can you provide an example?

Data Analysis Procedures

Each practitioner participated in two in-depth interviews, which I analyzed to identify themes and patterns. I shared my transcripts and thematic synthesis with them for review and feedback, ensuring that the interpretations felt accurate, resonated, and respected their privacy before including it in my research document.

After conducting interviews, I engaged in Authentic Movement to process my own sensory and emotional responses. This was followed by expressive art—drawing and spontaneous writing—an approach that deepened the research's authenticity, as it honored my own embodied experience and kept me connected to the essence of the inquiry, rather than analyzing purely on a cognitive level.

I then consolidated the findings into 13 meta-themes, using a visual chart to clarify focal points and variations. My process included documenting dreams, bodily sensations, and insights, with examples illustrating the evolution of my understanding. Interviews with a colleague further explored my shifting perspectives throughout the study. I revisited relevant literature to contextualize the findings and propose avenues for future research.

The Researcher's Body

In line with Organic Research Methodology, I remained mindful that my own life events could influence the study's trajectory. By balancing action with reflection, I honored the research's heuristic nature. Organizing the data into a grid, I immersed myself in writing about the 13 themes, always referencing the co-researchers' insights without imposing psychological interpretations. Often, our discussions prompted reflections on "whose material is this?" This question frequently arises in the intersubjective space between mover and witness.

My research process echoed Marie-Louise von Franz's stages of active imagination: opening to the unconscious, giving it form, the ego's response/conscious reflection, and living the experience (Chodorow, 1997; von Franz, 1983/1980). This evolving consciousness not only facilitates healing and transformation but also integrates embodied wisdom into everyday life. Through this journey, I confronted the patriarchal influences embedded in me since childhood, which shaped my life on a cellular level. (By patriarchy, I mean the power principle, which, despite the imbalances in many cultures, is not limited to gender.) I had to frequently reconnect with my body's signals, resisting the urge to speed up or anticipate conclusions in order to meet academic expectations.

Internal and External Challenges

A significant challenge arose during a meeting with a dissertation committee member who kept altering requirements, unintentionally hindering my progress while appearing supportive. The stress culminated in a sudden injury: feeling "beside myself" as I stepped out of a shop onto a busy sidewalk, my foot inadvertently landed in a hole that had not been visible given the press of passersby—shades of Persephone! I had felt the sensation of having "the rug pulled out from under me" in the committee meeting, and now I heard a distinct "snap." As I lost my balance, my ankle fractured, and I sank to the pavement—a vivid embodiment of the turmoil I was experiencing.

I realized that I began the research with a compliance-driven mindset, still adhering to hierarchical academic standards and their fluctuating requirements. Yet, as I delved deeper, I had to shed this "good girl" persona. Despite investing immense effort into dissecting the themes, I felt drained and disconnected, transforming vibrant, intimate experiences into sterile facts. The work was exhausting, and my body reacted: not only did I break my ankle, but also my left eye and the left side of my face twitched, and my back ached from countless hours of typing and poor posture.

It was a wake-up call from my primary research instrument—my body. Realizing the irony of writing about body wisdom while disregarding my own, I turned to Authentic Movement, drawing, and active imagination dialogue. A tension between my intuitive, creative side and my academically conditioned, results-driven side became clear. Seeking guidance through active imagination, I engaged in a dialogue between my left and right hands.

"What are you *doing*?!" my intuitive side (left hand) asked as I began to dialogue with her. "You're *killing* me!"

"Oh, please don't do this to me," my rational side (dominant right hand) begged. "I'll never finish the dissertation by the deadline. I'm in debt, time is running out, and I've done so much hard work already!"

"But I can't go on this way," my intuitive side said firmly, "and you're spoiling the feeling and undermining the whole reason for your inquiry."

"Do you have any better ideas?" my rational side finally conceded.

"Yes," she said. "Write stories."

This was revolutionary, providing a breakthrough in what had felt like an in-surmountable deadlock. Now, after dissecting the material and differentiating it into themes (using my "masculine"/*logos* side), I could return to relating to the women themselves through weaving the essential strands into their stories (a more "feminine"/*eros*–intuitive feeling approach). By the time I brought it all together, the Conclusions chapter caught fire, seeming to write itself in one sitting in a deeply satisfying and integrative synthesis (or "inner marriage"). Their process, and mine, followed the four stages of the transformative journey: (a) opening to the unconscious and the descent into the underworld; (b) retrieving the treasure, giving it form; (c) bringing it to consciousness and response by the ego; and (d) living it, offering back to the community. Owning unconscious "shadow" material, harnessing the critic, and developing healthier internal masculine energies allowed my feminine spirit, too, to find expression in my body and in my voice. Bringing these fundamental energies and perspectives together moved the process toward the sacred marriage that integrates the two within each of us in a more conscious union (Jung, 1981, CW 8, p. 208).

Findings: Meta-Themes in Transformation as a Path of Descent and Return

Thirteen meta-themes emerged, each representing a facet of the transformative journey:

1 **Attitude toward the Female Body**: Initial perceptions and the healing of trauma or illness.
2 **Strength of the Body Ego**: Heightened body awareness and reflective consciousness.
3 **Triggering Events**: Key life and cultural experiences shaping growth.
4 **Guiding Lights**: Supportive, influential relationships.
5 **Creating a Safe Container**: Providing a secure space for exploring the unconscious.
6 **Will, Surrender, and Sacrifice**: Embracing vulnerability and ego dissolution.
7 **Growth of the Inner Witness**: Developing self-compassion and reflective awareness.
8 **Integration of the Shadow**: Embracing and transforming hidden aspects of the self.
9 **Animus Development**: Transforming inner masculine energy into an ally.
10 **Presence of the Sacred**: Experiencing spiritual or divine connection.
11 **Conscious Feminine Principle**: Embodying presence and feeling values.
12 **Finding One's Voice**: Authentically expressing your true self, overcoming barriers that hold you back, and sharing your unique perspective with others.
13 **Community and Collective Body**: The importance of connection and collective healing.

I discovered that these 13 themes were not isolated descriptions of elements but formed a natural sequence, illustrating a developmental path of descent into the body and psyche, followed by a return to grounded awareness with offerings for the community. To my amazement, the process mirrored the timeless mythic and shamanic journeys of transformation, emphasizing the importance of individual pace and unique expression. It also became clear that the journey was not only about personal development, but also the enhancement of consciousness in the collective as a whole.

Healing and Transformation

Curing often implies a return to a former state of functioning, whereas healing and transformation involve profound, meaningful change. Marion Woodman summarized the distinction when she said, "Healing for me [is] soul work. I could be cured and live, and not be healed. And I may die, but I will be healed" (Woodman, 1996). Throughout my research, the Western focus on *curing* became less relevant, with *change* emerging as a key theme—from the micro level of nerve pathway alterations to the macro level of shifts in identity. Interviews with my co-researchers added depth to these concepts, highlighting their nuanced differences. Their experiences exemplify this, moving from body-felt density and lack of differentiation to greater embodiment and self-awareness.

Irma Dosamantes-Beaudry highlighted the resonance between movers and witnesses, emphasizing the group's power to hold and amplify healing experiences. Janet Adler described transformative Kundalini experiences and the wisdom in embracing wounds as ongoing sources of insight.

Re-Creating Wombs: Birthing the Unmothered Woman

As I see it, Authentic Movement creates a "safe enough" space, akin to a womb, for rebirth. It allows for shedding old defenses and rediscovering a sense of self within an interconnected community. In this container, women confront and transform past traumas, emerging with new strength and purpose. Authentic Movement invites a return to bodily wisdom, offering a path to integration and healing that is as profound as it is personal. My co-researchers' journeys, and my own, illustrate that deep transformation requires both honoring the wound and embracing the body's wisdom to live a more integrated, embodied life.

Transformative Stories

Irma Dosamantes-Beaudry: Flamenco

Irma Dosamantes-Beaudry shared a story about her psychoanalyst, Hedda, who typically refrained from offering specific advice. However, one day Hedda strongly encouraged Irma to watch the Spanish film *Carmen*, which featured breathtaking scenes of flamenco dancing set against a passionate yet tragic love story. For Irma, who had years of modern dance training through her childhood, college, and graduate school, this experience was transformative. It was her first time seeing a Latina movie star who looked like her, embodying sensuality and strength in dance. As Irma watched, tears streamed down her face, and she felt a powerful identification with the star dancer.

Inspired by the film, Irma let down her long, tightly coiled hair, allowing it to cascade to her waist. She began to feel the movement of her hips and the swing of her body in a new, freeing way through flamenco. For a time, she adopted the dancer's style, from her clothing to her posture, until she could internalize these qualities. This experience was profoundly transformative, helping Irma reclaim and embrace her Mexican heritage, connecting her to a sense of pride, rage, and sexuality.

Irma later had a dream that signaled she had received what she needed from flamenco. In the dream, *the flamenco dancer danced so hard and so fast and so fiery that she burnt herself to ashes, and then there was nothing left but a naked little pint-sized Amazon.* "For me," she said, "that was a very transformative dream because it had to do with giving up the narcissism involved in being the flamenca. Being a 'flamenca' is very dramatic; it's all about 'me'! [feigning a gesture of waving her plumage]. So to relinquish the flamenca in me meant getting ready to give up the grandiosity connected with it while retaining and internalizing its good qualities—pride, strength, and fire. The Amazon aspect was about being strong without having to be a giant. It taught me that I could be strong and powerful, and yet be more life-sized."

This experience also contributed in a fundamental way to the ongoing development of Irma's awareness, teaching, research, and support for people from different races and cultural backgrounds in her roles as a psychologist, researcher, author, department chair, and one of the leaders in the field of dance/movement therapy. Her participation in the study enhanced her interest in sacred female healing traditions and the role of the body as an instrument of consciousness.

Janet Adler: Kundalini

Janet, too, drew from her personal experiences to foster healing and transformation in her students. Her early trauma, involving a prolonged separation from her mother due to hospitalization as an infant, together with her family background as one of only two Jewish families in their post–World War II (WWII) Midwest community, shaped her understanding of the mind–body connection. This led her to explore how emotions and memories are stored in the body, influencing her further development of Authentic Movement.

Her teaching initially focused on healing and personal development, addressing unconscious material through movement. In later years, her work shifted from dance/movement therapy to spiritual growth, influenced by Kundalini energy and Jewish mysticism. She viewed Authentic Movement as a discipline that "invites and enables transformation," integrating masculine and feminine energies toward whole-ness. Her focus later evolved to helping others connect directly with their sacred source, mirroring her journey from personal history to exploring deeper mysteries.

Here, Janet recounts an experience from the beginning of her Kundalini awak-ening, detailed in her book *Arching Backward: The Mystical Initiation of a Con-temporary Woman* (1995). Kundalini, a spiritual energy arising from the base of the spine, is understood as the divine feminine in Hinduism and can be awakened through practices like Kundalini yoga and energetic openings in other forms of embodied depth work. For some, the density of matter in the unconscious areas of the body—blockages in the chakras as this vital energy travels from the base of the spine to the crown of the head—is experienced literally through physical pain; for others, it may be expressed primarily through images or both. When practiced by individuals with a strong body container, discerning ego, and disciplined practice, it can be integrated into daily life, enhancing personal and spiritual growth.

What follows is Janet's description of one of these experiences. In a studio over-looking a pond, she longed to move. Through the windows, the gray morning mist surrounded her, and she returned to Authentic Movement, her only vessel for hold-ing life's complexities. While she wished for a witness to hold consciousness, she did not want any verbal exchange afterward. Rosa, a visual artist and her compan-ion in the practice, agreed to be her silent witness, sketching as Janet moved. Janet recounts:

> I step in. This space, open and empty, invites me. There are no other people in this space or nearby. There is no need to fill it. Moving through it slowly, in such awe, it is hard to believe how clear, how free it is. This space is mine. Putting my cheek in my hand, I sink slowly toward the floor.

> I lie down on my back, knees bent, feet flat. I feel warm, the gray wet of the morning surrounding me. I sink slowly into my body, receiving my weight, receiving myself. I am opening. An energy field appears between my legs, push-ing them apart. The movement is infinitesimal, slow, until my legs fall open wide. With eyes closed, I see images.

> My hands reach toward my *yoni* [vulva], pulling out a long, long rope laden with *lingams* [phalluses]. Hand over hand I pull. Under the last lingam is a vibrant sphere, textured and beautiful. As it opens, a baby falls out. She glides back into me now, becoming a pubescent girl, released with utter joy and freedom to explore my entire pelvic cavity. It is open in there, pink and wet, free of organs. She moves as if swim-ming, with big and full strokes. She is home, returning home (Adler, 1995, pp. 2–3).

Janet felt a profound sense of homecoming, perhaps a fuller healing of her early infant trauma together with an experience of rebirth. When she opened her eyes, Rosa handed her a drawing. They exchanged silent gratitude and walked home together.

Women and Research: Embodied Paradigms

Embracing an embodied, feminine perspective in research brings unique insights to the field. Using the Organic Research Method allowed me to stay attuned to the lived experiences of my co-researchers and my own process. The word *re-search* truly became about finding anew, deepening my trust in Authentic Movement as a discovery modality.

A woman's sense of self is powerfully shaped by her family background, cultural roots, and the spirit of the times. Western culture's mechanistic, overspecialized worldview often divides the sacred from the secular and the spiritual from the physical, causing fragmentation and spiritual impoverishment. Though our technological advancements have brought material benefits, they have also devastated nature and eroded human connectedness.

Traditional, cognitively focused therapeutic approaches often mirror this divide, favoring mental insights over embodied experiences. However, a new paradigm is emerging, with people increasingly seeking holistic healing methods. The shift is slow, however, and the Western medical model remains dominant. This often alienates individuals from their bodies, especially women, who have historically internalized negative self-images and patriarchal attitudes. Though conventional medicine is essential for surgeries and other therapies and procedures, more integrative methods are necessary, bringing allopathic and complementary medical approaches together to empower individuals in their healing process.

Over the centuries women have devalued their innate wisdom, prioritizing the needs of others over their own and surrendering their power for protection and love. Reconnecting with this feminine knowing is vital, and movement practices like Authentic Movement facilitate this reconnection. The Organic Research Method enabled me to trust this embodied wisdom, revealing how it transforms a woman's sense of self and permeates all aspects of her life.

Healing the Split

Our ravaged bodies and psyches call for a new understanding, drawing from ancient indigenous practices. Reintegrating mind, body, and spirit with community and Earth remains a significant challenge. While this study focused on women's experiences, I have seen Authentic Movement profoundly transform men and individuals with fluid gender identities as well. In workshops and classes, I have witnessed men open to their vulnerability, strength, and love, transforming their relationships with themselves, others, and society. All people need ways to heal the body–soul split, which leads to projecting shadow material onto others, perpetuating conflict and violence.

In this depth-oriented practice, individuals are invited to listen to their bodies' callings and to give shape to the feelings and images that surface from underground wellsprings toward consciousness. Gathering in circles, like around a fire, movers and witnesses articulate these deeper truths, discovering energies that can guide us. Here, they make the transition from body to word, sharing experiences and images that are trying to speak through them from the Self and have much to contribute to the development of embodied consciousness. Authentic Movement touches the physical, psychological, spiritual, social, aesthetic, and ecological realms, offering a holistic approach. Witnesses are enriched by the transformations they observe, and movers are supported in their healing journeys. Together, we move toward a future where embodied wisdom nourishes our relationships with ourselves, each other, and the Earth, answering the call to live the love and wisdom that we come to know in our bodies. Poet Jan Richardson speaks of this process in her poem "How the Light Comes" (Richardson, 2015):

How the Light Comes

I cannot tell you
how the light comes.

What I know
is that it is more ancient
than imagining.

That it travels
across an astounding expanse
to reach us.

That it loves
searching out
what is hidden,
what is lost,
what is forgotten
or in peril
or in pain.

That it has a fondness
for the body,
for finding its way
toward flesh,
for tracing the edges
of form,
for shining forth
through the eye,
the hand,
the heart.

I cannot tell you
how the light comes,
but that it does.
That it will.
That it works its way
into the deepest dark
that enfolds you,
though it may seem
long ages in coming
or arrive in a shape
you did not foresee.

And so
may we this day
turn ourselves toward it.
May we lift our faces
to let it find us.
May we bend our bodies
to follow the arc it makes.
May we open
and open more
and open still

to the blessed light
that comes.
                              Jan Richardson

References

Adler, J. (1995). *Arching backward: The mystical initiation of a contemporary woman.* Inner Traditions.

Adler, J. (2002). *Offering from the conscious body: The discipline of Authentic Movement.* Inner Traditions.

Adler, J. (2022). *Intimacy in emptiness: An evolution of embodied consciousness* (B. Morrissey & P. Sager, Eds., with commentary). Inner Traditions.

Chodorow, J. (Ed.). (1997). *Jung on active imagination.* Princeton University Press.

Clements, J., Ettling, D., Jennet, D., & Shields, L. (1998). If research were sacred: An organic approach. In W. Braud & R. Anderson (Eds.), *Transpersonal research methods for the social sciences: Honoring human experience* (pp. 114–127). Sage Publications.

Creswell, J. W. (1994). *Research design: Qualitative and quantitative approaches.* Sage Publications.

Dosamantes-Alperson, I. (1974, Fall). Carrying experiencing forward through Authentic Body Movement. *Psychotherapy: Theory, Research and Practice, 11*(3), 211–214.

Dosamantes-Alperson, I. (1983). Experiential movement psychotherapy. Unpublished manuscript.

Dosamantes-Alperson, I. (1986). A current perspective of imagery in psychoanalysis. *Imagination, Cognition and Personality, 5*(3), 199–209.

Dosamantes-Alperson, I. (1987). Transference and counter-transference issues in movement psychotherapy. *The Arts in Psychotherapy, 4*, 209–214.

Dosamantes, I. (1992a). Body-image: Repository for cultural idealizations and denigrations of the self. *The Arts in Psychotherapy, 19*, 257–267.

Dosamantes, I. (1992b). The intersubjective relationship between therapist and patient: A key to understanding denied and denigrated aspects of the patient's self. *The Arts in Psychotherapy, 19*, 359–365.

Dosamantes, I. (Ed.) (1993). *Body image in cultural context*. UCLA DMT Publications.

Dosamantes-Beaudry, I. (1997a). Embodying a cultural identity. *The Arts in Psychotherapy, 24*(2), 129–135.

Dosamantes-Beaudry, I. (1997b). Somatic experience in psychoanalysis. *Psychoanalytic Psychology Journal, 14*(4), 521–534.

Dosamantes-Beaudry, I. (1998). Regression-reintegration: Central psychodynamic principle in rituals of transition. *The Arts in Psychotherapy, 25*(2), 79–84.

Dosamantes-Beaudry, I. (2003). *The arts in contemporary healing*. Praeger.

Dosamantes-Beaudry, I. (2024). *Irma Dosamantes-Beaudry, Professor Emerita*. UCLA School of the Arts and Architecture: World Arts and Cultures/Dance. https://www.wacd.ucla.edu/people/retired-faculty/irma-dosamantes-beaudry

Fairweather, P. (1994). An interview with Irma Dosamantes. *American Journal of Dance Therapy, 16*, 13–19.

Jung, C. G. (1961). *Memories, dreams, reflections*. (A. Jaffé, Ed.). Vintage Books.

Jung, C. G. (1981). On the nature of the psyche. In *Structure and dynamics of the psyche* (Vol. 8). Princeton University Press. (Original work published 1947.)

Moustakas, C. (1990). *Heuristic research: Design, methodology, and applications*. Sage Publications, Inc.

Patton, M. Q. (1990). *Qualitative evaluation and research methods* (2nd ed.). Sage Publications, Inc.

Richardson, J. (2015). How the light comes. In *Circle of grace: A book of blessings for the seasons*. Wanton Gospeller Press.

Stromsted, T. (2025). Meeting Joan Chodorow: Dancing in the depths. *IAAP News Bulletin* (36), January 2025.

Von Franz, M.-L. (1983). On active imagination. In *Inward journey: Art as therapy* (pp. 125–133). Open Court. (Original work published 1980.)

Woodman, M. (1980). *The owl was a baker's daughter: Obesity, anorexia nervosa, and the repressed feminine*. Inner City Books.

Woodman, M. (1996, February). BodySoul Rhythms Intensive [Conference]. University of California, Santa Cruz, Pajaro Dunes, Watsonville, California.

Part III

Movement in Practice

Chapter 8

The Moving Body in Psychotherapy

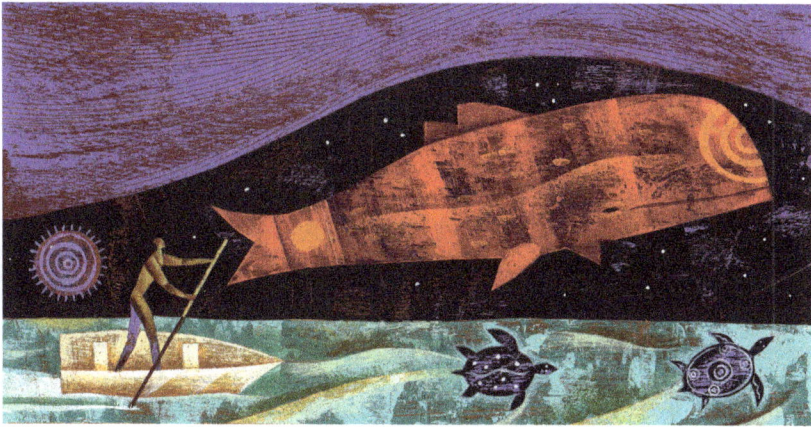

Figure 8.1 The Fisherman © 2007 by Rafael Lopez @ https://rafaellopez.com/.

The body is the home of feelings, the house of memory; it's where we experience joy, wonder, suffering, and awe. As Jung noted, "The symbols of the self arise in the depths of the body" (Jung, 1940/1959, CW 9i, para. 291). To heal, we need to connect with this physical realm. Body-oriented psychotherapy addresses a wide range of issues—physiological, psychological, emotional, relational, and spiritual. It helps us express a broader range of feelings, and reconnect with our healthy instincts, creativity, and intuition. By becoming aware of physical sensations, we can better regulate our nervous systems, leading to a greater sense of safety, resilience, and self-awareness. In therapy, this process fosters healthier boundaries, a stronger sense of identity, and improved relationships, reducing fear of intimacy and enhancing sensual experiences of the world in the here and now. It also equips individuals with skills to handle stress and life's challenges, opening them to new potentials and helping them live by their deepest values and thrive in community.

Through this journey, people often develop a more realistic body image, learn self-love, and connect with a deeper life force. Body-oriented psychotherapy

DOI: 10.4324/9781003538356-12

supports creative living and a sense of wholeness. Some clients begin this process after years of traditional, verbally oriented psychotherapy or analysis, which has provided great insights. However, these insights may remain stuck in the intellect, making it difficult to act on them. Others start their journey seeking to resolve conflicts, work through trauma, ease pain, grieve losses, and embrace conscious change.

Unresolved physical and emotional trauma is often held in the body until it can be consciously addressed (see Chapter 9). As an analyst and dance and somatic psychotherapist, I help clients reconnect with their bodies through sensing, movement, relaxation, breath, sound, dreamwork, art, writing, and other forms of body-oriented and creative work. This process allows deep-seated feelings and beliefs to surface, be safely explored, and integrated into the client's current awareness.

In this chapter, I explore somatic psychotherapy, focusing on dance/movement therapy and Authentic Movement (Stromsted, 2001–2002). Through two case studies, I demonstrate how these methods differ in structure but similarly facilitate transformative experiences. I also discuss key aspects of body-oriented therapy, including client assessment, readiness, and the role of the body-attuned analyst or therapist.

Elements of the Work

Dance/Movement, Somatic Therapy, and Authentic Movement

There are many approaches to dance/movement and somatic psychotherapy; here, I categorize them into two main types: structured and directive, and unstructured and self-directed, like Authentic Movement. The choice of method depends on the client's ego strength and readiness for deeper work (Chodorow, 1991; Lewis, 1993).

Authentic Movement as a form of active imagination is an approach that helps people access their unconscious thoughts and feelings, especially if they have a strong sense of self and are suitable for deep psychological therapy. It's best for people with neurotic disorders, rather than severe personality disorders or psychosis. This method is particularly useful for those who tend to intellectualize or focus on physical symptoms, or who have difficulty accessing and addressing their emotions in therapy. Additionally, Authentic Movement can be effective in therapies that explore spiritual or universal human experiences.

As clients develop a stronger sense of self, therapy may transition from structured to more open and self-directed approaches. Over time, clients learn to distinguish between movement directed by the ego ("I am moving") and movement that arises from the unconscious ("I am being moved") (Whitehouse, 1979, p. 57; Whitehouse, 1995, p. 243). Similarly, the types of verbal interventions I use as a psychotherapist may change throughout the therapy process.

Generally, structured movement interventions help clients feel safer as they become more aware of previously unknown or forbidden bodily sensations. When a client's ego is fragile, structured movement can help them manage overwhelming emotions and stimuli, expanding their emotional range and empowering them to engage with the world more effectively.

On the other hand, Authentic Movement requires a certain level of ego strength and is ideal for individuals who seek a deeper connection with their inner life and wish to relate to others in more genuine and spontaneous ways. This process allows them to connect with their feelings, body sensations, and creative imagination. With no music, choreography, agenda, or "right" or "wrong" way to move, they can explore their feelings, rhythms, and authentic responses, fostering genuine self-expression (Whitehouse, 1999).

As detailed in Chapter 5, during this process, the therapist, or "witness," sits to the side of the space. Although her eyes are open, she is not "looking at" the person moving. Instead, she is witnessing and listening, bringing a special quality of attention or presence to the mover's experiences (Adler, 1989; 1999, p. 21; 2002). If invited, the witness responds to what she has seen, felt, and imagined, without judgment or interpretation. Given the level of *embodied* reflection, this role differs in some significant ways from traditional verbal therapy. Her task is to be present for the mover and to her own experience as she observes. This includes being aware of and managing any personal reactions or projections to ensure the therapy remains clear and effective.

Somatic Assessment of Clients

As an analyst and somatic psychotherapist, I often spend extended periods talking with clients to understand their backgrounds, what brought them to therapy, their conflicts, and how they've tried to address them. I often integrate movement and somatic interventions to deepen the work, acting as the client's primary therapist. Sometimes, other analysts and therapists refer their clients to me as a "movement specialist" to help open pathways that can be further explored with their primary therapist and to assist clients in embodying the insights they gain from verbal therapy.

When a client enters my office, I start with an assessment based on what I observe and sense in their body. The body tells its story through posture, gait, sure-footedness, gestures, breath flow, muscle tonus, and complexion. Each body uniquely reflects how someone has shaped themselves to live with their history. As somatic pioneer Stanley Keleman says, "I have embodied my encounters with the world and they have left their mark" (personal communication). Our history is encoded in our body, including genetic inheritance and environmental influences— epigenetic factors in our early formative years and subsequent significant life experiences (Masterpasqua, 2009). While each person's presentation is unique— and I appreciate what somatics educator Don Hanlon Johnson calls the "somatic genius" [personal communication] of each person's way of coping with challenges— certain patterns can indicate the nature and extent of their wounds.

While working with clients, I carefully watch for feedback to guide the direction and pace of our work. Gradual, structured body awareness and movement explorations can be helpful during the early assessment and rapport-building phases of therapy (Brooks, 1986; Johnson, 1995). Depending on the situation, starting with large or strongly expressive movements might overwhelm or disorient the client. Similarly, diving too quickly into self-directed Authentic Movement may flood them with feelings or recovered memories. It's crucial to have "resourcing" skills as Peter Levine (2012) calls them—grounding, orienting, centering, noting safer areas in the body, and so forth—to help clients process these experiences safely. Timing is essential, as is creating a safe environment where clients can lower their defenses enough to experience their body-felt sensations, images, memories, and associations, connecting these with appropriate emotions. The next step may include expressing them through movement, painting, drawing, collage, sandplay, sound, or poetry—creative outlets that help clients create new, healthier, more embodied images and experiences of themselves. In doing so, they access deeper resources, explore new behavioral possibilities, develop better ways of relating to others, and become more fully who they are.

The Healing Relationship

Wounding happens in relationships, and it's within relationships that healing is most effective. Sensitivity, emotional honesty, intuition, and trust in our own feelings are the foundation of therapeutic work. Somatic psychotherapy explores the connections between a client's current relationship experiences and patterns established early in life, often rooted in the preverbal dynamics between the mother or caregiver and infant, and later with the father or secondary caregiver. These early attachment patterns significantly impact an individual's embodied experience, sense of self, and ability to relate to others in healthy ways.

Neuropsychologist Allan Schore highlights how early social environments influence all later adaptive functions. He notes that "attachment processes lie at the center of all human emotional and social functions," and that "the real relationships of the earliest stage of life indelibly shape us in basic ways, and, for the rest of the life span" (Schore & Schore, 2012, p. 27). Neuropsychologist Daniel Siegel discusses how this affects the developing brain and body, citing studies in attachment theory that show how communication patterns with parents shape the child's nervous system development (Siegel, 1999, p. 245).

Decades earlier, Stanley Keleman offered an embodied perspective on this process: "We do not grow up entirely by ourselves, but as bodies in a particular environment or matrix" (Keleman, 1984, p. 116). The way we are treated and how we respond, the shapes of our bodies, and the messages we receive about them all influence the images we carry of ourselves, the identities we create, and our lifestyle. An embodied therapeutic approach can access these deep structures, facilitating healing and growth beyond what verbal methods alone can achieve. This allows client and therapist to work on deeper, often nonverbal levels, including sensations, emotions, and the meanings derived from their experiences.

As discussed in Chapter 4, shadow elements often appear spontaneously through unconscious movements, gestures, voice tones, verbal expressions, breathing patterns, and moods. Over time and with rapport, the therapist can reflect these back to the client, helping them become more conscious of these elements. This is sensitive work, as the client must be ready to acknowledge these feelings without distancing themselves further. Exploring body-level responses provides a bridge to the unconscious, frees life energy essential for growth, and connects the client to a deeper sense of knowing, creativity, and wholeness.

Therapeutic Use of Touch

Embodied experience is often overlooked or marginalized in psychotherapy. As we begin our work, I let my clients know that therapy may involve touch, as its conscious and appropriate use can amplify and support feelings. The sensitive use of touch—with the right timing and skill, involving only safe areas of the body, and with the client's permission—can be invaluable when developing genuine self-contact, healthy boundaries, and an appropriate sense of intimacy.

Sadly, the issue of touch has become clouded by confusion, fear, and controversy, especially in the current climate of abuse. As discussed in Chapter 6, in patriarchal cultures, the body is often associated with so-called baser instincts or seen as a commodity to be perfected. As a result, this vital aspect of existence is often relegated to the shadows, separated from the cognitive, emotional, and "higher" spiritual aspects of our lives. Safe, discerning touch can help with integration, but it must be done by a trained clinician within their professional scope. In the absence of training or during telehealth sessions, clients can use self-touch to increase awareness and grounding, helping them manage uncomfortable emotions (Selvam, 2022). Examples of self-touch include placing a hand on the heart, the back of the neck, solar plexus, or belly, while feeling grounded in the chair with feet firmly on the floor. These interventions can help expand their "window of tolerance"—their capacity for emotional regulation and experiencing a wider range of feelings (Siegel, 1999)—the foundation for a richer and more meaningful life.

Unfortunately, some therapists have crossed boundaries, using touch in ways that are invasive or an abuse of power (Greene, 1980, 1999, 2001; Paula Koepke, personal communication). Before using touch, I carefully assess a client's attachment history, any indication of past abuse, transference dynamics, gender, and developmental level at that time. Touch is always used with client consent, focusing on less intimate areas, and with a deep awareness of its potential impact.

Working with Dance/Movement Therapy

Though I see a wide range of clients, I work with women who have a possible history of sexual abuse and other traumatizing earlier experiences in depth-oriented somatic psychotherapy, and this is the subject of the first case example.

When meeting a client, I assess her access to spontaneity, range of movement and feeling, and how connected different parts of her body are. I look for areas that seem isolated or cut off from her overall expression. I observe how she "holds" herself, which often reflects how she has been supported and how she continues to "carry" her experiences. I also ask about any medical issues, physical symptoms, injuries, or traumas, as well as any pleasurable physical memories and current experiences.

I listen not only to what she says but also to how she talks about her body. One woman might speak with cold, scientific precision, as if examining her body under a microscope. Another might speak vaguely, inaccurately, or with disgust. Some clients may become annoyed with my focus on their bodily experience, whereas others might provide detailed somatic information with incongruent emotions. Traditional therapy might see these as "resistance," but I view them as the body's attempt to tell its story, reflecting the unconscious nature of the wound or the result of years of secrecy, shame, or silence.

Some clients may have genuine difficulty talking, in which case gently working to support, encourage, and perhaps amplify what the body is already expressing can be instrumental in building a sense of trust (Mindell, 1985). This can be done through bringing attention to the breath, or by asking for any images, sensations, or feelings the client may have.

Ultimately, allowing the client to share her story of abuse, as much as she knows, is crucial for healing. When she speaks, I listen to her voice's tone and volume and the images and metaphors she uses. What is the feeling in her voice? What age does she seem to be? What kind of music does her voice suggest, and how does it relate to her story?

When sexual abuse is an issue, I often notice certain physical and emotional patterns. The pelvis might be stiff or frozen, and the arms can appear either weak and powerless or overly muscular from a subconscious need to maintain control or keep others at bay. The eyes might appear glassy, frozen with fear, lifeless, seductive, or disconnected, often not matching the rest of the body's expression. The chest may be collapsed or underdeveloped, as if trying to hide, deprived of the breath and blood flow that would draw attention to the breasts or bring more feeling to the heart. Alternatively, the chest might be defensively pushed forward, yet the woman might feel emotionally detached. Hands might feel lifeless and numb, flutter like lost birds, or engage in anxious behaviors like wringing, washing, or tearing tissues. In somatic therapy, body-image drawings often reveal a contrast: for example, a little-girl face with wide eyes and innocence paired with a voluptuous, adult woman's body, or the reverse—a figure entirely covered, giving a childlike, shapeless impression. Or there may be images of dismemberment, such as a torso lacking arms or feet. The mouth might be depicted as a single line or absent, symbolizing the inability to speak out about the abuse, or it might be exaggerated, possibly indicating the trauma's focal point.

As I assess my client over time, I gain insights into the severity of her wound, her awareness of body sensations (Gendlin, 1978), the strength of her boundaries, and how effective movement or body-oriented interventions might be. This helps determine the pace of therapy. Building rapport, trust, and comfort gradually is crucial, especially when dealing with trauma or abuse—be it sexual, physical, emotional, or psychological. I am mindful that some women who have experienced abuse may be compliant, which can lead to feeling pressured in therapy.

I often start by inviting the client to look around the room to help them orient to the space and stay present (Porges, 2011). I encourage her to become aware of her physical responses, asking her to notice sensations in her body with eyes open or closed, based on her comfort (Bainbridge-Cohen, 1997; Gendlin, 1978). I may draw her attention to the quality of her breathing (which may be held high up in the chest in a kind of panic response) and the meaningful expressiveness of her own natural gestures, postures, stance, and characteristic motility patterns. If her speech has taken on an intellectualized or runaway quality, I may ask her to slow her pace, letting her know that "it seemed like something important was being expressed through her body," encouraging her to "tune in" or "listen to" what she's experiencing internally at that moment. In an effort to lay the foundation for her to pay attention to and reinhabit herself, I may ask: "If this image, incident, dream, or story were 'living' or residing anywhere in your body, where would it be?"

Another method I sometimes use is "mirroring" my client's postures, gestures, and breathing to acknowledge, sense, and bring awareness to her nonverbal expressions (Chaiklin & Wengrower, 2009; Sandel et al., 1993). In so doing, I must be careful not to mimic, judge, or patronize her through this method of offering back what I see. If I sense that we have adequate rapport and that my client has the strength and willingness to try, I may ask her to amplify or exaggerate gestures she is making, letting her know that these movements are already going on in her body and that, in making them consciously, we are working toward discovering the meaning in their expression. This may also involve helping her complete gestures that were blocked during an assault. This step usually comes later, once she has built the internal scaffolding to tolerate the feelings that arise (Levine, 1997; Schoop, 1974). Throughout, I encourage her to trust her feelings and sensations and not dismiss them.

The body tells its story. Furthermore, the body remembers, as we can see and feel when a wound reopens for a client, or in our own lives.

Case Vignette: Lydia Blossoms

The following case illustrates the use of a relatively structured somatic movement approach with a woman whom I will call "Lydia." Our work was conducted in my private psychotherapy office, a spacious and warm room with ample natural light. Here, comfortable chairs are moved in for verbal work and off to the side to clear the space for movement. A futon folds out for work on the floor. There are percussion instruments and a sound system with a wide range of music. Paper, pens, and colors are available for writing and drawing. Fresh flowers add their beauty to the space.

Lydia was twenty-eight-years old with green eyes, thick wavy black hair, and pale skin. A beautiful woman, she covered her lower body with full-length skirts and tall boots, a dramatic juxtaposition to the plunging necklines of her blouses. Depressed and anxious, she'd been referred to me by a physician at a women's health clinic.

In our first session, Lydia shared her struggles with panic attacks and relentless nightmares. She spoke about her marriage to a much older, demanding, and possessive husband, whom she felt had "saved her" from her past life. Before marrying, she worked as a cocktail waitress in a jazz club, battled drug abuse, and often brought men home. Since marrying five years ago, she'd been stuck in an unfulfilling office job, with her husband forbidding her from leaving the house alone except for work. He stayed home, not working, and expected her to manage the household, cook, and meet his sexual needs without reciprocation. Any sign of resistance would result in one of two responses. Either he would slap her and pull her around the bedroom by the hair, showering her with humiliating insults about how she was "soiled goods," or he would collapse and, in a baby voice, whine for her affection and care.

During her early visits, Lydia mounted the stairs to my office with "frozen hips," swinging her legs in the manner of an elderly woman with two peg legs. On other occasions, when I invited her to stand and walk in a way that felt comfortable to her, she took on the demeanor of what she began to call "Daddy's little princess," swinging her hips in a sashay style, her pelvis tilted back and broken off from the vertical line of her body, with her nose and jaw lifted into the air. These embodied compromises had contributed to pressed-disc problems in her neck and back that had further hobbled her ability to move into the world. Lydia also complained of eczema, swollen lymph nodes, and multiple yeast and vaginal infections, which she reported "saved her from intercourse" with her husband. Additionally, she showed me rashes that sprang up around her jewelry, most notably her wedding ring and her watch.

Over time, we worked with a number of approaches to exploring what might be meaningful to her in these skin problems. They were not only "irritating and embarrassing" to her but also painful, as she could not refrain from scratching and tearing at them, making them bleed when no one was looking. Noticing the scabs one day, I asked her about them, and when she began to tear at them in response, I asked if I could see them. At first, she became angry and then began to cry, telling me she'd been doing this for years. As Lydia held her hands out, I asked if I could touch them. Cupping them in my hands, I explored their wounded surfaces tenderly and carefully. I thought of the Grimms' fairytale *The Handless Maiden* (Chapter 6). As I did so we talked about how important her hands were—for her work, for grappling with difficulties, for pushing away what she didn't want, for taking care of herself, and for reaching for what she wanted and needed in the world.

I told Lydia that I was glad that she was able to show me and tell me how painful this was for her and how sorry I was that things were so difficult. Then I encouraged her to express the pain and irritation on safer surfaces, such as by scratching pillows and wringing towels. As she made these movements, I asked her to exhale, make sounds, and eventually statements about how she was feeling. Some of the words that emerged were *vulnerable, raw, bleeding, too open, red, violent, body-crying*. Her relationship with her husband left her feeling weak, hopeless, and ashamed. We talked about her feelings about being at home, alternative places for her to stay, and ways to set boundaries and limits with her husband. She had come into therapy wanting to leave him but did not feel strong enough to do so. Nor did she feel capable of living on her own in what she perceived as a hostile world. I urged her to call the police if the abuse continued and to call me if she felt in danger or despair. After a month of working continuously in this way, these body symptoms disappeared.

Soon after this, Lydia and I began to work with "grounding" exercises (Keleman, 1975a, 1975b). Placing both feet firmly on the floor, about shoulder-width apart and with knees gently bent, Lydia began to feel her connection to the ground and to develop a sense of having her own legs to stand on. Her husband was frightening to her yet he also provided some source of security, though tentative at best. She had grown up with an alcoholic mother, her father having left when she was three years old. Her mother had remarried "someone she didn't love in order to get a roof over their heads," and Lydia had often been in charge of tending to her stepfather's needs. "At least he won't leave me," she said of her husband, caught in the old trap.

One week Lydia had a horrible nightmare about cats with severed heads. She was beginning to sense the disconnection and wounding she felt and wrote this poem:

> *Woman:*
> *the only flower*
> *that doesn't have the sense*
> *to stay shut*
> *when the sun's not out.*

As she became more aware of her body and trusted it to support her, Lydia's feelings arose. She suppressed them by grimacing with her mouth and "unscrewing" her head from her neck with a series of quick "no"-like shakes. When I asked her what she was feeling and whether she was aware of her movements, she was silent. "Real feelings," she finally said, "are not permitted and even dangerous." She felt worthless and explained how other people's needs were more important than hers. If she was being punished, somehow, she must deserve it. During her worst moments at home, she would sometimes, without knowing why, break something of her own or fantasize about running a knife through her hand—self-harm that could shift the locus of the overwhelming emotional pain she was experiencing to something physical (Frewen & Lanius, 2015, p. 186). As she spoke, I noted the childlike quality of her voice; this was followed by the pulling up of her body, with a stern and rigid expression. I sensed she was identifying with the child who had assumed blame for the parents' actions. Instead of learning that an awareness of her own perceptions and feelings could help her to care for herself, she had learned that her sense of self was out of her control.

As we began to access these feelings, there were times when Lydia would call to cancel her appointment, making up excuses not to come. "The work was going nowhere," she said, and "the pain was too great." She began to feel depressed and described suicidal fantasies. I asked if she had a plan, and when she nodded no, I reflected the fear and pain she was feeling back to her, acknowledging her desperate wish to stop the pain, though perhaps not to literally end her life. "Yes!" she said, but I can't bear it anymore." With further exploration I learned she had considered taking more of the sleeping pills she kept by her bed and referred her to a psychiatrist for an assessment, which made her feel I was acknowledging the seriousness of her fears. She realized that her impulses were a call for help. She kept her appointments with me and began writing me letters in between sessions to help her maintain a sense of contact. Her letters were powerful, revealing feelings that she had not been able to speak aloud. They often served as a beginning place for our work in the sessions that followed. In this way, over time, Lydia began to let her feelings, dreams, and imagination take the lead.

In one session, she came in saying there was "no escape." She felt trapped both at home and at work and was too anxious to sit down. I paced with her as she spoke about how frightening it was for her to make boundaries for herself. Then, coming to a standstill, I joined her in the grounding work that we had done and invited her to make the sound of how she was feeling, or to hear it inside. The cry of a wounded animal emerged, an anguish that touched me deeply. Then I invited her to say "no" by pressing into the ground first one heel, then the other, and then both while shaking her hands which then formed into fists. In previous movement explorations, her hands had hung limply from her wrists. Looking broken or cut off, they gave rise to feelings of helplessness as well as to images of women—many of them midwives, herbalists, and healers—who were once placed in stocks and accused of being witches, a literal expression of the Handless Maiden at the zealous hands of the patriarchal church of that time. Here, natural movement had reached a depth in Lydia's soul and the collective world of the psyche.

After first tentatively exploring this new movement, Lydia was able to do it more fully and eventually to say "no" aloud. "See if you can recruit as much of your body as possible into this expression of 'no,'" I encouraged her, "from the ground up and all the way to the sensations in your mouth and out through your eyes. Look at me and say it. Or, if that doesn't feel right, look at the empty chair or at an object of your choosing in the room. If possible, see if you can really hear the sound of your own voice and your heels landing on the ground!"

Lydia practiced the movement several times, connecting with her breath and her voice while looking at a tiny black panther that I had on my bookshelf, stopping when she felt satisfied. As she left my office that day, she asked if she could take the panther home with her for a while, along with the gold lion that stood next to it.

I agreed, wishing her well with these dark and light animal allies who were capable of natural responsiveness, fierce protectiveness, and moments of tenderness. She growled playfully as she left my office, showing her teeth and swiping her "claws" in the air.

Over time, Lydia and I worked along a continuum of gentle to strongly expressive gestures. We engaged various body parts to music, exploring issues and conflicts she presented verbally. At first, I moved with her, mirroring her gestures and offering support with my presence and modeling. Gradually I began to move back to allow her to find her own movement and to take her own space more fully. Through finding the particular rhythm, shape, and tension in the movement she began to feel more of her own body and was able to experience her own feelings and to communicate them. These were messages from the body that sought recognition, voice, and consciousness, rehearsals for new action that wanted to come into form in her life. Not long afterward, she reported being surprised to find that people at work said she looked and sounded different, and they began to treat her with respect.

Earlier in our work, Lydia had reported feeling terrified of relaxing, as a flood of bad feelings threatened to drown her. Vigilant since childhood, I sensed that her life had been driven by her sympathetic nervous system, with little access to the recuperative "rest and digest" capacity of her parasympathetic nervous system (Schore, 2009–2017). Though she knew that this frantic activity could not last forever, she had felt that it was the only way to protect herself and to siphon off some of the tension she felt in her body. Frequently, she arrived dressed up and pressured, pressing the boundaries of the hour with stories about her experiences at home and at work, sharing her fears and fantasies with me. On the heels of the assertive boundary work, however, she came in saying that she was too exhausted even to talk, eyeing the futon in my office. My sense was that shadow material was beginning to emerge; she was softening her outer vigilance and was genuinely tired from the energy it had taken to keep it intact. However, she also feared she lacked the inner support structure and resources she needed. Following her cue, I asked her if she would like to lie down and rest. She could talk to me if she wanted or simply attend to her own experience.

After some quiet time, Lydia began reporting sensations in various parts of her body. I directed her to see if she could stay with them a bit longer, bringing her breath to them and perhaps placing her hand on that part of her body for contact and support. At one point, she put her knees up and began gently rocking her pelvis from side to side. I asked her if she could feel the movement and whether she was aware of how her head was twisted away and to the side. Slowly she eased the muscles in her neck, bringing her head into alignment with the rest of her body. Her lips and chest began to tremble, and her breath dropped into her belly. I encouraged her to place one hand on her heart and the other on her belly. When she did, her lips gave way and a great howl emerged, followed by a long period of sobbing. A dam had broken. Her earlier cat nightmares came spontaneously to mind, and we talked about how they seemed connected to the twisting-off movements in her neck and the sense of her feminine nature, symbolized by the cats, which had been so profoundly wounded.

In the following weeks, Lydia's work grew more self-directed. She continued to ask to lie down, and we worked with her breath and body awareness. At one point, her feet began to fidget and paw the futon. When I encouraged her to amplify these gestures, little kicks began to emerge and grow more forceful, taking on a steady rhythm. Seeing her hands flail, I invited her to make fists and pound the futon with them as well as with her legs, supported by her breath and the firmness of the floor beneath her. "Let the force of your contact travel through your bones," I encouraged. We were building a body container for her feelings (Barlin & Greenberg, 1980). Sounds began to emerge. Gradually, I encouraged her to see if there were any words. "Stop," she yelled, "get away from me!" I had her spread her palms and make pushing-away movements on her exhalation. At one point, I put my hands up in the air above hers and invited her to push against them if the contact felt comfortable for her. As she did so, Lydia began to feel the strength in her hands and arms and was able to meet the pressure in my hands with her own.

After several rounds of assertive movement, she placed her palms against mine and left them there. "I can feel the warmth of your hands," she said, "and in mine." This was unusual for her as it began to replace the cold numbness she often felt there. Pausing to allow her to feel the sensation, I asked how far down her arms she could let this warmth travel. After a moment she reported being able to feel it trickle down her forearms and into her chest, where it pulsed and swirled. "It's touching my heart," she said, placing her hand there to feel her heartbeat. As she did so, her face flushed pink and her eyes brightened. "I feel powerful, and ... whole," she said. Indeed, she was radiant.

Following this experience, Lydia shared her memories of several men whom she felt had used her, and her shame at having had sex with them. We spoke about the rivalry for her stepfather that had been created between her and her mother while she was growing up. Her mother had "taken off" for months at a time, leaving her "in charge" of her stepfather. In the following weeks, Lydia began to have memories of sitting on his lap and feeling uncomfortable, describing how she had learned that the only way she could experience her power, or any sense of contact, was through her sexuality. She began to see how many of her relationships had been sexualized, substituting seduction for a genuine sense of contact, care, and empowerment.

After working on this material for several sessions, Lydia reported a dream *in which she had been riding an earth-colored horse with a firm saddle. Her hair flying in the wind, she had made her way into a circle of redwoods. There she had dismounted and, tying her horse to a tree, lay down in the streams of sunlight that filtered through. Feeling comforted and safe, she had fallen asleep there, awakening to find her grandmother sitting quietly by her side, smiling. Lydia returned the smile. "I love you," she said, putting her head in her grandmother's lap. Her grandmother nodded and began brushing Lydia's hair.*

As she shared the dream with me, Lydia said that she couldn't remember ever having felt this peaceful before, or so loved. She told me that she didn't own a car and rarely left the city. She had heard about these circles of redwoods but had never actually seen them. Sensing her longing, we wondered about how she might ask a friend to join her, taking a car or a bus to the woods. Though this remained a fantasy for a while, one week Lydia arrived beaming, saying that she and a friend had rented a car and made an outing to Muir Woods National Monument, north of San Francisco. There she had felt the magnificent presence and power of the tall, ancient redwoods, and recognized the roots she experienced in herself.

Following this experience, Lydia realized that she could no longer continue to "split off" parts of herself. She reported feeling a new sense of confidence that allowed her to act. Months before, she had reported that her husband was no longer abusing her, nor insisting on having sex with her, stopped by her ability to say "no" in a congruent, full-bodied way. Indeed, her voice, which had once been by turns childlike and then seductive, had a stronger, more resonant timber, emanating from a deeper part of herself. Though her husband's intentionally hurtful behavior had stopped, Lydia realized that she did not love him and could not remain in the marriage. "I guess he's been more like a protector for me," she said, "but at quite a cost. I realize now that I thought he would rescue me from my mother's neglect and the destructive sex with the other men." In a café near my office, she composed a letter to her husband, voicing her feelings, stating that she wanted a divorce, and would be spending the next few nights at a friend's house. Later they talked and she packed up her things, moving in with her friend until she could make other arrangements.

A month later Lydia found a full-time job leading arts and crafts groups with teenage girls. She realized that her work was bringing her full circle, as she supported the girls in a way that she wished she had been supported herself. The change also allowed her to expand her relationships, spending time with other staff members whom she liked and by whom she felt valued. And it enabled her to reclaim her hands and develop skills to manifest her artistic talent. Although creative herself, Lydia had stopped drawing as a child. She now began to paint self-portraits and brought them in to share with me, learning to witness herself through this process. Discovering her own ability to create filled Lydia with a sense of well-being and gave her another outlet for expressing her feelings—both the difficult ones as well as her newer sense of self. "For the first time in my life, I feel like I have a future," she said.

After looking around for the right medium, Lydia began taking African dance classes. These allowed her to experience her relationship to the earth and to her healthy sexuality and to feel a sense of belonging in a multiethnic community. She loved watching the man and woman who took turns leading the class. "Through them I can see a totally new way to relate to a man," she said. "Respectful, sensual, and fun. I'm not sure that I can manage that quite yet, but I look forward to it." She befriended another woman in the class who was new to town, and the two found a spacious apartment to share in a safer neighborhood.

Before leaving therapy, Lydia began selecting music from our sessions to support her in creating grieving, empowering, sensual, and joyous dances in her new home as she continued to develop a life of her own. Though she acknowledged that she still felt afraid or "down" sometimes, her life was much better, and she had confidence that she could now take care of herself. We agreed that it was a good time to stop the therapy. We spent the last few sessions going over the changes she had accomplished in the course of the work and confirmed that she could call me for some follow-up sessions, should she ever feel the need.

In our last session, I marveled at Lydia's spontaneity and access to her feelings. Laughter, tears, tenderness, movement, stillness, strength—all were reflected in her face and body and in her ability to relate in the moment.

Following this session, I sat quietly and closed my eyes briefly as I often do. There I saw a vision of a man's clenched fist releasing a woman's face into the river. As I watched, the face became a reflection of the full moon in the water.

Working with Authentic Movement

In cases like Lydia's, moving slowly is often an important way to begin, particularly when there is a history of trauma and a fragile ego that is not yet strong enough to withstand the energies from the unconscious that a more inner-sourced active imagination approach such as Authentic Movement can evoke. In what follows I describe the use of Authentic Movement in the treatment of a young woman whom I'll call Sofia whose ego structure was strong enough to engage her unconscious through being moved from an inner source.

Case Vignette: Sofia Emerges from Behind the Sofa

"Sofia" was a twenty-three-year-old Venezuelan woman who recently came to the United States to study sociology in graduate school. She had striking features—wide cheekbones, rich brown hair, a strong, straight nose, dark olive skin, and hazel eyes flecked with gold—yet she felt ugly and out of place. She referred to herself as Mestiza; her father was of Spanish descent, and her mother was from indigenous ancestors in Venezuela. Sofia's dark smocks hung on her wide frame, with leggings that covered her strong legs and ankles and utilitarian black shoes. Many of her friends in Caracas had already married and had at least one child. Most had had "work done on their faces and bodies." Sofia seemed relieved that "at least she had managed to avoid both."

Her father worked in oil industry management and had made a good living during the boom, decades before the country began to suffer from soaring inflation, escalating crime rates, and a growing economic and humanitarian crisis. As her father's work took him into the business world, he had numerous affairs. Her mother refused to divorce him, fearing social stigma, and having a limited capacity to earn a good income working as a seamstress or providing childcare—"the only skills she had."

Sofia described her older brother as "handsome, with light skin, the light of my mother's eyes." Their father, too, was proud of him as he worked in his office and was learning the business. Though Sofia sensed her father loved her, his guilt about his affairs and growing distance from his wife, who had Mestiza features like hers, "made him turn his eyes away." Sofia had earned good grades and loved reading, yet her mother didn't value this, having not gone to college herself. Instead, she expected Sofia to do chores around the house, "not do anything that would make us ashamed of you," and find a husband so she could move out and no longer be a financial burden.

"My Mom said more than once that if I hadn't been born, she could have 'left my father while she was still young and beautiful.'" Looking down, she added, "She'd always wanted to be a singer, a dream that never came true." Sofia knew this was not her fault, but her mother's rejection burned under her skin. She felt guilty for being alive, a "passion baby" who wasn't wanted in real life. Constantly reminded of her failings, having tried to make a living in Caracas, Sofia emigrated to the United States against her parents' wishes, obtaining an educational visa to continue her professional preparation. Although she had succeeded in getting into a graduate school program with a partial scholarship, she had had to reduce her course load during her first year due to limited funds and found an office job in a tech company in San Francisco's flourishing financial district.

Though lovely and bright, Sofia's superpower was in becoming invisible; she was afraid to shine. She had developed a crush on a young man who worked in the same tech company. James had initially seemed kind, laughing and talking with her freely when they met in the hall, and then taking her out for drinks after work, until she invited him into her bed. Soon, however, he began flirting with the new receptionist and turned his back when Sofia approached. The hurt shot through her, piercing the heart she "didn't know was still there." "Was I only a conquest?" she deliberated. "I thought he cared for me and that I'd found love in San Francisco; how could I be so wrong?" Her chest began to ache, and she developed shortness of breath, feeling there was "no room for her heart."

Suddenly, she felt the shame and loneliness she had been pushing away for many years. She wanted to cry, though no tears came. "Was I dead inside?" she wondered. Her belief in herself collapsed, and she felt there was no one to confide in in her new, adopted country. Now, when she returned home, after a cursory greeting of her beloved dog, Macuto, she began to pour herself a rum drink, numbing the pain. As she continued drinking and felt tired in the mornings at work, she realized she needed help and went to the Women's Building in San Francisco, where they provide services and advocacy for women and girls. When a counselor heard her speaking disparagingly about her body and learned she spoke fluent English, she gave her my name as a possible therapy referral. Sofia felt uneasy as this was her first therapy experience. As I learned later, she was afraid I might not take her seriously or that, as a Caucasian American woman, I might not value her or be able to understand her, let alone help her. However, she had heard about Authentic

Movement in one of her graduate school classes. Though unsettling, it sounded natural and drew her more than "talk therapy" alone.

During her first visit to my office, I invited her to sit where she felt comfortable—either in the big chair facing me or on the floor in a folding chair. She sunk to the floor, and I joined her, sitting across from her. She was polite, yet her eyes darted around the space before looking down; her feet jiggled nervously. I felt a hovering sensation in my solar plexus. Noting that it was hard for her to settle, I invited her to look around the room or walk around to take a closer look at things and even touch them if they interested her. Visibly relieved, she got up and went to the books in the large bookcase. After studying their titles, she paused when she saw a basket of rattles, drums, and rhythm sticks in the corner of the room; tapping on a small drum, she looked at me sheepishly.

Having circled the circumference of my office as if making it her own, she returned to the chair on the floor. "Tell me about yourself," I said. "What brings you here at this time?" Sofia spoke of her parents, her brother, and of her sense of feeling awkward growing up and now out of place at graduate school. "Was there a friend you could talk to growing up?" I asked. "Were there any subjects you especially liked at school? Any books, movies, dreams?" She related how they had lived in a small town before her family relocated to Caracas for her father's job. Her maternal grandmother had lived there, too. She was nurturing and kind and there had often been music at events in the square and in the community building. "I didn't expect to find a drum in your office," she said. "Touching it brings back the memory of the curious girl I used to be who was lost so many years ago."

Hesitantly, she showed me a brooch her grandmother had given her—a deep blue lapis set in gold, a family heirloom the older woman had pressed into her hand when they left the village. Sofia hadn't dared to wear it as it called too much attention to herself, though she kept it in the pockets of her skirts, turning it over in her hand when she was anxious. Slowly, she told me about her growing-up years, how strict the nuns had been. She had "disappointed her parents" and felt "less than" her friends. Having summoned all her courage to leave her country, she had trouble affording both tuition and her living expenses—the reason she'd come to the US. It wasn't until some months later, when she felt safer, that I learned about the young man at her office.

Each time we met, a strange sensation came over me: my body felt heavy, and it was hard to clearly see the contours of her face and body. I felt a leaden weight in my belly and blinked repeatedly to try to clear my vision so I could see her more clearly. Sometime later, after a few experiences of this kind with women who had a trauma background and were new to healing work, I heard Marion Woodman reflect on the impact of the mover on the witness and vice versa—the physics of the observer/observed relationship and how one affected the embodied experience of the other. Having worked for years in psychiatric hospitals and as a supervisor at a community mental health clinic, I had begun integrating Authentic Movement into my work with individual patients. Over time, I learned that when there's a history of neglect, abuse, or unattended-to unconscious feelings that have been stored in the body, in some cases this can have the effect of "knocking out" the witness/ therapist—a kind of somatic countertransference (Bernstein, 1984; Dosamantes-Beaudry, 2007; Pallaro, 1994/2007). The witness can feel sleepy or otherwise foggy in her capacity to see the mover clearly, struggling to stay more alert at her usual level of consciousness.

While growing up, Sofia had either felt like an eyesore, or judged and controlled so she had become an expert at pulling a cloak of invisibility over herself whenever she needed to. This way, she avoided potential harm, but it also left her feeling alone and unseen. Was I falling into the experience others in her life had had? Her pain might also have been touching some of my own early family experiences; much as I had worked on them, my body still remembered. I journaled about my experiences with her and sought consultation.

In our sessions, Sofia talked distractedly about her job and her little dog, Macuto, who, apart from her grandmother, she loved most in the world. Although I continued to try to draw her back to the issues that troubled her and had brought her into therapy, her stories wandered away each time. I decided to simply listen and let her speak freely during the hour, providing a steady interest and noninvasive presence as she filled the room and the hour with what felt like the torn scraps of paper, paperclips, tacks, and gum that had been holding her life together.

After meeting for several weeks and with more of a sense of her background and readiness, remembering her original request, I quietly asked if she would like to explore some Authentic Movement. She looked down, as a cascade of emotions quickly passed over her face—fear, excitement, hope, sadness, and shame. Thinking it might help ground her in her legs and perhaps even find some expression for her feelings, I asked, "How about if we stretch and warm up a little bit to music first, and then explore some Authentic Movement for a few minutes?"

Standing up, I made small rotating movements of the joints, slowly reaching my arms out to the sides and gradually engaging more of my body. Sofia looked down initially, saying she felt too shy. But when I let my body shake a bit—"shaking off any icky things that are still stuck to me"—she joined me and then followed my lead as I first stretched tall toward the ceiling and then curled up small toward the floor. I could see she was holding her breath, so I released mine with a sigh, encouraging her to do the same with the sound of how she was feeling.

Then I put on some Latin music. Sofia smiled in recognition and then looked sad as the melody touched her. Seeing this, I asked if she would like to continue with the music or begin her Authentic Movement. She nodded at the latter, and I gently turned down the music. Then I stepped back to sit at the edge of the room, leaving the space open for her to move on the soft, salmon-colored carpet, hoping this could be a safe and free space.

I shared the Authentic Movement guidelines with her—letting her know she could move with her eyes closed (or slightly open, maintaining an inner focus) in any way that felt comfortable, following her body's lead and noticing what she experienced, including any sensations, emotions, or images. "I'll be sitting to the side, 'holding space'—witnessing your movements, sensing what I'm feeling in my body, and tending to the time," I said. I invited her to draw afterward, write, or join me to talk, sharing whatever she would like to, letting her know I could offer feedback afterward without judgment or interpretation.

"How much time would you like?" I asked. "Five minutes, ten?"

"Five," she said, her eyes searching the space.

Holding up a Tibetan singing bowl, I said, "I'll ring the bell once to begin, and three times to end." Then, to my surprise, she slid behind the folded futon, squeezing between it and the wall! No part of her was visible, and she remained there until the end of the movement session.

I couldn't see her and battled an urge to move closer. "Am I offering her anything?" I wondered. "Should I even be charging her; what can she be getting from this?"

When it was time to move the next week, she again took her place behind the futon. And then the next, and the next. Following each movement session, she spoke simply about waiting to feel her body, and then returned to talking about her experiences at school and at work. At one point, I asked her how the movement explorations were working for her, and she said she wanted to continue. I wondered if it was a way for her to not talk about important things, but my gut told me to wait and trust the process. Several weeks later, I heard a scraping noise and felt startled to see her left foot emerge from behind the futon, remaining still until it was time to ring the bell.

Each week, after some initial sharing, as in a ritual, we took our places: she was wedged between the folded futon and the wall; I sat to the side of the space, my back to the wall of books. She now asked to move for more extended periods. One day, I noticed that I could see her ankle and foot bending, her toes pointing and wiggling like a baby exploring its movements for the first time. Her left calf and thigh emerged the following week, revealing the black leggings under her dark brown skirt.

Over a series of weeks, her leg, torso, arm, and hand emerged. Then her shoulder, neck, and finally her head, her long hair falling over her face. Then, one day, her body fully emerged. I was startled and speechless and could see the contours and details of her face and body clearly for the first time. Her solid and womanly shape was clearly defined now, with a sense of grounded presence—connected to the earth and a sense of place. The color in her forest green pants and a deep burgundy shirt popped! And there was a lightness of being in my body, a warmth in my heart, and a clarity of thought. I felt present, quiet, and grateful to share the space with her in this deeply earned experience of embodied consciousness—a kind of birth neither of us could have anticipated or planned. As I rang the bell three times, she opened her eyes and gazed at me, smiling, with tears streaming down her face. I returned her gaze and felt warmth spreading through my heart, my spine strong, with a shimmer running through me. She was alive, present, here, and so was I. She was allowing me to *see* her, and perhaps she saw *herself* for the first time.

Pulling our cushions closer on the floor, I invited her to share whatever she would like from what she experienced in her movement exploration, and any feelings, images, or associations that may have come to her.

She began with how scared she'd been to "show up." "I was afraid you wouldn't be able to see me," she said. "Or you wouldn't like what you saw, and I would hate myself in what I saw through your eyes. I've felt so worthless most of my life, and if you couldn't see me, there would be no chance for me." Nodding my head in understanding, I tell her how deeply moved I am by the honesty, courage, and beauty I feel in her presence.

When I asked if she wanted witnessing, I described how I first saw her wiggling toes emerge, and then her ankle, her calf, her thigh, and finally her hip, torso, arm, hand, neck, and face—first hidden behind her hair and then emergent, soft, and radiant with tears. How she had reached and crawled along the floor to explore the space, making her way to the mandala at the center of the carpet. How, with her eyes still closed, she had found her way to the center of it, coming to a seated position surrounded by the floral patterns on its borders. I let her know I felt peaceful and centered seeing her there, my breath easy and my body settled comfortably on the floor.

One week she came in flushed and told me she had *a dream of her grandmother's face, with the faces of other women growing clearer behind it.* When I asked what she made of it she said, "They were dark skinned and beautiful. Their mouths were moving, and I wanted to hear them. I have a sense they are my ancestors; their arms were waving in unison."

Her dream gave her a sense of inner support—a connection to Mother Earth in the lands of pre-Hispanic Venezuela, a place with which she had a long, deep connection. While split off from her body, shrouded in shame and a sense of being less than men or others with more privilege, she had not been able to access this. Now, however, it was beginning to feel more like a part of her.

Sofia soon left her job at the tech company, finding better work as a writer and administrator at a Spanish-speaking magazine. "It's a relief to be away from that guy," she confided. She felt a new sense of agency in her work and was coming into her own voice in her writing. The women in her new job were different, too—a mixture of locals and women from several Latin American countries. She began making friends, played with Macuto more often, and no longer needed the rum. One day she joined the Sierra Club, enjoying hikes with people of different backgrounds and ages and the natural beauty of the mountains, valleys, forests, and beaches surrounding the Bay Area. The birdsongs and wildflowers delighted her, and they saw a herd of elk one day and a raft of sea lions the following week! Manuel was a biologist in the group who shared her fascination with nature and learning. She loved talking with him, and he made her laugh. Soon they began alternating outings with the group with adventures of their own.

Sofia began to talk about feeling more connected to herself, to nature, and to others, and how she was better able to set boundaries and hold her own standpoint, instead of needing to collapse or flee when she felt uncomfortable. After two years of work, she told me she felt better and more whole. She was more tender with the parts of herself she had once rejected, and was ready to complete her analysis. Together, we reflected on her experiences from childhood, adult life, related dreams, and her present and future path. She thanked me for my care, patience, respect, and steady presence, letting me know how deeply she appreciated that I hadn't made her feel she had to be like anyone else but rather discover who she was. She wore red more often now. In our last session, I noted she was wearing her grandmother's brooch on a necklace, its striking deep blue lapis flanked by small gold leaves on her blouse that brought out the light in her eyes.

In our final session, Sofia surprised me with a gift of a CD—*Al Norte Del Sur* (*To the North of the South*) by Franco de Vita. She told he had been her favorite singer when she was growing up in the village before moving to the city. Touched by the meaning of this gift, I asked what her favorite song was. "*Te Amo*," she said. "It's about love; can we play it?" As de Vita's voice filled the space, she asked, "Can we dance together this time, like before?" This time, I invited her to lead. She swayed gently, whirling through the space with delight! There was a feistiness in her dance and a firmness in her steps; her hair, released from her bun, flowed freely.

Her confidence and joy were infectious! Simultaneously I remembered an old Zen koan I had learned about in my twenties during my Buddhist practice: "Show me your original face before you were born." Sofia's experience gave me a renewed sense of the deeply personal ways we grow into our real, authentic self—the face we are and were "before we were born." She taught me many things, including a deep trust in the waiting—the soul's timing in the process of conscious embodiment. An alchemical process, this was the "cooking" of the dense lead of the *prima materia* that was needed to transform the heavy, unconscious material into something lighter, that is, the unconscious body weighted with painful, unspoken feelings that was now changing form (see Chapter 13). Sofia had taken the risk and the painstaking time to allow her authentic self to cocoon, form, and then emerge, inch by inch, from behind the sofa.

"Individuation is the product of a personal struggle for consciousness" (Stein, 2015, p. 88), "an unfolding of [our] original, potential wholeness" (Jung, 1953, CW 7, para. 186)—a personal journey that contributes to evolution on our planet. In the process of finding herself, her heart, her voice, and more of her value in the world, Sofia had reconnected with the land of her ancestors and had learned to find guidance in her dreams, drawing from a deeper archetypal source. As Jung said, "The meeting of two personalities is like the contact of two chemical substances: if there is any reaction, both are transformed" (Jung, 1955, p. 49). Clearing the chairs in my office for the evening, I turned up the music and continued to dance. "*Te amo*," I sang, as I touched my heart and then opened my arms to the starry, evening sky.

Reflections for Further Inquiry

Many people enter analysis because they haven't felt seen or heard. They've tried their best to please others in a materialistic culture that fosters curated images and values power and material wealth over genuine relationship and matters of the soul.

How can we, as therapists, increase our awareness and comfort with our own bodies, so that we can model this with our clients and not unconsciously impose limitations on the depth and direction of the work? As we engage in healing work, it is essential to remember that there are not only two psyches in the room but two bodies, two souls seeking incarnation—a critical element that may often be overlooked in verbally oriented psychotherapy. Becoming aware of the impact of the work on the therapist's body is an important step in this direction (Adler, 1987/1999; Atwood & Stolorow, 1993; Bernstein, 1984; Pallaro, 1999; Stromsted, 2001; Woodman, 1984). In working with a client, my intention is to attend to the music of the work as it plays through the bodies and imaginations of both people, deepening my ability to listen for the many voices—the cellular resonance through which the Self seeks expression.

As I reflect on the developments in the field of somatic psychotherapy and of Authentic Movement, there are many other important elements and areas of application such as age, gender, race, culture, physical or psychological limitations, sociopolitical and environmental elements, and more that are beyond the scope of this chapter. Advances in the fields of trauma work, neuroscience, pre- and perinatal psychology, attachment theory, polyvagal work, and ecopsychology are deepening our understanding of the relationship between body, psyche, spirit, and nature within the intricate dance of self and other (see Chapters 16 and 17 for further reflections). This, in turn, offers new hope for the prevention and treatment of developmental impasses, including traumas that occurred before the acquisition of language—a deeply formative time in the development of the brain–mind–body continuum (Pert, 1997; Rothschild, 2000; Sieff, 2009; Wilkinson, 2010). Notably, given current advances in neuroimaging studies we are now even able to track areas of interest in the brain related to the neuroanatomy of consciousness of the body (Frewen & Lanius, 2015, p. 171). Though in-depth training is essential, psyche and body can no longer be distinctly separated but should rather be considered as essential partners in the process of healing, growth, and transformation.

In the medical arena, as was suggested in the work with Lydia's physical symptoms, movement can also offer a great deal for people struggling with a range of illnesses. My experience in working with postmastectomy women has given me great respect for the power of Authentic Movement in assisting women in reinhabiting the body, which they often feel has betrayed them (Dibbell-Hope, 1989, 1992). Somatics practitioners, dance therapists, analysts, and medical professionals could learn a great deal from one another and work more effectively by communicating along these deep interfaces.

My nearly five decades of experience in a variety of clinical settings continues to teach me how movement psychotherapy, whether structured or inner-directed, is a process of soul-making and body-making. Together, body and psyche, matter and spirit, find union and generate new form. The work helps people access their unconscious thoughts and feelings more directly than verbal therapy, offering a deeply felt and experienced process toward individuation and integration.

This unfolding, creative process yields enriched access to the self, enhances relationship, assists in building community, and supports our sense of connection with other living beings in the more than human world. What moves me most has to do with embodied presence, and how it awakens and grows. I find wonder in the richness of life as we experience it through our senses. And I trust the power of this wisdom to inform our spirited participation with one another in the natural world. Shall we dance?

The Unbroken

There is a brokenness
out of which comes the unbroken,
a shatteredness
out of which blooms the unshatterable.
There is a sorrow
beyond all grief which leads to joy
and a fragility
out of whose depths emerges strength.

There is a hollow space
too vast for words
through which we pass with each loss,
out of whose darkness
we are sanctioned into being.

There is a cry deeper than all sound
whose serrated edges cut the heart
as we break open to the place inside
which is unbreakable and whole,
while learning to sing.

Rashani Réa
Written in 1991 after the 5th death in her family.
https://www.rashani.com

References

Adler, J. (1989). Still looking. [Videotape and 16mm film]. (Available through University of California Extension Media Center, 2176 Shattuck Ave., Berkeley, CA. 94704.)

Adler, J. (1999). Who is the witness? In P. Pallaro, (Ed.). *Authentic Movement: Essays by Mary Starks Whitehouse, Janet Adler, and Joan Chodorow*. Jessica Kingsley Publishers. (Original work published 1987.)

Adler, J. (2002). *Offering from the conscious body: The discipline of Authentic Movement*. Inner Traditions.

Atwood, G. E. & Stolorow, R. D. (1993). *Faces in a cloud: Intersubjectivity in personality theory*. Jason Aronson, Inc.

Bainbridge Cohen, B. (1997). Body-mind centering. In D. H. Johnson (Ed.), *Groundworks: Narratives of embodiment* (pp. 15–26). North Atlantic Books & The California Institute of Integral Studies.

Barlin, A. L. & Greenberg, T. R. (1980). *Move and be moved: A practical approach to movement with meaning*. Learning Through Movement.

Bernstein, P. L. (1984). The somatic countertransference: The inner pas de deux. In *Theoretical approaches in dance-movement therapy* (Vol. 2) (pp. 321–342). Kendall/Hunt Publishing Company).

Brooks, C. (1986). *Sensory awareness: Rediscovering of experiencing through the workshops of Charlotte Selver*. Felix Morrow.

Chaiklin, S. & Wengrower, H. (Eds). (2009). *The art and science of dance/movement therapy: Life is dance*. Routledge.

Chodorow, J. (1991). *Dance therapy and depth psychology: The moving imagination*. Routledge.

Chodorow, J. (Ed.). (1997). *Encountering Jung: Jung on active imagination*. Princeton University Press.

Dibbell-Hope, S. (1989). *Moving toward health: A study of the use of dance-movement therapy in the psychological adaptation to breast cancer* [Unpublished doctoral dissertation]. The California School of Professional Psychology.

Dibbell-Hope, S. (Director). (1992). Moving toward health [video]. (Available from University of California Extension, Center for Media & Independent Learning, 2176 Shattuck Ave., Berkeley, CA 94704).

Dosamantes-Beaudry, I. (2007). Somatic transference and countertransference in psychoanalytic intersubjective dance/movement therapy. *American Journal of Dance Therapy*, *29*(2), 73–89. https://doi.org/10.1007/s10465-007-9035-6

Frewen, P. & Lanius, R. (2015). *Healing the traumatized self: Consciousness, neuroscience, treatment*. W. W. Norton & Company.

Gendlin, E. (1978). *Focusing*. Bantam Books, Inc.

Greene, A. (1980). *The use of touch in analytic psychotherapy: A case study* [Unpublished thesis]. New York C. G. Jung Training Center.

Greene, A. (1999). *Conscious body—conscious mind* [Unpublished doctoral dissertation]. The Union Institute, College of Graduate Studies, School of Interdisciplinary Arts and Sciences.

Greene, A. (2001). Conscious mind-conscious body. *The Journal of Analytical Psychology*, *46*(4), 565–590.

Johnson, D. (1995). *Bone, breath, and gesture: Practices of embodiment*. North Atlantic Books.

Jung, C. G. (1940/1959). *The collected works of C. G. Jung: Vol. 9i. The psychology of the child archetype*. Pantheon Books Inc.

Jung, C. G. (1953). *The collected works of C. G. Jung: Vol. 7. Two essays on analytical psychology*. Pantheon Books.

Jung, C. G. (1955). *Modern man in search of a soul*. Harcourt.

Keleman, S. (1975a) *Your body speaks its mind*. Simon and Schuster.

Keleman, S. (1975b). *The human ground: Sexuality, self, and survival*. Science and Behavior Books.

Keleman, S. (1984). Interview with Tina Stromsted. In Dreamdancing: The use of dance/movement therapy in dreamwork [Unpublished master's thesis]. John F. Kennedy University.

Lewis, P. (1993). *Creative transformation: The healing power of the arts*. Chiron Publications.

Levine, P. (1997). *Waking the tiger: Healing trauma*. North Atlantic Books.

Levine, P. (2012). *In an unspoken voice: How the body releases trauma and restores goodness*. North Atlantic Books.

Masterpasqua, F. (2009). Psychology and epigenetics. *Review of General Psychology, 13*(3), 194–201. https://doi.org/10.1037/a0016301

Mindell, A. (1985). *Working with the dreaming body*. Routledge & Kegan Paul.

Pallaro, P. (Ed.). (1999). *Authentic Movement: Essays by Mary Starks Whitehouse, Janet Adler, and Joan Chodorow*. Jessica Kingsley Publishers.

Pallaro, P. (2007). Somatic countertransference: The therapist in relationship. In P. Pallaro (Ed.), *Authentic Movement: Moving the body, moving the self, being moved* (pp. 176–193). Jessica Kingsley. (Originally published 1994.)

Pert, C. (1997). *Molecules of emotion: The science behind mind-body medicine*. Touchstone.

Porges, S. (2011). *The polyvagal theory*. W. W. Norton & Company.

Rothschild, B. (2000). *The body remembers: The psychophysiology of trauma and trauma treatment*. W. W. Norton & Company.

Sandel, S., Chaiklin, S., & Lohn, A. (Eds.). (1993). *Foundations of dance movement therapy: The life and work of Marian Chace*. Marian Chace Memorial Fund of the American Dance Therapy Association.

Schoop, T. (with Mitchell, P.). (1974). *Won't you join the dance?* National Press Books.

Schore, A. (2009–2017). Neuroscience and attachment theory seminar series for clinicians, Berkeley, California.

Schore, A. & Schore, J. (2012). Modern attachment theory: The central role of affect regulation in development and treatment. In Schore, A. (Ed.), *The science of the art of psychotherapy* (pp. 27–51). W. W. Norton & Company.

Selvam, R. (2022). *The practice of embodying emotions: A guide for improving cognitive, emotional, and behavioral outcomes*. North Atlantic Books.

Sieff, D. (2009). Confronting death mother: An interview with Marion Woodman. *Spring: A Journal of Archetype & Culture, 81*, 327–348.

Siegel, D. (1999). *The developing mind: Toward a neurobiology of interpersonal experience*. Guilford Press.

Stein, M. (2015). *Jung's map of the soul: An introduction*. Open Court.

Stromsted, T. (2001). Re-inhabiting the female body: Authentic Movement as a gateway to transformation. *The Arts in Psychotherapy, 28*(1), 39–55.

Stromsted, T. (2001–02). Dancing literature: Authentic Movement and re-inhabiting the female body. *Somatics: Magazine-Journal of the Mind/Body Arts and Sciences, XIII*(3), 20–31.

Whitehouse, M. (1979). C.G. Jung and dance therapy: Two major principles. In P.L. Bernstein, (Ed.), *Eight theoretical approaches in dance/movement therapy* (pp. 51–70). Kendall-Hunt. (Original work published 1977.)

Whitehouse, M. (1995). The Tao of the body. In D. H. Johnson (Ed.), *Bone, breath, & gesture: Practices of embodiment*. North Atlantic Books & The California Institute of Integral Studies. (Original work published 1958.)

Whitehouse, M. (1999). Physical movement and personality. In P. Pallaro, (Ed.), *Authentic Movement: Essays by Mary Starks Whitehouse, Janet Adler, and Joan Chodorow*. Jessica Kingsley Publishers. (Original work published 1963.)

Woodman, M. (1984). Psyche/soma awareness. *Quadrant*, 17(2), 25–37.

Wilkinson, M. (2010). *Changing minds in therapy: Emotion, attachment, trauma, and neurobiology*. W. W. Norton & Company, Inc.

Chapter 9

Working with Trauma
Awakening Psyche and Soma

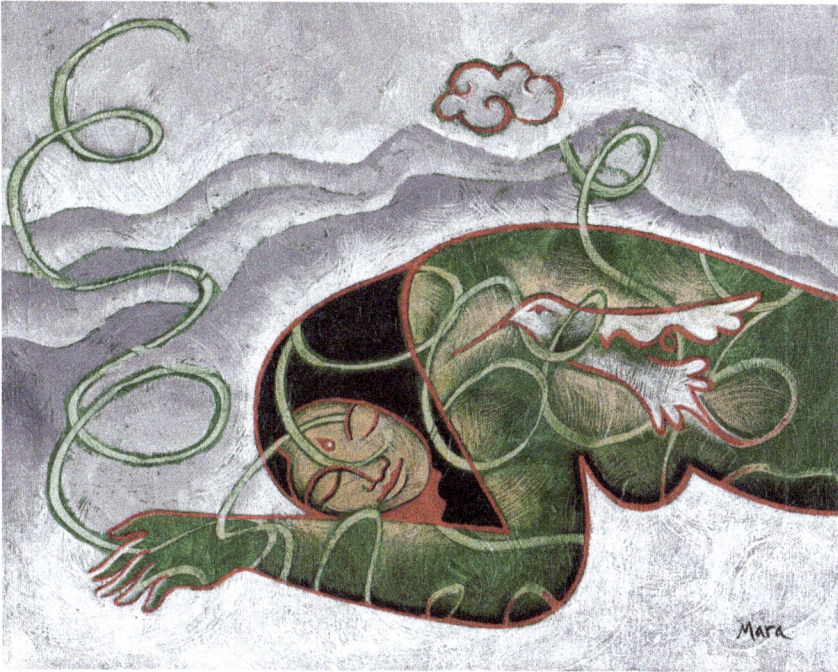

Figure 9.1 Waiting © 2005, by Mara Berendt Friedman
@ www.newmoonvisions.com.

Our journey through life is encoded in our bodies just as the rings of a tree encode the life-story of that tree. If we grow up in an emotionally supportive environment—barring other environmental or genetic difficulties—our posture will be more secure, our movements fluid, and our speech expressive. We're more likely to be at ease with our bodies and enjoy an open connection between body and psyche.

DOI: 10.4324/9781003538356-13

If we grow up in the wake of emotional trauma, it is a different story. Our bodies take on the postures, movements, and ways of speaking that seem to offer us protection: we may puff ourselves up or make ourselves small, overeat or starve, yell or stutter. Once established, these bodily defenses limit our experience of ourselves and the world. Additionally, they often create painful physical symptoms.

Equally damaging is the disembodiment that accompanies childhood trauma. Emotions are deeply rooted in bodily responses, so by cutting off from our bodies we can distance ourselves from unbearable pain. We are not necessarily conscious of our disembodiment, but there are consequences. We cannot pick up the subtle feelings that reflect our bodies' emotional states and which could act as a compass during life. We have little access to the images that arise in our bodies, which could help to guide our journey. We see our bodies as objects and tend to blame at least some of our pain on their imagined inadequacy.

This chapter is adapted from a conversation with Daniela Sieff, an independent writer and scholar, with a background in biological anthropology and an active interest in the psyche. In the book *Understanding and Healing Emotional Trauma: Conversations with Pioneering Clinicians and Researchers,* she engages with experts in psychology, neurobiology, and evolutionary studies about trauma and transformation. Our conversation focused on healing trauma by working directly with our bodies to release what they hold, and forging the connections between body and psyche that will enable us to live an embodied life. There are many creative ways to do this work, including Authentic Movement, voicework, embodied dreamwork, yoga, and working with masks.

Daniela: Why should we pay attention to the body when we work with trauma?

Tina: Our journey through life is not simply psychological or spiritual; it is also *concretely* experienced and recorded in the body. As a result, trauma is written into our physical bodies as well as into our minds. It literally shapes our nervous and hormonal systems, our musculature, posture, and our movements.

Trauma, which is often defined as deep and lasting wounding resulting from overwhelming pain, can also sever our sense of connection with our bodies. Sensations and emotions arise in the body and then "make their way" up through the ancient parts of the brain to the oldest parts of the right hemisphere—which, as Allan Schore (2022) tells us, is the side of the brain that is primarily responsible for our emotional life. From there, from what we understand at this time, information passes to the more recently evolved areas of the right brain, which is where we become conscious of emotions and, with more involvement from the left hemisphere, we can start to put words to them. However, when pain is too great for us to bear, we block its journey into consciousness and into words, dissociatively trapping it in our bodies and in the lower regions of the right brain, where the survival-oriented fight/flight/freeze/appease defense mechanisms are organized. However, we still need to make sense of our experiences, so we create substitute narratives, often self-critical ones, to help us understand what is happening beneath our awareness. This is often our only option at the time, but it means that our pain cannot be metabolized. It also means that we end up living half a life, inhabiting our minds and the critical stories we were told or came to believe, but not our bodies. What is more, when we dissociate from our bodies, we have no access to the emotions that normally guide our actions, and so we find ourselves without a compass.

Unable to draw on our bodies' natural wisdom or to reach out for needed support from others, we may feel "orphaned," deflated, or mistreated, slow to trust, or powerless. Some may inflate their importance in an effort to make up for a profound sense of impotence and emptiness. Others may become abusers, repeating the crime in trauma cycles that are passed down from one generation to the next, often nonverbally, in the earliest phases of life.

Trauma also shapes the way we think about our bodies. All too often, we mistakenly see our bodies as the source of our wounding and consequently despise them.

Despite the impact of trauma on our bodies, Western culture has, until very recently, paid little attention to the body when working with emotional trauma. However, we only have to look at common metaphors to realize that we implicitly know that our emotional life is deeply connected to the life embodied in our flesh and bones: "I need to get something off my chest," "I've had to shoulder that secret for so long," "This is a pain in the neck," and "I feel torn in two directions" are familiar examples.

Ancient healing practitioners viewed the body as essential. The Greeks valued body development but separated it from abstract, cognitive intelligence, which they elevated. Later, Christianity saw the body as the repository of sin, encouraging people to transcend their "animal flesh" and reside in spirit. Other major religions also express difficulties in reconciling this split.

We will not heal trauma if we reside in spirit—quite the opposite. To heal trauma, we must bridge the dissociation between body and psyche, pay careful attention to what our body holds, and re-inhabit it. To achieve that we have to work directly with our bodies, rather than seeing them as second-class citizens compared to our psyches.

Creating a Healthy Relationship with the Body

Daniela: What would a healthy relationship with our body entail?

Tina: First and foremost, we would treat our bodies with respect and love. We would foster appreciation for their natural shapes, listen to their needs, and develop a sense of their intrinsic rhythms. We would feed our bodies with wholesome food and find a nourishing and sustainable balance between activity and rest, stimulating experiences and soothing ones, social relating and inner time. We would give ourselves time to walk, swim, dance, and sing, engage in loving relationships, and fill our senses with the sights, sounds, smells, and textures of the natural world. We would create opportunities to experience ourselves as embodied creatures that are a vital part of the web of life.

We would be connected to our bodies and allow their feelings and sensations to flow freely through us. We value our bodily experiences just as much as our thoughts. We would inhabit our bodies as fully as we inhabit our minds, taking restorative time in nature to reconnect with *all* living beings (as described in Chapter 16).

Because emotions are interconnected with bodily states, a healthy relationship with our bodies also requires that we are able to regulate our emotions and soothe ourselves when distressed, so that our bodies do not have to suffer prolonged periods of either stressful hyperarousal or flattened hypoarousal. To do that, we need to be able to tolerate strong emotions when they sweep through us, finding ways to express or contain them, depending on the situation. Otherwise, we have no choice but to try to escape from those emotions by splitting mind from body, by entering a flattened depressive state, or by turning to an addiction. Additionally, when we are unable to tolerate our emotions, our musculature, organs, and nervous system are left carrying our emotions for us, possibly contributing to a disease process over time.

We are born with the potential to have a healthy relationship with our bodies, yet realizing this potential is deeply impacted by our early relationships. Our parents' attitudes about and treatment of their bodies, and ours, make a lasting impression. If there's trauma involved from a deeply troubled childhood, it will take patient, sensitive work to bring the dissociated parts—the split-off embodied sensations, emotions, and memories—back together so we can experience a sense of wholeness and well-being.

Cultural Body

Daniela: In terms of objectifying our bodies, it seems that in the Greco-Christian belief-system we needed to tame and shape our bodies in order to secure the love of God, whereas in today's world we believe we need to tame and shape our bodies to secure the love of other humans. That belief seems to be particularly strong in those who, as a result of troubled early relationships, grow up believing they are inadequate and unlovable.

Tina: Absolutely. As children, if our parents and caretakers mistreat, neglect, or in other ways fail to attune to and love us in the way that we need to be loved, then we seek to understand why. The conclusion we invariably draw is that there is something wrong with us that makes us unlovable, and given the culture's emphasis on having the "perfect body" it is all too easy to imagine that it is our bodies that don't "measure up." This is partly due to our culture and partly because it gives us hope that we can "fix" or control what is "wrong" with us.

A client who, as an adult, had surgery to reshape her nose, was about twelve years old when, looking at herself in a mirror, her mother happened to walk by. In a kindly tone, her mother said, *"It's too bad about your nose, honey, but when you get older you could do something about that."* The mother, unable to love her own body and wanting her daughter to be happy, sincerely believed her child would have more happiness if her nose was of a different shape. But unfortunately what this mother ultimately gave her daughter was not the opportunity for happiness, but a deeply held belief that she was unattractive and that only surgery could change that.

Daniela: It is not only our attitude about our bodies that can become distorted with childhood trauma, but the physical body itself can become distorted too.

Tina: Yes, through posture, gait, gestures, movement, and muscular tone, our bodies record how we have shaped ourselves in response to our emotional environment. If we were held with love and attuned attentiveness as infants—barring later damaging experiences—that memory would be embodied, allowing us to become adults who hold ourselves securely and move in a strong, lyrical, flexible, coherent way. If we were held with ambivalence or cold detachment, parts of our bodies might become stiff, frozen, rigid, and deadened. If we were held with a mix of neediness, anger, and detachment, our bodies might move in disorganized and conflicting ways. When reaching for something or someone, our arms might stretch forward while our pelvis pulls back.

Body Armoring

Additionally, the forms our bodies take encompass more than just a simple reflection of our experience; they can also be protective. In response to physical or emotional trauma, we learn to take up certain postures in an attempt to protect ourselves. Wilhelm Reich was one of the first people to articulate this in the 1930s, and he called the process "body armoring." For example, we might push our chest forward and puff it out, having learned that we can intimidate others into leaving us alone. Conversely, we might collapse our chest and make ourselves small, having discovered that the less threatening we appear, the more chance we have of averting attacks, or perhaps eliciting caretaking responses from others. Animals are experts at this, instinctually changing their shape to improve their chances of survival.

When we *repeatedly* have to take on a posture in order to protect our self, that posture becomes part of who we are, shaping how we move in the world and ultimately how we experience it. If a childhood need to disconnect from unbearable pain left us with a head position that is set apart from the body and angled upward, as adults we may find it easier to have lofty thoughts than to connect to our needs and our emotions. Others may also think we're aloof, rather than simply doing what we can to cope with vulnerability. When the helplessness of our childhood becomes enshrouded in sunken shoulders, a collapsed chest, and withdrawn limbs, then it is incredibly hard to reach out into the world, and others tend to look like "parents" who are going to be critical. Worse still, with such a posture we are more likely to behave in ways that *draw* that critical energy to us. So our body's early attempts to protect us unwittingly become a conduit for re-creating our painful early experiences, eventually producing a belief that the world is an unkind or dangerous place.

A woman I worked with, whom I will call Kate, suffered childhood sexual abuse. Her terror and pain were held in her clenched and frozen pelvis and in her arms, which were permanently tensed in an unconscious attempt to "keep a grip on herself" and in the hope that she might be able to push her abuser away. Kate also binged on food because she believed that if she became large enough, then she would no longer be subject to abusive sexual attention.

However, the costs were severe. Kate's frozen pelvis left her with chronic lower-back pain, and her tensed arms resulted in persistent pain in her shoulders and neck. Her binges left her feeling terrifyingly out of control, and that was an unconscious reminder of her childhood trauma, when as an abused child she had had no control over what happened to her. In addition, she hated herself for being fat because a younger part of Kate secretly hoped a prince would rescue her from her pain and take care of her, while the fat part believed that no man would be attracted to her. So, as a result of her physical response to early abuse, Kate was left in chronic pain and at war with herself. Kate's situation is not unusual. Many who suffer some kind of childhood trauma end up with their own unique set of emotionally and physically painful embodied consequences.

Daniela: Donald Kalsched (1996, 2013) describes how the defenses that we develop to protect ourselves as wounded children become so determined to prevent us from being retraumatized that they become self-persecuting. Can the protector-persecutor be written into our bodies as well as into our psyches?

Tina: Very much so, and Don's work has made profound inroads in deepening our understanding of these internalized dynamics. Imagine that as a child, whenever we started to cry, our parent said something like, *"If you don't stop I'll give you something to cry about."* It would not be long before we learned to bite our lip or clench our jaw to inhibit our tears. In doing so, we would not only protect our self from overt criticism but also incorporate that inhibiting, critical parent into the musculature of our face.

I had a patient who grew up in a Calvinistic household where pleasure was severely frowned upon. As a result, whenever he planned something that might be enjoyable, his body did whatever was necessary to keep him away from that supposedly unacceptable emotion. By way of examples, three days before leaving for a holiday in Hawaii, he lifted something that was far too heavy and damaged his back so badly that he could not go; he signed up for music lessons, but fell and broke his wrist so that he could not play; the day before going on a weekend hike with friends, he sprained his ankle. In short, this man's intense fear of pleasure—instilled in his unconscious during his childhood—was played out through his body, which was trying to protect him from going into forbidden territory.

It is not uncommon for our speaking voice to be physically constrained by an embodied "protector-persecutor." Growing up in a healthy emotional environment our voices are rooted in the deep resonators in our bodies. But in the case of childhood trauma, that can't happen because it is too dangerous to speak our truth—so we may stutter or talk with the voice of an unthreatening little girl, or speak with a restricted, thin sound. Although these ways of speaking may protect us as children, as adults they prevent us from expressing our truth, sticking up for our values, and being heard.

Daniela: Does trauma affect our breathing?

Tina: It does. If we have had a secure childhood, and have not experienced trauma at birth or in later life, then we are more likely to breathe deeply and easily, taking in life in a natural, effortless way. However, if we have suffered emotional wounding and lived in fear, then we are likely to constrict our breath, keeping it high in our chest, with our diaphragm held tight. This not only perpetuates our state of fear; it also contributes to the process of separating us from our bodies and prevents our emotions from reaching awareness. Neurologically speaking, when we constrict our breath, the part of the brain that is able to reflect and process what is happening (the orbitofrontal cortex) is dampened down; whereas the emotional limbic brain, which mediates our defense system, takes over.

Daniela: Can you speak to the need to work directly with our bodies as part of the process of healing trauma?

Tina: As I mentioned, one of the common consequences of early trauma is that we become dissociated from our bodies. If we speak our trauma story without attending directly to our bodies, we are at risk of perpetuating that dissociation rather than healing it. We also need to work with our bodies because, as we have discussed, many of the consequences of trauma are lodged in our bodies, and we simply can't get at them through words alone.

Equally important is what Allan Schore (2022) teaches us: early trauma is typically stored in the right hemisphere of our brains, and the primary language of the right brain is images, metaphor, sensations, and bodily emotions rather than words. Thus, to access what the right hemisphere holds and to rediscover the aspects of ourselves that lie dormant, injured, or silenced, we need to work in its nonverbal vocabulary.

Working with the Body

Daniela: How do we go about working with our bodies?

Tina: The "animal body" is instinctual and loyal. It longs to communicate its inner truth, but it will hold tight until it is safe enough to do so. Thus, it is essential that we find an environment in which our body's truth can be received in an attuned, respectful, and nonjudgmental way. Generally, that means finding a therapist who is attuned to their own body and who can be present to our emotional experiences and resonate with them. Such an attitude helps us to culti-vate acceptance and curiosity about the meaning of our bodily communications. These are typically expressed through nonverbal channels, such as body posture, spontaneous gestures, breathing patterns, tone of voice, quality of eye contact, rhythm, and more. A sense of natural embodiment on the part of the therapist also invites the aliveness of our body into the space.

Once a sense of safety is established, we (as clients) can start to tell our story while reconnecting to the embodied aspects of our experience. To do that we need to slow down and pay deliberate attention to the sensations, feelings, movements, and postures that may be present. The very act of pausing and bringing our embod-ied reality into awareness can change the anatomy of our brains as this interrupts our habitual journey down well-established neural pathways and begins to build new pathways that offer us different options.

The next step might involve exploring a specific movement or posture that has come into awareness. For example, if we notice we are tapping our feet, we can exaggerate that movement to see what it reveals. Perhaps our foot-tapping stems from an unconscious desire to kick away emotional attacks. We might realize that, as children, trying to kick away emotional attacks would have caused more trouble, so we hid that energy in our feet. However, as adults on a healing journey, that kicking energy can be transformative. Allowing the kick to become as big as it wants can help us integrate that energy and use it to fuel change.

Daniela: Once we discover what our bodies carry, how can we take the next step?

Tina: We need to work with our bodies to build the resources that will allow us to free our bodies of their burdens. This involves learning to do what was once too dangerous for us to do. Now changing how we stand, or altering other as-pects of our posture, does not magically bring psychological change, but unless we change our muscular patterning, we physically limit what we can experience and the changes that can be made.

Daniela: Is there a role in healing trauma for movement practices that follow an established form such as Yoga or Tai Chi?

Tina: Forms like Yoga and Tai Chi can be fantastic when we are beginning to connect to our bodies in the wake of trauma. They can ease the breath and offer us a safe and containing framework in which we can start to become aware of both bodily sensations and how we hold ourselves. They help us to develop mental discipline and to become more mindful of our bodies. Their repetitiveness can be wonderfully comforting, enabling us to hold our self together when the chaos feels like too much. They teach us new movements, thus helping us to move beyond the physically embodied defenses that we have developed. And they are often done in a class, which offers us a feeling of community.

However, in terms of healing embodied trauma there are limitations to these practices; because they are directed by someone else, we are maneuvering our bodies into someone else's standardized movements, rather than finding our own reality. Free-form movement practices, in contrast, offer us the opportunity to open to movements that spontaneously emerge, often from a deeper unconscious source.

Ultimately, it is important to have a range of bodily practices: structured and predictable forms when we are feeling fragile, and freer forms when we are feeling strong enough to explore the unknowns that we hold in our bodies and in our unconscious minds.

Authentic Movement

Daniela: Can you describe some of the freer forms of bodywork?

Tina: One of the most potent practices that I have discovered is Authentic Movement as developed by Mary Starks Whitehouse (1963/1999). This approach facilitates a descent into the body and into the inner world of the psyche through unstructured, natural movement. It encourages us to surrender our habitual reliance on the verbal, rational, linear, time-bound properties of the left hemisphere and, instead, to inhabit the nonverbal, affective right hemisphere and the body itself. With practice, unconscious emotions and gestures find words. The left and right hemispheres become more integrated, and we experience a more spirited sense of embodied aliveness, coming home to the body in the context of a supportive relationship.

Through this process, we create gateways to our unprocessed trauma. Often that will involve literal re-enactments of the movement patterns surrounding our wounds. These are the places where resources ran out and we had to cower, freeze, or puff ourselves up to survive. If we can return to the site of the wound, with the additional resources of adulthood and embodied, depth-oriented therapeutic practices, we can heal ourselves. (By way of example, see Keith's experience when he released his structured Tai Chi movements and entered an inner-directed Authentic Movement process, described in Chapter 3.)

Authentic Movement does not just help us integrate our old trauma; it can also help us form a bridge to our unconscious. Through the practice, we can discover and develop parts of our potential that we could not live when we were growing up, either because of trauma or because we simply did not have any opportunities to do so. In Authentic Movement, these hidden or less developed parts often emerge spontaneously through unconscious movements, gestures, voice tone, verbal expressions, and breathing patterns. Paying attention to what emerges, we become conscious of these parts and can explore, integrate, and practice living them. In so doing, we foster our growth, connect to our creativity, and gain a deeper sense of wholeness.

What is more, because in Authentic Movement we listen to our bodies with non-judgmental acceptance and respect, we move into our bodies and begin to inhabit them more fully. Then, instead of thinking of our bodies as "objects" to be tamed and perfected, we begin to think of them as partners and teachers, and we start to see how much we can learn from them.

Role of the Witness

Daniela: Can you talk more about the role of the witness?

Tina: The witness attends to the mover with an attitude of nonjudgmental compassion. Witnessing is very different from "observing" or "looking at"; looking can be quite objectifying, but witnessing means being actively present with the mover. A witness brings awareness not only to the mover's experience but also to what is happening in their own body as they attend to the mover. As a mover, knowing we are witnessed allows us to descend deeper into our psyche and open to the mysteries held in the body.

Moreover, in having a witness who is attending to us with nonjudgmental presence, we can begin to heal some of the damage caused by troubled early relationships. As Allan Schore (2022) and others have shown, it is our caretakers' ability to attune to us in an empathetic and nonjudgmental way that enables us to develop an awareness of our inner states and to experience, contain, and express the full range of our emotions. If our caretakers can't attune to us in that way, then our bodies are inhibited, and our psychological development is impaired. The relationship between witness and mover can contribute to repair.

Typically, the witness's role goes beyond silent observation. When, as mover, our movement comes to its natural conclusion, we may speak to our witness about our experience in order to reflect on and begin integrating what has arisen in us. Then, if we wish, we can ask the witness to describe the movements that she has seen us make. That helps us remember the movements, sensations, emotions, and memories we have just lived. When a witness is invited to share her experience, the task is to stick to what she saw, taking care not to judge the mover in any way or to project her own feelings onto the mover.

That said, it can also be helpful for a witness to share what she experienced in her own body when being present to the mover, so long as she owns those experiences as her own. For example, if the witness is strongly affected when we wrap our arms around our body and let our head drop, the witness might say, *"I see your arms wrap around your body and your head drop, and I feel comforted and contained."* By owning her feelings, the witness is not imposing her history on us but giving us the opportunity to experience somebody being with us in a way that is very different from the original critical watcher.

Mind you, things are not always what they seem and sometimes what happens in the witness's body can open up the hidden reality. I am remembering an analytic client I will call Sarah who cried a lot as she moved. However, whenever I witnessed Sarah's crying, I did not feel sadness in my own body as I often do when witnessing other movers who are in pain. Instead, I felt itchy; I wanted to scratch and noticed that I was really irritated. When Sarah asked for my authentic response, I shared my sensations and feelings with her, saying that I did not know what to make of them. Sarah's instant response was *"I'm not angry"* and she stormed off, slamming the door to my consulting room behind her. When Sarah turned up for her next therapy session, she said, "*I have been so mad at you; I wasn't angry, and I don't know why you were suggesting that!*" I was interested in her reaction and asked Sarah what else she had felt. Eventually, it emerged that in Sarah's family, it was okay to cry but not to be angry—that was too threatening. And so Sarah had learned to substitute crying for anger. While witnessing Sarah, my body picked that up, despite the words she was using to describe her experience.

Daniela: In my experience, we can learn just as much from witnessing as we can from moving.

Tina: That is true. In particular, witnessing can be very powerful in helping us to develop empathy. If we had a difficult childhood, we may have shut down our empathic self in an attempt to put distance between ourselves and the negativity that others were directing toward us. Witnessing encourages us to take the risk of opening to receive another's experience.

Additionally, empathy requires that we resonate with another's experience, and resonance happens through the mirror neuron system of the brain and through the sensations and feelings that we experience in our bodies. If we are cut off from our bodies as a result of trauma, then our capacity for empathy is limited. Witnessing, in encouraging us to pay attention to our own body's experience, helps us connect to our bodies and so fosters empathy. At the same time, witnessing can help us learn that there is a distinction between our own feelings and those that belong to another person. It teaches us not to impose our reality on others, paving the way for us to create increasingly conscious and respectful relationships.

Thus, for both witness and mover, the process can help us move beyond our isolated sense of self and experience what it is like to meet with another from a place of authenticity, relatedness, and compassion.

Additionally, through witnessing we often discover aspects of what we hold unconsciously in our bodies—the shadow material I mentioned earlier. As witness, we continually bring awareness and curiosity to questions such as these: *"What body sensations am I becoming aware of as I open to the mover's experience? Do I feel my own grief, or my own shutting down, or my own joy?"* Witnessing will activate our own mirror neuron system, so that we too may begin to feel aspects of ourselves that have long been shut away.

Authentic Movement and Mindfulness

Daniela: When you talk about Authentic Movement, it sounds like a mindfulness meditation practice—do you see it in that way?

Tina: Authentic Movement is a form of mindfulness, when mindfulness is taken to mean paying attention to our emotions, our bodies, our hearts, and our souls. However, the mindfulness of Authentic Movement is different from the mindfulness practices of traditions like Zen meditation that involve impartial observation of what is happening without entering the subjective feelings.

Authentic Movement helps us to develop a body that is strong enough and flexible enough to experience sensations and express emotions in healthy ways so that we no longer have to dissociate. In my understanding, Zen meditation encourages us to notice the sensations and emotions that are happening in our inner world, without attachment or engagement. In some cases, this can enhance a capacity for self-reflection, containment, and emotional regulation; whereas in others, it may exacerbate dissociative tendencies.

Crucial to Authentic Movement is the relationship between mover and witness, and that human connection offers us the opportunity to heal the relational part of ourselves that got damaged when we were children. With Zen meditation, we may sit in a room with other people but explicitly relating to them is generally not part of the practice, so there may be fewer opportunities to develop our relational capacity.

In other words, although becoming mindful of what is happening in the body and psyche is at the core of Authentic Movement, it is a different type of mindfulness than what is fostered by some of the sitting meditation traditions, such as Zazen. The former helps heal attachment wounds and encompasses attunement to bodily experience; the latter emphasizes self-management and an attitude of "nonattachment" to emotions that arise. Each practice can be good, depending on what we need at a given time. For example, I would not advise Authentic Movement practice for someone in crisis whose ego is already being flooded with material from the unconscious. At such times, more structured body/mind practices are best, until the person's ego is strong enough to contain and channel the upwelling of emotional energy.

Creative Energy

Daniela: In Authentic Movement groups, when people stop moving, you often encourage them to allow the energy to continue to unfold through painting, modeling clay, writing, or coming into voice? Why?

Tina: If we go from Authentic Movement directly into spoken words, we risk imposing our old, familiar story onto our experience, so the new energy that is ready to emerge closes down. However, if we go from moving to painting or sculpting or writing, we create an open space in which the new energy can continue to unfold and be received. It also allows the mover to linger a bit longer in the nonverbal right brain, rather than attempt to make meaning prematurely.

That said, for drawing or sculpting to be effective, it is best not to think about how we want an image to look, but rather to let the body, in concert with the right brain, continue to move through its use of colors, the marks it puts on paper, and the shape it molds out of clay. Then, once the body has finished creating its image, we can sit back and see what comes to mind: we may notice a lot of black or red, or a rainbow of pastel colors; the lines may be jagged or geometrical, or they may be soft and voluptuous. Seeing those things with an attitude of open curiosity can help us become increasingly conscious of the energy that first started to emerge when we moved.

We can do something similar with other creative forms, one of which is "free-writing" (Goldberg, 1986). We put pen to paper and do not let up until ten minutes have passed; we do not cross out; we do not write complete sentences or worry about grammar; we are not polite and there is no censorship. We simply let the words tumble out and do our best to get out of their way. Coming out of an experience of moving, or indeed out of witnessing, we might start with a question like *"How did I feel?"* or *"What touched me?"* or *"What moved me?"* (Using body-based questions can be particularly potent). Once we have our starting point, if we can keep our hand moving, then we will begin to express a little more of what is ready to come into consciousness.

Moving between modalities is not only relevant to Authentic Movement, but can be very valuable in more conventional therapeutic settings too. When working with a dream, if there is a character that we are drawn to, it can be very enlightening to ask: *"How does he stand? How does she hold herself?"* Taking that stance, we might see what movement or feelings emerge, or we might let a sound come out, noticing how it feels to make those kinds of sounds. Eventually, if this character speaks in words, we might see what comments it makes, again noticing how we feel when we hear ourselves say these things. Alternatively, we might do some free-writing, taking on the perspective of the dream figure. Our images and dreams spring from our unconscious, so we can learn much more about ourselves if we embody our images by imaginatively inhabiting them with awareness, rather than just talking about them from a place of intellectual curiosity.

Working with Masks

Daniela: Working with masks is another medium through which we can become aware of what we carry. You and I have both done mask work in the context of BodySoulRhythms® workshops led by Marion Woodman, Ann Skinner, and Mary Hamilton and now you teach it. Can you describe this work?

Tina: BodySoulRhythms® work is profoundly creative and deeply integrative. It is generally done in residential workshops that take place over several days, and working with masks, which give form to "shadow" energies, is an important part of the process.

Working silently, in groups of three, a mask is made on the face using strips of Plaster of Paris. As we lie down and surrender to the process, and to the intimacy of others touching our face, we begin to descend into the unconscious. The following day, we complete the shape of the mask and "decorate" it. As with other forms of bodywork, it is not our ego that makes these choices—rather we see what shapes, colors, and textures call to us. Maybe the mask wants to be painted black on one side and gold on the other. Maybe it wants a spiral of string circling its cheek and a zigzag of sequins across its forehead. Maybe the mask wants to be covered with dirt and twigs. We do not need to be an artist—the mask gets made on our face and then finds its own way to express what is currently alive in our unconscious.

Once its form settles, guided by a facilitator, we start to wear the mask. We come to this with no preconceptions and simply explore how we feel in our mask, how we move, and what kind of sounds we make. Maybe we are a needy baby. Maybe we are a child, petrified by the stare of an abuser. Maybe we are catlike, curious, independent, and playful. Maybe we are a young boy who wants to climb fences, steal apples, and see the world. Maybe we are a sexy, sensual woman. Maybe a wise old woman, who says outrageous things and does not care about what others think. Maybe we are a tree rooted in the ground. Maybe we are a fish swimming deep in the sea.

Wearing our mask, we meet other masks, and within the confines of what is safe, we have permission to engage with those other energies in whatever way is initiated by the energy of our own mask. That allows us to go beyond our normal ways of relating, maybe to be silly or playful, funny or angry, sexual or powerful. At the same time, the other masks may relate to us in ways that nobody has treated us before.

One of the advantages of a mask is that it gives us explicit permission to be something other than our familiar, well-practiced everyday self. When we wear our mask, we step into an unfamiliar shadow aspect of ourselves and explore it freely. What is more, we live that previously unknown aspect in a fully embodied way. It can be a very powerful and transformative experience.

These creative methods to bring previously unlived parts of ourselves into consciousness are all part of what Jung called "active imagination." The steps include relaxing the ego to allow the unconscious to take the lead; giving it form through creative expression; reflecting on what emerges; and gradually integrating what we have learned through practicing it in our daily life (Chodorow, 1997). Mask work is one form of active imagination; Authentic Movement is another.

Challenges

Daniela: Bodywork can create powerfully intense experiences; whereas bringing the emerging energy into daily life is a tough process that takes perseverance and hard work. As a result, one danger is that we seek one intense experience after the next, instead of striving to live what we have discovered in these experiences.

Tina: Yes, this can be a danger. Insights that come through imaginative body-work can be exciting, freeing, and full of adrenaline. We can get habituated to the neurochemical rush evoked by intense experiences. That may set off an addictive hunger for more such experiences, whereas the real work lies in integrating our insights.

What is more, in certain social worlds, going into altered states and having sacred experiences garners praise and leaves us feeling special. If we have been wounded during childhood, carry shame, and do not feel good about ourselves, then the social cachet and feelings of being special can be addictive in and of themselves. When that happens, we are at risk for doing the work not to fuel the hard, slow grind involved in change, but for the narcissistic reward. That does not bring healing; it is important not to identify with transpersonal energies but to relate to and integrate them.

Jung said that once we have been informed by the unconscious, we have an ethical obligation to *live* what we have learned. He was right but making the changes that will allow us to live our insights is often easier said than done!

Daniela: Why is it so difficult to make those changes?

Tina: Change is frightening. People often prefer to live with the "terrible familiars" than to navigate the "possible unknowns." When old defenses are challenged, our knee-jerk reaction is to put ourselves back together in the old way because we do not know how to live the new. Sometimes, when previously forbidden feelings enter our lives, we are so scared that we try to numb them out by reverting to old addictions and toxic behaviors. Or even worse, the new way of living is attacked by our old defense system. An inner voice may say something like, *"I don't take up space like this—this is NOT all right"* or *"My voice doesn't usually sound like that—speaking like this will get me into trouble"* and so on and so on.

It is particularly hard when the attack from our old defenses comes not as an inner voice, but via the musculature of the body. Suppose we have been speaking from a more embodied place and saying things that we have never before allowed ourselves to say; we might start to get a stiff neck that physically prevents us from speaking in the new way. However, because there is no obvious voice that comes with our stiff neck, we will have to work patiently to discover what underlies it. We might dialogue with the stiffness to see if a voice emerges; at the same time, we might work very gently with our neck to slowly loosen it up; or we might allow it to take the lead in Authentic Movement and see what emerges.

Nonetheless, there is often truth in what the defense system is telling us. It is one thing to live a new energy with a trusted therapist or in the safety of a workshop, but quite another to live it with family, parents, and colleagues who have not wit-nessed our transition and might feel unsure about the new "us." After all, many of the people in our world—including family and friends—will expect us to behave in particular ways. Indeed, if they are wounded themselves, then they will need us to behave according to our shared script; when we depart from the script and respond in new ways, they are likely to feel lost and uncomfortable. As a consequence, they will try to push us back into the old shape or may even walk away from the rela-tionship. We have to be prepared for that, and we have to have a system of support that will hold us if and when it happens.

The Spiritual Journey

Daniela: You see body-oriented practices such as Authentic Movement as en-riching our lives not only through helping us to heal our trauma, but also through what they can contribute to a lifelong spiritual journey. Perhaps, to conclude, you could talk about what you mean by that.

Tina: Yes, the spiritual journey is an essential dimension, as the practice be-comes part of our life. We follow it not just to heal, but so that we can continue to develop and grow. We practice it because we want to remain open to the unknown within ourselves. The process helps us deepen our relationship with our bodies, with our unconscious minds, with others, and with life's mysteries. The body holds our vital essence, the divine animating spirit that gives us life! We practice because we long to feel that essence, the shimmer of spirit in the body, the life force at the center that can inspire and nourish us. When this happens we feel "at one" with the universe, reconnected to the larger life force that animates all living beings. It is that deeper intelligence that can guide us and give purpose and meaning to our lives. Conscious embodiment practices can awaken us to our deepest values and teach us how to embody them. In the process, we discover more creative and au-thentic ways of living that unfold within us as we grow and change.

In addition, engaging with a practice that enables us to come home to our bodies inspires us to enter into a healthier relationship with the rest of the living world. Our bodies are a microcosm of the macrocosm; when we stop blaming them for our pain, starving them, shoving junk food into them, shutting them down in an effort to protect us from unbearable suffering, or extracting every last ounce of energy from them through overdoing, then we are also much more likely to change how we relate to our animal cousins and to the planet.

Body-oriented practices such as Authentic Movement are soul work; they al-low us to contact the spirit in the body, the light in dark matter; they awaken an embodied consciousness that can guide our life's path and support the fulfillment of our destiny.

The body pulses with the oldest language and contains a deep historical memory. We strive for an intellectual understanding of its language through neuroscience, genetics, attachment theory, evolutionary anthropology, somatic psychology, and quantum physics. That intellectual understanding needs to be matched with the understanding that comes from *lived* experience. We engage in body-oriented practices to reconnect with our instincts, affirm our feelings, heal childhood wounds, and develop healthier relationships with our bodies, ourselves, and other people. We come to know and love who we are; we embrace life and are embraced by it!

The Moment that Mattered

In the midst of a gnarled aspen grove
where the tree trunks were contorted,
distorted and knobby, my husband,
hiking behind me, joked,
These trees have been through a lot.
And they're still here.
And I stopped mid trail
and turned to face him.
We've been through a lot,
I said. *And we're still here.*
And there beneath the misshapen
trees with their leaves still green
and trembling in the wind,
we hugged and cried and cried
and hugged, knowing the full weight
of everything that might have kept us
from this moment.
Surrounded by aspen
and fields of purple asters,
I knew full body that this
was the moment that mattered.
                    Rosemerry Wahtola Trommer

References

Chodorow, J. (Ed.). (1997). *Jung on active imagination*. Princeton University Press.

Goldberg, N. (1986). *Writing down the bones: Freeing the writer within*. Shambhala Publications.

Kalsched, D. (1996). *The inner world of trauma: Archetypal defenses of the personal spirit*. Routledge.

Kalsched, D. (2013). *Trauma and the soul: A psycho-spiritual approach to human development and its interruption*. Routledge.

Schore, A. (2022). Right brain-to-right brain psychotherapy: Recent scientific and clinical advances. *Annals of General Psychiatry, 21*(46). https://doi.org/10.1186/s12991-022-00420-3.

Whitehouse, M. S. (1999). Physical movement and personality. In P. Pallaro (Ed.), *Authentic Movement: Essays by Mary Starks Whitehouse, Janet Adler, and Joan Chodorow* (Vol. 1) (pp. 51–57). Jessica Kingsley Publishers (Original work presented 1963, Analytical Psychology Club of Los Angeles).

Chapter 10

Transforming Life

Movement as Meditation, Medicine, and Artistic Expression

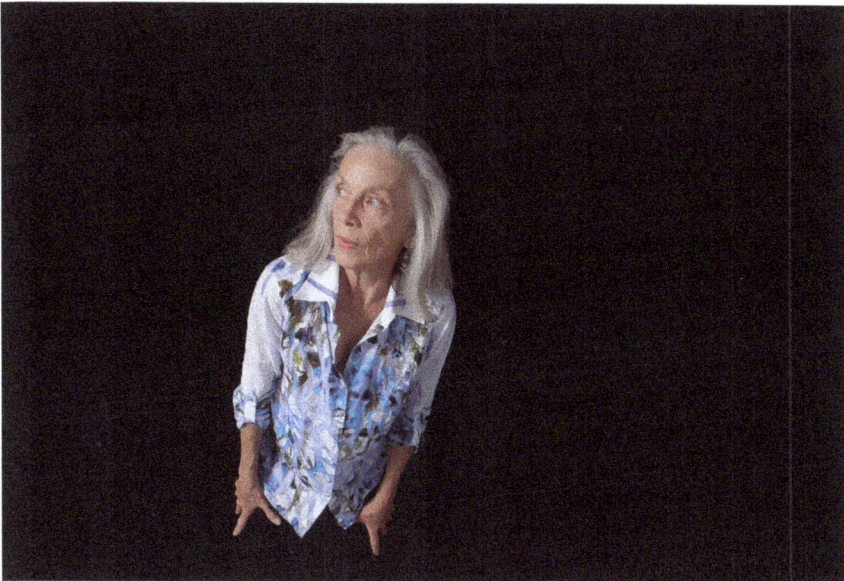

Figure 10.1 Andrea Olsen. Photo by Alan Kimara Dixon of evening-length solo Dancing In Wild Places: Seaweed and Ocean Health, 2014, courtesy of Andrea Olsen.

Authentic Movement helps us deepen our trust in the intrinsic wisdom of the body. It is the practice of being true to who we are in the presence of others.

Andrea Olsen

DOI: 10.4324/9781003538356-14

Background and Contributions

Andrea Olsen is a writer, modern and improvisational dancer, and choreographer who teaches and performs internationally. Although I had heard of Andrea's work through Janet Adler from their collaborations in Northampton, it wasn't until she came to teach "Authentic Movement and Performance" at our Authentic Movement Institute in Berkeley that we met. Slim, blonde, limber, and humorous, she was also creative, thoughtful, wise, and articulate. Tremendously informed on a variety of subjects, she was also a good listener who was quick to question her own ideas as well as others' ideas.

The middle child of three girls, Andrea was raised on a farm in the Midwest. Her development as an artist began at an early age, inspired by her father, a painter and professor of art, and mother, a primary school teacher and musician. Her work is deeply integrative, bringing together the disciplines of art, science, and education. Professor Emerita of Dance at Middlebury College in Vermont, she is also a certified instructor of Holden QiGong and Embodyoga. As an educator, she is committed to courses that communicate feminine values, such as feeling, sensing, inductive learning, respect for the inherent wisdom of the body, and human and other species' interrelatedness and responsibility within the earth's ecosystem. Her teaching, writing, and performing explore experiential anatomy, creativity, and the relationship between body and place.

She is author of a quartet of books on embodiment: *Bodystories: A Guide to Experiential Anatomy*; *Body and Earth: An Experiential Guide*; *The Place of Dance: A Somatic Guide to Dancing and Dance Making,* with colleague Caryn McHose; and *Moving Between Worlds: A Guide to Embodied Living and Communicating.* Andrea has continued her explorations in writing, performing, and film with a focus on global communication. Beginning in 2003, a decade of Body and Earth International annual workshops with Caryn McHose were hosted by Eeva-Maria Mutka and Andy Paget at Pen Pynfarch in Wales. This project has continued in various settings, and she is currently celebrating the twentieth anniversary of this body of work with a two-year tour. New books, websites, and articles reflect this period, including, in 2022, a multi-award-winning film made in Finland, *Matkalla* (*On The Journey*), with Eeva-Maria Mutka, by filmmaker Scotty Hardwig. Authentic Movement continues to be an essential resource, with consistent sessions in Northampton, Massachusetts, with her original group from 1979, as well as workshop offerings and ongoing sessions with local and international dance colleagues.

The Feminine Body

Playing in the fields and with animals as a child on her family's farm on the plains of Illinois formed the foundation for Andrea's passion for nature and "place." Both Andrea's mother and father loved and defended nature, spending outdoor time together during their courtship and later, with their three children, camping, traveling, ice boating, sailing, and sharing breakfasts in the park. Andrea's father was an introvert who, as a painter, "looked closely at the land" and felt a spiritual relation-ship to it.

Many of Andrea's dances, interwoven with stories, have grown out of these early experiences. She continues to dance outdoors in a variety of natural en-vironments to discover how "place" affects movement. As we talked about the relationship between body and place, Andrea re-called the discrepancy she felt between the movement of running, climbing, and being physical outdoors, with the highly refined Russian classical ballet teaching that she received. Beginning at the age of seven, Andrea remembers her ballet teacher encouraging the chil-dren to "perform" movement, accompanied by inspiring music in a beautiful dance studio.

"There I learned to put my natural movement into an abstract vocabulary. This distanced me from place because the language of the body reflected the studio and the demands of a proscenium theater. Many ballerinas would say the same thing— you become awkward in the real world."

Though she majored in painting as an undergraduate (Indiana University, Millikin University, and Institute of European Studies [Paris]), Andrea participated in four years of training at major summer dance festivals at Connecticut College with Martha Graham, José Limón, and other "greats" of modern dance—people who dramatized the role and expression of the body.

Her father was a professor of art at the college where both he and her mother received their degrees. He painted prolifically and took Andrea to art museums, childhood experiences that had a profound impact. Her mother was a violinist and an international traveler, and had confidence in navigating the world. Through them, Andrea learned "that the arts were essential to being human, not superflu-ous." When I interviewed her in Northampton, Massachusetts, Andrea generously invited me to attend a rehearsal of *Our Fathers' Daughters,* a theater piece she had co-created with five other women with whom she'd been in a writing group for many years. Through writing, moving, and music, these six women told the sto-ries of their relationships with their fathers, culminating in the experience of their fathers' deaths.

The stories I'd heard about Andrea's early life had circled around her father; her mother seemed conspicuously absent. When I asked about her, Andrea de-scribed her mother as a first grade teacher, a musician, and a cultured woman with a close group of high-powered women friends—president of the Women's Club and the Parent Teacher Association (PTA), "a doer." Early in the marriage, her mother had also "stayed home for seventeen years to raise her three girls and grow vegetables on the farm." Andrea added, "She was also beautiful and was the Queen—homecoming queen, and Miss Saturnia on the boat when she crossed the ocean to Europe. So from my childhood on I participated in beauty contests."

During this time, Andrea rejected her mother and this image or "outer shell" of womanhood. "She was a brilliant educator, receiving three government grants for innovative teaching ... but I didn't really respect what she did, or who she was ...

I felt overwhelmed by her extraverted energy, and bonded with my father." Though her mother bought Andrea dolls, she also communicated the message that there was no limitation to being female, and that she needn't be expected to be a mother herself. Because of her mother's stature and confidence in the world, Andrea never thought of women as being "under" men.

The farm belonged to her mother, and her parents had something of a role reversal. Her mother was well-off, professional, Republican, independent, and comfortable in the world. Andrea's father was a Democrat, an artist from a poorer background whose father had deserted his family; he also was more introverted, although he taught painting at the university and in workshops and exhibited in art fairs in the Midwest and in Florida. "He built boats and did unusual things. All three girls were bonded to him," she said. "Mother was Presbyterian, believed in church, and in helping people. Dad was spiritual; Mother, religious." Reflecting on this, I wondered how challenging it might have been for a woman of her mother's generation to be otherwise, given the cultural pressure to adorn themselves for patriarchy, rather than having their own direct access to the feminine face of God through embodied spirituality. Andrea's early emotional environment was shaped by these experiences. "Mother described their marriage 'more as parallel tracks than as a team.' They each went their own way a lot. Got together for meals. After their first year together, he never gave her presents. He wasn't very 'honoring' of her, and didn't often call when he was away." Yet, their connection was strong. Andrea describes an Authentic Movement experience that captures some of the flavor of that time.

Control

For weeks, I would lie on the studio floor and find myself reaching with my right arm, wiping it horizontally in front of my body. I recognized this movement as a gesture I had incorporated in many of my dances, combining it with turns or leaps, or bringing it to the floor. But I was surprised it was so determined to appear in my Authentic Movement sessions. (Later Janet [Adler] said, there is no need to 'remember' movement from one session to the next. If a gesture wants to be recognized, it will return again and again until it is brought to consciousness.) One day when this movement appeared, I got the image of myself as a little girl in our farmhouse in Illinois. We had a long countertop in our kitchen which collected objects, and it was always a mess in the usual family way. Whenever my parents would argue, I would clear the counter. It was my way of controlling, quieting, bringing order to what I perceived as chaos. The movement pattern in my body was sourced in this childhood activity. And I was still using it in the same way, to bring order and calm (and the safety of the Illinois landscape) to the dynamics of performance.

The work in Authentic Movement is valuable in many ways. In this situation, it gave me choice about the use of a movement in choreography. The hand-wiping was not a particularly interesting gesture to watch, and I probably didn't need it in all of my dances. It was compelling to both the audience and to myself primarily because of my investment in its content. As I brought awareness to this language of the body. I began to listen for other patterns based in my personal history.

(Olsen, 1991, pp. 71–72)

I asked Andrea about her mother as her first witness, and how that may have played a role in her attraction to Authentic Movement. Andrea reflected that although her mother placed an emphasis on decorating—how things looked—and on status, she also communicated to Andrea that she could do anything that she wanted to when she grew up.

"I was witnessed by opposites. Although I always felt safer with my father, my mother taught me about independence and how to be successful in the world. I feel like she gave me a global perspective; travel was very much part of understanding what it means to be human on the Earth. What I had to reject in her was the image of correctness, of 'being good.'"

Masks

Reflecting on childhood, Andrea wrote: "I was raised in the era of Little Miss Sunbeam, the Jantzen Smile Girl, sororities, cheerleaders, and Miss America pageants. I participated in each of these from childhood to high school to college. The smile was an important asset, useful to monitor communication and response. The many tiny muscles of the face created a mask, with the smile a strange, dull reflex when disconnected from emotional response, sometimes dazzling as it worked to hide the same. At one such contest, I was wearing white gloves and a polka dot dress and was smiling at the judges in a small, close room. I remember thinking, 'What am I doing here?' And I stopped smiling. I felt it dissolve from the inside out. It was the first time that my face didn't work" (Olsen, 1991, p. 43).

In her twenties and thirties, Andrea supported herself by creating oil paintings on paper while on tour as a dancer. During our conversation, she reflected that she had stopped painting in Northampton about the same time that she started Authentic Movement. To continue both would have meant spending too many hours isolated in the studio. At that time, her paintings were psychological portraits of individuals looking in the mirror—a matador, an Amish farmer, a wide-eyed young lady. "Who's the mask and who's the woman?" she wondered.

"The questioning face of a young woman (who was the original inspiration for Lewis Carroll's *Alice in Wonderland*) continued to reappear. And then whole bodies emerged, which was exciting. It was a natural shift; I needed the emotional embodiment in dance of what I was doing on canvas."

Martha Graham had posed the question in Andrea's body: "How to go deeper than my experience of ballet, to contract and release in my core." Of Graham she said, "I was totally caught by her work because it was something I didn't understand.

I was drawn to the mystery of it—it was based on the dialogue between unconscious and conscious experience. I was awestruck by her performances. I wanted to take my paintings, which were two-dimensional and experience them. I wanted them in my body. I didn't want to be distant from them."

She was "hooked," and went on to graduate school in dance, earning her master of fine arts (MFA) at the University of Utah. Questions about the relationship between body and psyche and between art and culture continued to emerge. These were made more conscious in courses with John M. Wilson, her primary mentor in graduate school. He had been a student of dancer Margaret H'Doubler, the American pioneer of dance in education who carried a skeleton with her to every class to encourage a view of the intelligence of the human structure. Wilson's work offered Andrea a multilayered vision of the body—an interweaving of science, philosophy, ethics, and aesthetics rooted in "the understanding that human anatomy is based in our evolutionary history; the multidirectional efficiency of our skeleton is partnered by the complexity of the nervous system." His interdisciplinary approach to the training of the dancer had a profound impact on her thinking and the development of her work. Nature writers, poetry, and science books about the body offered further guides. Not surprisingly, Homer's *The Odyssey* was "the earliest book of significance—a journey!"

Andrea deepened her access to the unconscious through dance and choreography through five years of dream analysis with Jungian Mary Bowen. She further developed her ability to contact her emotions through the body in Authentic Movement, first with Janet Adler and then with her peer group of forty-five years, which continues to this day. Questions about the relationship between body and earth, dance and place have since become central to her and are the subject of her most recent books.

Training: Strengthening the Body Ego

Inspired by her summer experiences at the dance festival at Connecticut College, Andrea went on to form a modern dance company called Dance Gallery, presenting "a gallery of human portraits in dance," performing in Europe and New Zealand. Years later, when she settled in Northampton, Massachusetts, she had the opportunity to explore the relationship between Bonnie Bainbridge Cohen's Body-Mind Centering® work and Authentic Movement as it was introduced to her by Janet Adler. Janet had offered to work with the Dance Gallery, feeling that what she was witnessing in the Authentic Movement studio was more evocative than anything she was seeing on stage. Andrea worked collaboratively with both women, bringing her perspective as an artist and choreographer—an inspiring and creative time. Though Andrea subsequently moved to Vermont to teach at Middlebury College, she commuted twice a month to participate in her Authentic Movement peer group. Over the years, the work has become her spiritual practice, allowing for "deeply moving, intimate, physical and sacred dimensions." Vipassana meditation, environmental studies, experiential anatomy, Continuum, yoga, and T'ai Chi have further informed her life and work. Andrea's personal art practice revolves around creating performance pieces, stories, and writing, work that is deeply nourished by her time in nature, including daily walks with her husband.

Years of exploring her inner life have transformed the images of Little Miss Sunbeam and the women's faces who once looked for themselves in the mirror in her paintings. Today, Andrea has a natural look, often dressing in loose-fitting clothes that are comfortable for moving on the floor, through space, or for working with other's bodies. "I quit teaching dance and choreography at Mount Holyoke College [in 1978] because I was evoking material with students that I didn't know how to handle," she said. "I knew I needed more information before going on. Then I began Authentic Movement." Decades of Authentic Movement practice have transformed her relationship with the audience as well—"It's given me the opportunity to know myself better and to feel more grounded in who I am and what I have to offer," she reflected.

Now, Andrea invites students to create dances rooted in meaningful source material that emerges from their Authentic Movement explorations, rather than overemphasizing how something "looks." She also reminds them that "unlike the fast-food culture we live in, the dance we begin today is often the resource for the work we'll be making in twenty years. Most successful dances or paintings are preceded by an unfolding process that includes multiple attempts"—an attitude that is sure to reduce women's perfectionistic expectations about their bodies and their "performances."

Focus of the Work

Andrea describes herself as working from "three tracks: as an artist, a scientist, and an educator." Her mindset about the body is grounded in a "serious investigation of the body, studying the bones, muscles, the neurological connections, the evolutionary history." She cites growing up on a farm as part of her preparation for her "science track," "meaning you learn how things really work—you see cats born, you see corn grow, you see corn changing to flour, changing to what you eat—it's a very practical understanding of how the physical world works." Although her teaching often has a healing effect, she does not practice Authentic Movement within the context of psychotherapy, but with an artistic and educational focus, using the discipline as a resource for creative expression. In this context, students are encouraged to bring form to what they discover in the unconscious, coupling the movement with other mediums such as choreography, visual art, and writing. When I asked Andrea what elements of the practice she felt were fundamental to transformation, she responded:

"Changing one's attitude from thinking of the body as an object, as a commodity or possession, to the body as having intrinsic value is fundamental. This holds true for our relationship to the Earth as well. Many people consider that the Earth has no worth unless we are using it for something. For example, at a meeting about protecting the vast, forested land around our home in Maine, one man announced, 'The forest has no value unless there's a forester to harvest it.' Instead, Authentic Movement teaches us about intrinsic interconnectedness—at the level of the body and on a global environmental scale. I teach dancers, pre-med students, and environmental studies students to recognize that the body is an informative, miraculous entity; that the Earth has its own intelligence and order if we learn to listen.

"One athlete said, 'It's so interesting to pay attention to my body, because I've been abusing it all my life. I've been pushing, I've been ignoring pain, I've been winning for my coach, I've had thirteen operations already ...' Frequently in college you override the body to get ahead, pushing yourself for success. Especially at highly competitive liberal arts schools, you often have to ignore signals for rest, recovery, health to get your work done. So in the first week of Authentic Movement, a lot of what you hear is, 'I don't want to pay attention to my body, it hurts. It's been hurt.'"

Andrea's teaching emphasizes the dimensionality of the body, helping students explore profound levels of differentiation and interrelatedness of the mind and body, studying the parts to better understand the whole. She also finds it helpful to differentiate the two (thinking mind and body), asking "What's the dialogue between them?" She phrases it in a positive interactive way rather than the oppositional style characteristic of the old positivist paradigm.

When asked how her knowledge of anatomy assists in her practice of Authentic Movement, as mover or witness, Andrea responded, "I don't think of it at all while I'm doing Authentic Movement, or when I'm witnessing. But when you ask me to reflect on the transformative nature of Authentic Movement, I can speculate that when people are spinning, they are disorienting their nervous system. What they're doing is opening new pathways that aren't their familiar habits, allowing fresh connections to be made. It's like when you walk home from school one way your whole life, and someone shows you a shortcut. Then you have two choices. Once a pathway is open, it's available for your use. Initially, it may feel less familiar. Change, even if it's towards efficiency, can feel wrong or uncomfortable."

Andrea sees this as a crucial element in Authentic Movement, emphasizing that "what we want to practice is being familiar with the sensations of not knowing. It's a place in the brain, it's a place in the body. The amygdala (part of the limbic system in the brain) registers newness, alerting survival responses throughout our structure if something is surprising or out of the ordinary. In the practice of Authentic Movement we learn that not knowing is an okay way to feel, allowing the body to open toward further investigation."

I pointed out that this has a lot of implications around not having to be in control, to which Andrea nodded and added, "And the ability to change. That being disoriented in the process of change is an actual state in the body. It may be one step in a mystical experience; however it's still grounded in the laws of the body ..."

Cellular Knowing

Andrea feels that for something to be truly transformative, it must affect all of the cells. From an anatomical perspective, "change has to occur throughout the whole person. Movement patterns are stored primarily in the cerebellum of the brain as well as in the tissues of the body. As these are reexperienced and acknowledged, the possibility for whole-system change is engaged." Andrea describes her body's capacity for teaching and healing.

Holding

"I spent a week in an apartment in New York alone. Each day I would lie on the floor and do bodywork before venturing out into the city to explore. It seemed ironic, to be in a huge city and do such private work. I began working with the hip socket, circling each leg slowly, feeling the reactions as nerves and muscles released. One evening my leg began jerking uncontrollably. Somehow, I was more interested than afraid. My mind observed as I felt my whole body thrashing around from the vibrations in my leg. Thoughts passed in and out as the body did its own release: memories of crossing legs properly as a young lady should, daily classes since childhood developing rotation at the hips for classical ballet (with hip sockets not quite shaped for that activity), deep wide 'second positions' and hundreds of pelvic contractions in modem dance, sexual stories—warm and safe, cold and confusing. I started crying, more from relief than from pain or fear.

"When that side was exhausted, I slowly began the other side. A similar process occurred: the circling, then jerking, vibration, and extension out through the foot until the whole body was shaking. On and on the mind went in partnership with the body, on a floor in New York with people going about their multitude of activities. I repeated the work for the next few days, with less dramatic responses but still with a sense of releasing old tensions and of recognizing all that is stored in hips and thighs" (Olsen, 1991, p. 93).

Transformative Elements and Conditions in Authentic Movement: Creating a "Safe Enough" Container

Andrea begins her teaching by creating a "safe enough" learning environment. This enables her students to "get comfortable in their bodies so they can start to recognize how much is going on, how much intrinsic wisdom there is available." Andrea made the point that her work as an artist and teacher who trains dancers shifts the role of the witness somewhat. Instead of acting as the primary "container" or therapist for her students' discoveries, she acts instead as a facilitator, inviting them to transfer this energy onto their own creative work or to their visions of themselves as artists.

When I asked her what key elements she felt facilitated the process of transformation in the practice, she named five:

1 Establishing the safety of the environment—including the participants, the facilitator, and the place. This is essential so that each person's nervous system gradually can relax its protective role.
2 Shifting attitudes about the body toward "intrinsic intelligence, reinforcing that the body has much to teach us if we learn to listen. This includes articulating the possibility for three layers of experience that often arise through movement (as identified by Janet Adler): a) the physical, including personal story, b) the collective or group story, and c) transpersonal or archetypal elements. The process is nonhierarchical, emphasizing that all three levels play equal and important roles."
3 "Getting familiar with the perceptual system through which the body experiences and expresses itself—how it senses, how it perceives and interprets, how it responds to information and reports back to community." It helps to understand our own perceptual orientation as well, establishing the dialogue between the thinking, emotional, physical, intuitive, and spiritual aspects of the self.
4 Learning to phrase relationship in a way that is "positive and interactive, rather than oppositional. This helps the group understand that each person is unique and part of the whole."
5 Valuing the experience; "holding" the material respectfully without judgment.

Andrea fleshed the process out further, speaking about the importance of "engaging and negotiating mystery." At first, the process can feel "delightful and scary," yet "becoming familiar with fear" is an integral part of the process; practicing being comfortable with mystery.

"You're teaching people that you need a container to go where you've never gone before. The point is not that it's better to explore new depths, but what kind of support do you need to practice going into the unknown and coming back? In terms of allowing transformational experience, Authentic Movement practice trusts that your body will only go as far as you're safe going. But Authentic Movement teaches us about other dimensions. Time becomes its own reality. It's not about clock time; it's about dimensional time. And for students who are driven by the clock, it's a broadening perception: that there are ways to be guided beyond the cultural norm.

"One of the lessons in Authentic Movement for me is that things are unfolding all the time … The psyche knows how long you have in each session, and it takes you to a certain place. And that's as far as you can go. As you become familiar with this process, you begin understanding how the psyche works."

In this way, Authentic Movement provides a model for relationship—"ground rules" for how to live with oneself, with others, and in the culture. Andrea compared the climate established for facilitating deep work in Authentic Movement with the elements in churches that provide containment.

"In silent prayer, you are having a conversation. As you engage the process of individuation you realize that that conversation is with yourself, in relation to a larger entity or energy or sense of wholeness. I think that the church as a container satisfies the need to feel you are a participant in something beyond yourself most spectacularly through the space ... it's a space that's bigger than you. Music is bigger than you. Community is bigger than you."

Alternatives to Hierarchy

Andrea emphasizes the inherent political element in Authentic Movement that empowers individuals to come to know themselves and to trust their inherent body wisdom as an essential guide in their lives. It also offers an alternative to our current model of how thinking occurs, which places the head above all other parts of the body.

"Teaching asymmetrical movement, for example, in which no part of your body takes priority over any other, allows people to begin experiencing themselves in nonhierarchical ways. Valuing every body part equally shifts the paradigm from dominance to inclusiveness."

Andrea highlights the importance of the creative imagination in the process. "The creative imagination is integrative—it's the one place where you have access to all aspects of knowing. So if there were a visual image [of this process], maybe the creative imagination would be in the center—it brings you access to science, to the natural world, to relationship, to family, to ... It's the place where I experience the connection between all the different components. And that's where I put Authentic Movement in my life. As a creative resource. I go there to find truth. In writing, I say something, then close my eyes and move. Sometimes my body has an entirely different opinion about what I just said. It comes to me when I close my eyes, and it's very clear. It's a checking ground for my conscious experience. But part of that's based on knowing, as a teacher of anatomy, that the body is recording much more than we can be aware of at any moment—experience is larger than our conscious awareness."

Andrea's Jungian dreamwork taught her a good deal about the role of the unconscious and the role of the shadow, as well as teaching about the characteristics of Jung's psychological types—thinking, feeling, intuition, and sensation. She underscored the impact Authentic Movement practice can have in equalizing or dismantling the hierarchical ways of thinking inherent in much of our educational system. Coming to value different perceptual and learning styles has a direct impact on how we treat ourselves and others.

"For many dancers, it's a relief to realize that if you happen to be a feeling type, and can't articulate clearly, it does not mean that you're 'less than' the thinking type who can be very clear, very fast, and recognize overall form. In dance, the sensate person is often the stronger, more physically expressive dancer, but they may not be able to articulate experience. In contrast, the intuitive dancer perhaps can't remember the movement, yet there's a rich improvisational quality. So Authentic

Movement is an avenue for valuing different strengths of moving and perceiving movement.

"Another way that Authentic Movement challenges these hierarchies is to reveal that every person has a complex interesting story. So there's nothing 'special' about being a choreographer, except that you give form to the experience … And that's one place where the hierarchy dissolves. You become more comfortable with the ordinary and the extraordinary in yourself.

"Another equalizing element is the sharing of power as mover or witness. You realize that they are the same at some point, and that we each contribute to the picture at the moment. Someone has to be still for someone else to be wild, and you will change roles eventually. And that's transformative because it provides a different model of community."

Will and Surrender

"What I find in academic institutions, where the thinking mind dominates, is the profound fear of letting go of control," observed Andrea. "There's a surrender required with Authentic Movement that I think happens in many different layers through your advancing years." Andrea quotes her friend, the late Nancy Stark Smith, one of the early founders of Contact Improvisation, who says, "Replace fear with curiosity."

"The fundamental first step in the process is called 'bonding with gravity' in human developmental terms. A healthy baby bonds with ground by releasing weight to be held, with air on the first breath, and with mother by touch and nourishment on the first suckling. We have to release our weight down to lift the head up or have support for a reach or a step. Humans require connection to air, earth, and nourishment for survival, as well as touch, movement, and community.

"When you ask college students to relax their weight into the floor without doing anything—without protecting anything, without being smart or in control—you are saying they are enough simply as they are. It's like relearning a state of being. I experienced it myself after years of ballet. I didn't know how to let my weight release, because I had spent years lifting up, leaping off, creating an illusion of lightness. Reestablishing relationship to gravity and to weight is important.

"Another element is recognizing the role of the mind: starting to differentiate all of the different voices that are inside you offering information, judgment, advice, and confusing chatter. Once you get to know the terrain of your mind, you become less fearful.

"It's the same process with emotions. Closing your eyes, you may feel nausea and fear. You learn to recognize the role of the emotions: 'Oh, that's fear. That's what fear feels like.' 'Oh, this is what sexuality feels like.' 'This is what calmness feels like. I don't have to do anything except notice.' Just getting familiar with these layers is essential education, reeducation, similar to that offered in meditation."

Development of the Inner Masculine

Paradoxically, the development of a healthy "inner man" or *animus*, as Jung referred to this part of a woman's psyche, brings necessary support to the unfolding of her feminine sense of self or ego identification. Through the process, images of the masculine shift from a critical stance to a more open one, a transformation that gradually occurs both inwardly and in outer relationships. Andrea's struggle with this balance began early in life, as her strong bond with her father and rejection of many of her mother's values attracted her to the masculine elements in ballet.

Voyage

In my years of studying dance, I was always told that ballet is the epitome of femininity. The youthful sylph; the spiritual essence. In my own experience, ballet was the closest I could get to experiencing myself as a male in the world. The rigorous training, the concentration and competitive drive, the physicality and sweat gave me independence and distance from traditional girl responsibilities. I watched my father, as a watercolor painter, at his desk, focused for hours on his work. I went to ballet class daily after school and was required to focus equally as hard; school never provided that challenge. I was away from my small community, in the city, in the world alone, dealing with the challenges of mastering the body. And the occasional experience when the music and the dancing flowed together, moving the body by forces I never knew existed, felt like religion to me. Obviously, it was an escape as well as a goal. My image was not to be a dancer, not to be feminine, it was to be free.

(Olsen, 1991, p. 141)

While sitting in the office at Thorne's Gallery, Northampton, following *Our Fathers' Daughters* rehearsal, Andrea told me that her travels to Asia began following her breakup with her previous partner and colleague of thirteen years. Though enormously creative, their relationship had become painful and had broken up many years back when their artistic paths diverged, a separation that she said was partly made possible by the direct and practical style of the Freudian analyst she was seeing at that time.

In her early days as a professional dancer, when she would perform new work, she often would dream of a large, threatening man who would come on his raging horse and want to kill her. Her work in analysis had helped her recognize the power of her own *animus*, bringing more of her feminine self in at these times. Eventually, Andrea was able to develop and rally more of her own positive inner masculine energy, taking the risk to marry Steve and buy a house in Vermont. Years of practicing Authentic Movement helped deepen her capacity for intimacy. "I've also gotten more connection to the natural world by partnering. He's taken me further into nature than I would go myself—long wilderness trips; I was never willing to do these solo. He went to the woods the way I went to ballet school—to find meaning."

Body Symptoms, Illness, and Healing

Injury and depression can be the shadow side of the dancer. Andrea tells the story about how she found that she "just wanted to lie around on the floor" when she began to do Authentic Movement. As a dancer she first thought this meant that she was in the wrong profession, but then soon realized that she was simply exhausted from her high-pressured rehearsal and performing schedule. Once she could admit this, she was able to move on, discovering micro-movements that were alive in her body. These pointed the way toward more natural movement that wanted to emerge.

"Many dancers exhaust their bodies. In those days, I had an injury—numbness passing through my body that started with my right arm, which is related to control. And then it traveled through my body, and my leg went numb. I was performing, trying to land from leaps without being able to feel the floor. I was doing Jungian dream work at the time, and it was also pretty clear that I didn't 'have a leg to stand on' emotionally, and that I was numb in my relationship.

"Authentic Movement gives you a place to move in ways that allow healing. You can't express it in the outer world, but you've got all these micro-movements that are about releasing the pattern. Working with that injury was the first time I found that the body does know how to unwind places where the nerves are damaged or restricted from tension. If you just attend, the body will find stretches or movements that are very hard to get at through exercise. Bodywork techniques like Trager, Feldenkrais, and cranial sacral work are similar, but in Authentic Movement the motions come up naturally, on their own."

This point has larger cultural implications as well.

"Many people in our culture are exhausted in their autonomic nervous systems. We're constantly in the somatic, the outer, the conscious—while simultaneously on guard (protecting ourselves) through the sympathetic portion of the autonomic nervous systems. And we exhaust our resources. The digestive, integrative part of our bodies, the parasympathetic division of the autonomic nervous system, needs support. ... Physical therapists that I've talked to affirm that often what they do first in a session is calm down the sympathetic nervous system, which is locked into the fight, flight, freeze, friendly 'action' response. Authentic Movement offers tremendous rest for the body, and in that way, it's inherently healing—offering a balance to our culture."

Ancient Fish Patterns: Changes in the Body

As we get to know and value the body and its dimensions, and continue to differentiate how the layers of the self interact, transformation becomes more possible.

"For most people I've witnessed, the body gets clearer in its neurological pathways, movement gets more efficient, both in life and in Authentic Movement. It's something I call a house-cleaning effect. Old scored memories, traumas, attitudes, conflicts ... a lot of cleaning and clearing and simplifying happens simply by giving attention to your moving body."

In her own case as a ballerina, Andrea had a very tight lower back. "My ribs were stuck out. I did Rolfing, massage, different kinds of analysis. Once I started doing Authentic Movement the emotional work cleared out some of the patterns."

As a thinking type, exploring and expressing emotions had not come easily to her. "I didn't have a lot of places to explore that track in my own life ... But Authentic Movement gave me a place for some of the emotional history to come up. I remember feeling every vertebra of my spine moving for the first time. Very deep, ancient fish patterns and reflexive nervous system patterns that are under my ballet training came back. They just come. You find yourself doing wave movement or rolling in ways where the whole spine spirals. I did a headstand for the first time, even though I'd never been able to do that before. If someone told me in a class to spiral my spine, or stand on my head, I would force it with big muscle work. In Authentic Movement, it simply emerges, supported by archetypal, human developmental, or evolutionary patterns. Now my body is quite efficient. And teachers will say, 'Your iliopsoas is so clear, how did you ever do that?' It wasn't from dance technique. It was from Authentic Movement—with patterns getting simpler and clearer and cleaner in my body."

Student Case Example

Andrea's background in anatomy and dance informs the healing she facilitates through Authentic Movement. Here, she reiterates that "part of what's transformative has to do with becoming comfortable with fear itself. Shifting your relationship to fear produces change."

"For example, I have a student who was in a very serious car accident—almost severed her spinal cord. But now she's back dancing. When she begins the Authentic Movement work, she goes right into the pattern of the accident. She has no intention of going into that but her body goes right for it. And, generally in my experience people only go as far as they can go safely, but with her it's almost to the point of freezing in that pattern of the moment of almost death ... But as she becomes comfortable with going into the state and surviving it, she's able to go into that place of tremendous fear and start healing. I move with her sometimes now. I don't leave her alone in it much because it's too hard. And the healing is at the physical level as well as the psychological level—but there really are nerves that are still caught in trauma. The nice thing about the nervous system is that once a pattern is introduced, it's there. Then the body has two choices instantly. And so by working—revisiting this place—through conscious touch I can help her out of the trauma pattern. There's a lot of twitching and jumps where the trauma's directly being released from the body, and the movement starts to happen in a different way.

"Then specific images come back, like the moment that she hit the ceiling. Little flashes of memory. So this is an example of becoming comfortable with that state of fear, and how close you can go into it. My basic line on Authentic Movement is always, 'You don't have to do anything hard. Don't push into areas that are difficult.' But Authentic Movement offers a place where you can experiment with your relationship to fear that's safe. And every time that this woman and I have worked together there's change happening."

Personal Transformative Experience: Finding One's Voice

Though not "injury prone," voice has been a big challenge for Andrea, manifesting in numerous sore throats. She describes how she has spent a lot of time in Authentic Movement "trying to undercut the tendency to go into throat-raging coughs. Often if something is coming up, it just goes into my throat and into a cough. And I know it's psychological. So how do I work with that in Authentic Movement?" Her explorations have taught her repeatedly that the issues are about speaking, "about articulating honestly, without having to be in pain." She recalled a time when she moved in relationship to a powerful image of Joan of Arc burning at the stake.

Burned at the Stake

"This had something to do with my voice. Mouth, tongue, being killed for speaking. Being killed for having any vision that isn't the cultural one. It was not an intellectual experience at the time. I remember the mouth stretching wide, and an image of being burned, and the feeling of how dangerous it is—at a very deep level—to speak one's truth. That was the beginning of my writing, before *Bodystories* [her first book]. Once I experienced the 'burning at the stake' movement sequence in Authentic Movement, it was totally done. It wasn't anything I ever needed to repeat. Or to make a dance about. Or even to say out loud. … But I think what was meaningful was simply recognizing the actual danger of speaking, after a whole life as a young woman going through the educational systems saying 'all the right things.' I had fever blisters on my lips a lot. And then went into dance where you don't have to speak."

There were also some other inner figures that she began to incorporate into her performances—Little Red Riding Hood, a little girl sitting on a bench struggling with whether a black ball or seed was trying to go into her mouth or out, blocking her speech, or opening her voice. And a transitional figure, a Chinese woman, who sang in an "ancient distant voice," who was the first one to bring voice into what had previously been exclusively kinesthetic dances. Following these Authentic Movement explorations Andrea began to incorporate voice into her performances, and now moves with fluidity from movement to word.

"Certainly the voice is still coming, but it's changed from that almost strangled distant female to a very present, open air quality. As I'm becoming familiar with these particular characters, they're teaching me … I feel like they're growing in me. They were calls for attention and change. As I got more familiar with my own voice and my own writings as a woman, different images were allowed to emerge.

Paying attention allows change. In my life and work in Authentic Movement I can see a progression. Now I sing clear, strong tones and overtones."

Calling for the Nourishing Mother

Another powerful early image that had come in Andrea's Authentic Movement was the image of a hungry little bird and how starved she felt "in her mother's kitchen—the place of the feminine. Thirteen years later, I still put my head back and stretched my mouth open the way I did in the performance of *In My House* in 1986," she observed. "Now it's filled with all sorts of new dimensions, but it's the same image of either a starving or singing female. So the image grows with me." For Andrea, this movement pattern is accompanied by a mixture of celebration and grief.

"It's clear that the mother image is the one that I've put aside the longest. The movement that came was a baby bird waiting in a nest: 'Feed me, feed me, feed me …' I was starving for nourishment in the female place. This was the only movement image that came in the kitchen, in the womb of the house. And then I'd leave it in performance. With it comes a sense of emptiness—a hole in the psyche which makes me feel I want or need something—an incompleteness personal or female?

"Authentic Movement is a lifelong process. This year, when my mother suffered a dangerous stroke, I could hardly breathe. I didn't want to take in the news, to absorb it in my body, cell by cell. I felt the many ways I've been supported by her breath all these years. I touched her hand, caressed her cheek. As my mother's animus softens, I come closer. From her hospital bed, she looks directly in my eyes and says, 'I just wanted you to be your own original self.' She waves and adds, 'Parting is such sweet sorrow.' In Authentic Movement, my fingers wipe across my eyes, clearing my vision; a man in our group presses his hand into my back, then rolls over my body and down between my legs, birthed and free. Some part of myself has shifted in the process of seeing and being seen."

Shadow Dances and the Development of the Inferior Function

Andrea spoke of the capacities that can be developed through the practice of moving and witnessing.

As we begin Authentic Movement we may face basic fears: hatred of our body, fear of being empty inside, fear of stillness, fear of being alone, fear of not being loved. 'I'm too fat, I'm too thin. If I'm not moving, I don't exist. If I'm not seen, I'm nobody. If I don't do something good, nobody will love me.' Although these statements may seem harsh, they occur again and again in movement sessions. As we close our eyes and listen to our bodies, there is also the potential of accepting ourselves just as we are. (Olsen, 1993, p. 48)

As we replace fear with open waiting, we can learn how rich our inner world really is ... Generally we push into the unconscious what we consider to be negative—our sadness, our meanness, our fear. But below that layer of unexpressed movement is the wealth of human experience. That is the resource from which we draw in Authentic Movement and which we hope to bring to the stage [... and to life].

(Olsen, 1993, p. 48)

Can we trust ourselves? In personal/developmental work we have to know that a process of change can and will be supported. For example, if a difficult memory from childhood emerges in a movement session, the mover needs to trust that she has the resources and will take the time to integrate the experience into conscious awareness. Otherwise it is more appropriate for the memory to remain unconscious. By internalizing a nonjudgmental but discerning inner witness, we develop self-trust at a deep level.

(Olsen, 1993, p. 49)

As each person follows her own impulses, no one is 'responsible' for taking care of anyone else. [This is often a relief for women, who are generally trained to take care of others at the expense of their own needs. We don't have to be polite or nice.] We long to be seen for who we are in our totality, not for the limited view of who we present ourselves to be, or who others want us to be. The practice of Authentic Movement is the practice of being true to who we are in the presence of others.

(Olsen, 1993, p. 50)

As a thinking type, Andrea has also been helped by Authentic Movement to develop a more conscious relationship to her feeling function. "In my own early work with Authentic Movement, I felt that the practice gave me the emotional subtext for a dance. I could develop it any way I wanted, but the emotional and structural clarity had been established within me" (Olsen, 1993, p. 51). This in turn shifted what she was able to bring to her movers as a witness. Currently, the women in her groups are increasingly interested in their inner life and Andrea is leaving more time for emotional sharing and processing following the movement experience.

The Role of Community and Stages in the Transformative Experience

Andrea sees Authentic Movement as containing elements of the shaman's journey.

"I've always viewed performance as a shamanic activity: going back into an unknown place, bringing back what I've found, and sharing it with the community. Similarly, for me, Authentic Movement is about engaging mystery, following the movement as it unfolds, and reporting back to the witness and sharing within community through creative form. It isn't just about the individual, it's about how everything connects. It doesn't matter how far we go individually, if we can't bring back our findings."

This involves giving the energies you've awakened a shape and a place in the world—a sequence that also seems to reflect classic elements in the Buddha's story, Christ's experience in the desert, stories from other religious figures, and Native American vision quests.

"Your task is to do what you have to do as well as you can—as thoroughly as you can possibly do it—and hope that there's some piece of it that connects to others, because you can't intend to help other people. In my life, I've always used performance as the place where I embody what I've been working on before I can live it in life."

After decades of Authentic Movement practice, Andrea's focus as an artist is not in "trying to push for the high-end of critical attention, pushing to 'make it,' but rather intuiting how much the work itself can handle. This involves developing a heightened sensitivity, staying in close resonance with the integrity of the form that is being embodied rather than trying to perform for an outer, disembodied perfectionistic standard. Relationship is key: Authentic Movement points to a process of recognition between mover and witness, performer and audience. As we feel seen, we can see. As we feel heard, we can begin to hear others. As we develop an articulate and supportive inner witness, we can allow others their own experience of moving and being moved. The process of listening to the movement stories of our body encourages us to know ourselves and to bring this awareness to performance" (Olsen, 1993, p. 53).

Development of Feminine Ways of Knowing

Authentic Movement has assisted Andrea in forming, exploring, and nurturing relationships that are tremendously intimate, although she points out that they don't necessarily carry over into the verbal, social world. She credits Authentic Movement as providing a real education in intimacy whose depth and quality "make life feel like it's okay." Humility is also developed in this practice, especially for dancers who have specialized training, in recognizing that "everyone has a story. Everyone has beautiful movements." In fact, she points out how sad it is that we've separated out "the dancers" from the "non-dancers."

Overall, the practice gives her "a deep respect for humanity that [she] doesn't find elsewhere." Andrea also spoke about how her work in the academic world involves compromise. "Working responsibly in institutions requires an enormous amount of energy." She does, however, feel that "ethically I can stand behind my work, which is about recognizing the many ways our attitudes about our bodies affect our relationship to the Earth.

"Authentic Movement is transformational because you realize that your body represents a much larger schemata of life. You are not just your 'little processes.'

You engage the intelligence of your body—not through language, but through experience."

Dance, art, science, spirituality, embodied wisdom, and ecology continue to inform Andrea's practice and daily life. Whether spending relaxed time with her in conversation, or witnessing her on the dance floor, her pioneering gifts have an inspired, integrative effect. As Martha Graham said, "The body says what words cannot. Dance is the hidden language of the soul" (Graham, 1985/2002, p. 2734).

References

Graham, M. (2002). Martha Graham reflects on her art and a life in dance. Republished in *The New York Times Guide to the Arts of the 20th Century*. (Original work published March 31, 1985.)

Olsen, A. J. (in collaboration with McHose, C.). (1991). *Bodystories: A guide to experiential anatomy*. Station Hill Press.

Olsen, A. J. (1993, Winter/Spring). Being seen, being moved: Authentic Movement and performance. *Contact Quarterly, 18*(1), 46–53.

Chapter 11

Teaching Active Imagination in Movement

with Neala Haze

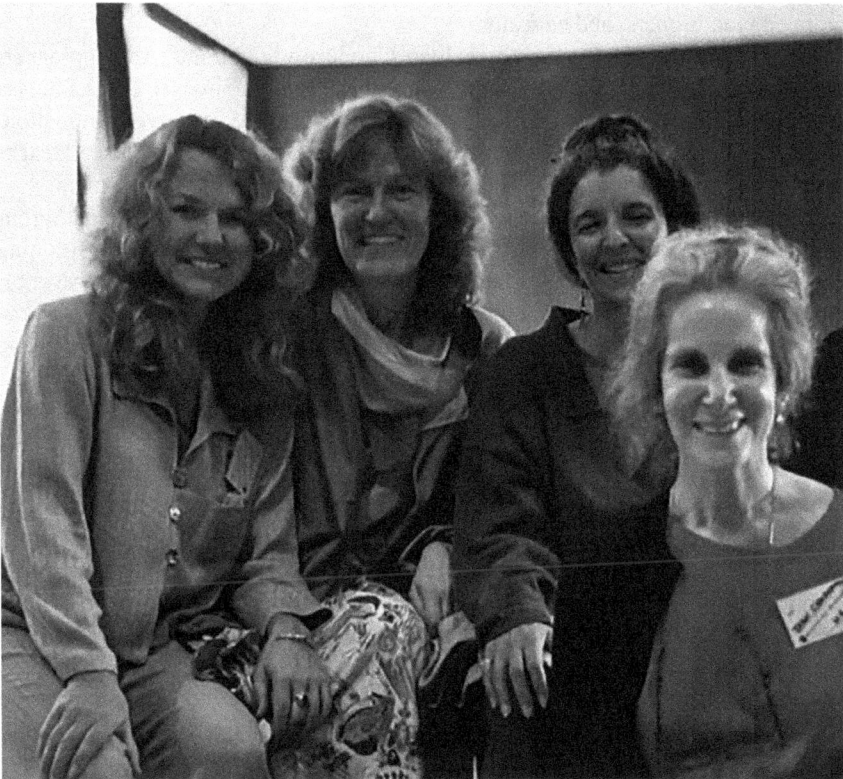

Figure 11.1 Tina Stromsted, Neala Haze, Janet Adler, & Joan Chodorow. First International Dance/Movement Therapy Conference, Berlin, Germany 1994. Photo courtesy of Maria Luise Oberem.

DOI: 10.4324/9781003538356-15

Authentic Movement is grounded in the idea that the mind and body are inseparable. In 1993, Neala Haze and I co-founded the Authentic Movement Institute (AMI) in Berkeley, California, to explore the connection between psyche and soma, engaging life's primary experiences as the foundation for our investigations. The Institute (1993–2004) offered an innovative curriculum that combined experiential and theoretical learning, exploring the interplay of creative, psychological, and sacred dimensions through the unique body-based process of Authentic Movement. Over three-year training programs, Neala Haze and I further developed and presented the fundamental elements of Authentic Movement, applying these concepts to psychotherapy, artistic endeavors, embodied spiritual practices, and the enhancement of daily life. The training included theoretical seminars, ongoing group movement sessions, supervision, peer practice sessions, personal exploration through external analysis and psychotherapy, and workshops tailored for therapists, artists, body-oriented practitioners, and educators.

Joined by core faculty members Joan Chodorow and Janet Adler, pioneering teachers of Authentic Movement, we invited Jungian analyst Louis Stewart (1986) as a faculty member, who contributed his expertise in active imagination, affect theory, and play therapy. Senior practitioners, authors, and respected teachers in the field, all contributed to the teaching and curriculum development.

In later years, we were joined by senior dance/movement therapist Linda Aaron-Cort, and Lysa Castro, an AMI graduate and Body Tales teacher. As the training expanded, we invited several guest teachers to share their expertise in ecopsychology, choreography, and performance. We further refined practice elements for various clinical populations, including breast cancer survivors and psychiatric patients. Techniques were also adapted for professionals interested in integrating core aspects into their work. This included analysts, psychotherapists, educators, medical professionals, bodyworkers, spiritual practitioners, graduate students, artists, ecopsychologists, choreographers, performers, and social activists.

Neala brought her experience in dance/movement therapy and elements from her background in Eastern thought, humanistic psychology, and creative, body-based healing methods. My work focused on Jungian psychology, essential practice skills, clinical applications, dreams in movement, elements derived from Arnold Mindell's Process-Oriented Psychology (Mindell, 1985), Marion Woodman's contributions, and the creative arts therapies. Together, core faculty and guest teachers enhanced the richness, depth, and integration of our curriculum and practice.

The Institute was not just a place to teach but a unique environment where we all learned so much from each other as we continued to develop and deepen the practice, becoming a creative hub for Authentic Movement in our local and international community.

In this chapter, Neala and I reflect on our theoretical framework, share examples of our multi-modal approach, and discuss the dyad practice—the essential "ground" from which our work begins, expands, and returns. We also offer resources for consideration when teaching Authentic Movement.

The Dyad: The Road In

"Inherent in being a person in the cultures of the West, is longing for a witness. We seem to want, deeply want, to be seen as we are by another" (Adler, 1987/1999a, p. 158). Authentic Movement recapitulates our first primary relationship in which being seen is inherent: the dyad of a mover (child/client) and a witness (mother [or caretaker, throughout this chapter]/therapist). The practice provides an explicit and secure space to explore "all that impedes us from our growth and wholeness but also all that can serve to heal the wounds, bring us to balance, transform inner relationships, and direct us on our unique life journeys" (Lewis, 1993, p. 3). In the process, learners develop skills such as listening, observation, reflection, and empathy; identify interpersonal themes, boundaries, and group dynamics; and acquire an understanding of the creative process and the multi-modal method of active imagination.

The first step in teaching is to introduce beginning movers to the fundamental elements of Authentic Movement that have therapeutic value and support safe practice. A basic tenet is that there isn't a "right" or "wrong" way to move. Some instructions are practical. For instance, even though most movement is done with the eyes closed, if a mover needs to move quickly or suddenly, it is important that they open their eyes for safety. Other guidelines have a psychological and developmental basis. For example, during the interaction following a movement session, both mover and witness learn to use self-referencing language as a means to distinguish self and other, inner and outer experience. In Chapter 12, I discuss the guidelines for working in groups in more detail.

Authentic Movement assumes all participants' equality, valuing the diverse experiences and perspectives of each (and when referring to the mover or witness as "she," I include men, women, and nonbinary individuals). The practice also encourages the simultaneous presence of the observing self and the preverbal and unconscious self and acknowledges the inner authority and interdependency of all participants. According to psychoanalyst Michael Balint, the aim is that the participant

> should be able to find himself, to accept himself, and to get on with himself, knowing all the time that there is a scar in himself, his basic fault, which cannot be "analyzed" out of existence; moreover, he must be allowed to discover his way to the world of objects [inner figures] and not be shown the "right" way by some profound or correct interpretation.
>
> (Balint, 1986, p. 280)

The process of recapitulation in Authentic Movement begins with a mover in a studio in the center of the space and a witness who sits to the side and watches their unfolding movement. One of the essential means of freeing the unconscious is for the mover to begin with closed eyes, turning their attention inward. In this receptive attitude of waiting, they stay alert for a sensation, feeling, image, mood, or an inner impulse to move.

The trainings at AMI took place in a lovely dance studio—a warm, clear space with a sprung wood floor for ease on the body and skylights for natural light and privacy. As the work began, we secured the door to the studio to prevent intrusions from outside and to create the experience of a safe and protected space.

Looking around the studio and exploring the surrounding space are important ways for movers to establish a sense of familiarity and safety before beginning the process, an orienting practice psychologist and neuroscientist Stephen Porges later described in his Polyvagal research (Porges, 2011, pp. 195–196; Porges, 2017, pp. 235–237).

The witness/leader may then suggest a structured activity that prepares the body for movement, including working with what Jung called "starting points" in the active imagination process (Jung, 1916/1958, CW 8, para. 167). Mary Whitehouse later adapted these to movement themes that explored polarities in the physical body and the personality such as open and closed, up and down, right and left, contracting and expanding the body, movements of assertion and surrender, stretching and rotating the joints (Whitehouse, 1979/1999b, pp. 79–83). Once they have had an opportunity to warm up and explore a starting point, movers are invited to close their eyes and continue their investigations, releasing the movement theme when spontaneous movement begins to emerge in a natural way from within. In this way the mover learns to experience the "difference between movement that is directed by the ego ('I am moving') and movement that comes from the unconscious ('I am being moved')" (Whitehouse, 1958/1999a, p. 43; 1979/1999b, p. 82). Exploring this differentiation remains central to the practice of Authentic Movement.

By closing her eyes, the mover embarks on a potentially transformative journey. Eliminating external visual information, she can begin to quiet the busy, controlling mind and focus on more primary stimuli. Softening her ego's grasp on the daily world, she connects to her embodied experience, past and present. As the mover surrenders to her inner experience, she is listening to and allowing herself to be moved by something greater than her sense of self. She does so in the presence of the group leader as witness, or within a group of movers and witnesses. For some, regression may occur as the physical action shifts from *distally initiated movement* (from the limbs) into *proximal sensing* (nearer the core of the body).

Closing the eyes facilitates a deep sensing experience, which can reach into the body's cellular intelligence and evoke imagery, emotion, body sensation, memory, and dreams. The conscious mind can take an active interest in and become receptive to the knowledge stored in the body. Chodorow, an expert in affect theory and active imagination, describes the process:

As the brain begins to receive an ongoing but diminished flow of sensory input, it may begin to create its own internal experience through increasingly vivid imagery and, at times, body image distortion. Such navigation through the nonrational world of the unconscious can facilitate profoundly important insights and new levels of integration for people who have already developed a strong ego position.

(1977/1999, p. 238)

Personal associations, stories, and, for some, mythic journeys arise in movement, sound, touch, and smell, sometimes even recapitulating birth experiences or other life passages where impasses occurred. Movers can physically re-experience and apprehend their past and present, bringing about more integrative healing. Meanwhile, "the body, which allows the impulse to manifest itself, remains firmly rooted in the fact of its own existence" (Chodorow, 1977/1999, p. 246).

"Dahlia", a student new to the practice, described her experience:

As I step into the movement space, I want to be brave. But my body is stiff, made of wood. The image of a warrior comes to mind; the "me" I have been. My forehead is crunched, my hands are in fists, and my jaw is tight. I am ready for battle. Though now I realize I must sheath my sword, lower my shield, shed my armor, and loosen the grip that chokes and binds me.

Walking toward the window, I close my eyes, feel the warm sun, and gently lower myself to the floor.

Wrapping my arms around my knees, I wait for an eternity until a recent scene from a dream reemerges, plunging me into darkness and a torrent of waves. Overcome with fear, I cling on desperately, only to realize that I must let go—something I don't know how to do. I practice the movement warm-up Tina guided us through—contracting and expanding, breathing deeply, and exhaling fully—until I finally feel my muscles and throat relax. Slowly, I release my weight into the support of the warm, wooden floor beneath my frightened body.

Unseen eyes watch as I wash past shrouded figures.

Am I cleansed? Pardoned? Banished? Ridiculed? Celebrated? Forgotten? Suddenly, I am free-falling into a brilliant light. The sky opens, and I splash into a breathtaking blue-green pool held in a floating copper-lined basin—colors I love, now cradling me far above an unknown planet. I dissolve, preparing to reconnect with what calls me to rise and be reborn.

I will need more time, but there is no rush. This practice connects me to my soul, the spirit of my ancestors, and the heartbeat of the world. I cry out and hear the sound of my voice for the first time.

As I open my eyes, I see witnesses holding space for me, their eyes soft. One puts her hand over her heart and smiles. I smile back, feeling welcomed into this new world.

Reflecting on her experience in her journal, Dahlia wrote:

I have felt like a person adrift at sea, valiantly trying to row my boat without the guidance and wisdom of my body. Traumatic experiences at a young age instilled a deep mistrust of my body and emotions, which became sources of shame and humiliation. Instead of risking punishment, I squeezed my brain and learned to rely on my intellect for trusted guidance, silencing and dismissing the voice of my body and its messages from my unconscious.

Now, some deep undercurrents are propelling me forward, urging me to step into this rowboat and set off from shore—a sacred journey. In this circle of movers and witnesses, I am beginning to trust that I can find new land—a place to be, maybe even a place to belong.

Says Jungian analyst Marion Woodman, "Good sailors ... build their ego strong enough to ride with the power of the wind and wave. And that ego can only be strong enough if it is supported by the wisdom of the body whose messages are directly in touch with the instincts" (Woodman, 1983, p. 16).

Yet, understanding does not come solely through self-awareness. It also emerges through the act of nonjudgmental "seeing" by the witness. The witness provides both a receptive mirror through quietly holding presence and space, and an active mirror through verbal response, playing a crucial role in the mover's journey.

To be mirrored is to be understood, to feel that someone empathetically follows our thoughts, feelings, and experiences. Yet to mirror another person requires a willingness to enter into his or her world, to suspend critical judgment and reflect what is being offered. The need for mirroring from another is lifelong.

(Schwartz-Salant, 1982, pp. 45–46)

While the mover's task is to allow her inner content to have expression, the witness's role is to accept the mover without critical analysis or direction and to speak only when the mover asks for a response. Her task is to bring a receptive quality of clear attention to her observation of the mover (Adler, personal communication). Janet Adler writes:

The witness practices the art of seeing. Seeing clearly is not about knowing what the mover needs or must do. The witness does not "look at" the mover, but instead, as she internalizes the mover, she attends to her own experiences of judgment, interpretation, and projection, in response to the mover as catalyst.

(1994/1999, p. 194)

As they learn to identify and contain their own experience and biases, movers and witnesses employ certain protocols, including a linguistic framework, to assist them in the challenging task of differentiating clear perception from projection. "Percept language," as developed by John Weir, one of the pioneers in the Human Potential Movement with whom Janet Adler studied, is a speaking practice she integrated into Authentic Movement as part of that protocol (Adler, cited in Haze & Stromsted, 1994/1999, p. 114). Its purpose is the creation of language that is neither judgmental nor interpretive. Witnesses make "I" statements that locate the perceptions (and the feelings that accompany them) in the speaker rather than in external objects (the movers). For example, a witness would say, "I felt full of sorrow watching the slow shuffling movements of your feet," rather than "you were full of sorrow when you made those slow shuffling movements with your feet."

The mutual intent to utilize percept language fosters an environment or "container" of trust and safety as it is an effective tool in working with projective material. The process is infinitely valuable and personally challenging for both the mover and the witness. Together, they can achieve a level of perception of self and others that evokes deep respect, empathy, and compassion for our humanity (Haze, 1994, p. 104).

Theoretical Framework

Movers and witnesses bring to Authentic Movement their whole being—mind and body, personal history, persona, sexual orientation, family of origin, culture, age, and race. With their ancestral lineage, they come as a member of society within the larger context of the historical and cultural evolution of the world.

At AMI, to better understand and hold this wide diversity of human experience, we drew on Jungian analyst Joseph Henderson's theory concerning the cultural unconscious for its theoretical frame. Henderson, who furthered Jung's work with his book *Cultural Attitudes in Psychological Perspective* (1984), described five cultural attitudes that singly or together shape an individual's way of seeing and being in the world: the social, the religious (spiritual), the aesthetic (artistic), the philosophic, and the psychological. Typically, one or two of these attitudes dominates the way a person perceives and values experience, although we are born with the potential to activate all five. In Authentic Movement the dominant cultural attitude of a mover shapes the realms they explore and the ways in which those realms are understood. A witness's response is similarly shaped by the cultural attitudes they bring to the act of seeing.

At the Authentic Movement Institute, our aim was to embrace all five perspectives separately or in tandem. We achieved artistic imagination through improvisation, choreography, the visual arts, and visualization. We explored the philosophic through theory, research, ethics, and language. We experienced the social through individual and group interactions with potential applications in clinical and multidisciplinary work. We observed the spiritual dimension through ritual and sacred dance. We embodied the psychological self-reflective function through the exploration of transference/countertransference dynamics, regression, remembering, and dreams. The psychological attitude has the capacity, as Henderson says, "to enrich and profitably modify" the other attitudes by bringing awareness to them (1984, p. 14).

Because of the complexities that arise in bringing awareness to unconscious material, our teaching began with the dyad of mover and witness and the self-reflective psychological attitude. The use of a psychological construct provided a structure for the relationship and a language for addressing elements that frequently emerged between the mover and the witness. This, in turn, allowed beginning movers to identify and work with projection, interpretation, and judgment (Adler, Haze, & Stromsted, personal communication, 1986). As the study and practice progressed, all of the other cultural attitudes came into play, enriching everyone's ways of seeing and experiencing.

Shadow elements arose as well. Memories of loss and grief, brokenness and wound-edness, and the affects of sorrow, joy, startle, shame, anger, fear, curiosity, and inter-est surfaced for mover and witness alike (Chodorow, 1991; Stewart, 1987). Devalued, repressed, or projected onto another, these shadow elements develop when one attitude dominates and another falls into unconsciousness. Exploring this hidden material is a crucial component of the work. As poet Robert Bly writes, "We notice that when sunlight hits the body, the body turns bright, but it throws a shadow, which is dark. The brighter the light, the darker the shadow" (Bly, 1988, p. 7).

Shadow elements often manifest through projection. People bring prior experi-ence to their present circumstances, which may distort or limit their realistic as-sessment of what is happening. Projection is an unconscious emotional response (Freud, 1915/1961; Jung, 1946/1975, CW 16). For example, a person who has had a negative experience of being criticized by a harsh parent may mistake even the gentlest instructor for a harsh critic. At AMI, in the mover witness-dyad and group, we sought to identify the projective filter of old memories that colored experience and worked to establish more accurate responses.

Not only are negative past experiences influential in our integration of what is going on in the moment, but positive memories are also active. These enter into the powerful unconscious bonds that develop in relationships and in the psychotherapeutic realm. It is also important to determine the client/mover's strongest cultural attitude and the response of the therapist/witness to it, given their own dominant cultural attitudes. If, on the one hand, both have the same "attitude," the pair may experience a comfortable sense of agreement. But this comfort can be misleading and create a mood of compla-cency and short-sightedness. On the other hand, if cultural attitudes are too different or unexpressed, participants in the mover/witness-dyad can meet unexpected resistances to each other and engage in mutually negative projections (Henderson, 1984).

This projective phenomenon includes somatic components, which operate pow-erfully in Authentic Movement. Pallaro advocates that "Authentic Movement is fundamental to sorting out and understanding the somatic countertransferential re-sponses" (Pallaro, 1994, p. 11). More specifically, she writes:

> This work enables the witness to separate his/her conscious and unconscious activities and own the inner kinesthetic, somatic or imaginal responses elicited in relationship to the mover. Verbalizations of such experiences by the mover and the witness often help clarify the experience itself for the mover and/or the witness, organizing such experiences into a meaningful framework and estab-lishing a strong "internal witness" [self-reflective consciousness] for both the mover and the witness.
>
> (1994, p. 9)

Our theoretical framework also integrated the concepts of Wilhelm Reich who, in the 1920s, pioneered studies on the body's role in storing emotional conflict, preverbally, in the musculature. He wrote, "The rigidity of the musculature is the somatic side of the process of repression and the basis for its continued existence" (1948, p. 236). Reich found that each character attitude had a corresponding physical attitude and began to work directly on relaxing muscular rigidity or "muscular armoring" in conjunction with his analytic work. He discovered that loosening the muscular armor freed considerable libidinal energy and aided the process of psychoanalysis. As time went on, Reich's psychiatric work increasingly dealt with freeing emotions, such as sadness, anxiety, rage, and pleasure, through work with the body. He found that this led to a far more intense experience of the infantile material uncovered in the analysis (Reich, 1961, pp. 92 and 169–187).

While Reich emphasized the role of muscular armoring, Trudi Schoop, through the healing power of dance and theater, helped complete actions of the body that had been frozen or interrupted through trauma. Schoop, a leading figure in dance therapy for four decades, began her clinical work in 1958 with patients at Camarillo Hospital in Southern California. Her objective was to use "every aspect of movement that will increase the individual's ability to adapt adequately to his environment and to experience himself as a whole, functioning human being" (Schoop, 1974, pp. 157–158).

Reich's and Schoop's concepts became embodied as learners deepened their movement practice. As movers "re-inhabited" themselves, they became aware of the emotional conflicts that existed within the musculature and in all of the cellular structures of the body (Stromsted, 1994/1995; 2001; 2007/1998). Our work at AMI emphasized the importance of this awakening in relationship to each individual's own timing—in peeling off and entering into the layers of their history—personal and transpersonal. In their own time, the mover discovered that it was "the fulfillment of action that makes the link to inner experience" and "throughout is woven the relationship of the body, the imagination and the emotions" (Chodorow, 1991, p. 23). Learners often took their experiences back to their outside analysts and psychotherapists for further exploration and integration.

Polarities: The Tension of Opposites

Polarities exist and are expressed in the body physically, emotionally, and "through the personality, into all the pairs of opposites, including the unconscious and the conscious mind. Life is never either/or but always a paradox of both/and" (Whitehouse, 1979/1999, p. 79). The myriads of pairs are extensive, for example love/hate, right/left, up/down, masculine/feminine, heavy/light, happy/sad, and anxious/peaceful.

Chodorow points out, "If we consciously attend to the simplest body movement, we will experience the interrelationship and interdependency of the opposites" (Chodorow, 1991, p. 12). For example, when a mover extends her arms wide, opening in the chest, her shoulder blades come together, closing in the back. Perhaps she might experience sadness, but slowly, as the motion extends, the feeling may transform into joyful love. Or motion upward may awaken feelings of lightness, hope, spaciousness and independence/confidence or at another time willfulness, rigidity, and aloneness. Moving downward may bring about sensations of feeling heavy, collapsed, and defeated; or alternately of surrendering, descending into herself, accepting the support of the ground, and experiencing her relationship to the earth.

Similarly, in the interpersonal realm, polarities find expression as conflicts that may arise during movement, most notably through touch and sound, that exist on a continuum. At one end of the spectrum are experiences with silence, sighs, and whispers; *proprioception* (the awareness of the body in space); light touch, leaning, and support. At the other end are urgent howls and wrestling. In the midrange are songs, melodies, toning, and gibberish, possibly building into loud vocalization and sounds. In contrast to touch, sound permeates the entire space, which can create tension within the group. Resolution may be negotiated through a variety of creative structures offered by the group leader, for example, experimenting with sound in one round of movement, with silence in another round, and inviting a choice in the third round to discover more about sound and silence.

Touch may occur within the circle, and it is up to movers whether they want to explore and engage in physical contact with each other as it may augment, challenge, or interfere with their experience. Often the leader will invite awareness of this dynamic as it emerges. Tactile exploration, if it occurs in the process of moving to one's own authentic response—for example leaning support, movers interweaving in group clusters, cradling, wrestling, or withdrawing—can create an awareness of patterns in relationship, levels of intimacy, and boundary-making. As touch is physically expressed (or not) and experienced through the body, patterns of contact and resolution of conflict can be more directly explored. What is essential is that learners set concrete limits and exercise individual choice. The choices in the studio regarding the expression of something or the containment of it evoke the dynamic relationship of the internal and external, actor and observer, and become a paradigm for life beyond the studio.

In journaling about her movement, a learner reflects on her experience with touch, which was initially negative.

Moving, I feel my fingertips on my rib cage. I hear another mover approaching me who then begins to touch my face, my hair, my mouth ... I freeze. I am unable to move or speak. My eyes fly open, and I see that it is a man who is touching my mouth. I remember when I was violated as a child. Later, in dialogue, he says, "I was just exploring your face." This was hard to hear, to take in—my stuff is activated. I feel helpless rage and tears. Slowly, over time, through practicing the form I learn how to stop contact, say no, and move away and also how to make contact, savor, touch and take in physical support. This is an enormous learning experience for me.

Before, I used to freeze. No words came, and I wasn't able to move away from the kind of touch I didn't want. Other people's needs overtook me, invading whatever space I had. Through months of work as a mover and witness I've been able to feel body sensations and emotions that weren't available to me before. Now I can create healthy boundaries. What I learned in the studio now permeates my life.

A woman attending an ongoing group comes to the circle and states: "I feel isolated. I want a sense of community and connection, but I feel conflicted because I'm afraid of being judged." After moving with the group for a few times she slowly ventures out and comes into contact.

> *My back lightly touches someone. I sit very still. I want so much to be held; I want her to touch my hair. Will she? I tentatively want ... I feel her torso move close against my back. I lean into her and begin to cry. I hate crying but her body feels so good. This other mover is strong. We begin to rock together. I feel safe, taken care of. I feel nurtured through the touch. We stay this way for a long time, and memories of my mother come back to me. She died when I was so young. Tears flow down my cheeks, and I begin to sob. My mover holds me and holds me, humming and rocking. Slowly I quiet. I melt into the mover's body, exhausted. Two days after this experience I write: "Thank you mover, group, Authentic Movement ... God. I found a piece of myself. I was held, I am held in community. I feel so seen."*

Movers can say "yes" or "no" to touch, and can move away or toward one another. Thus, we see how these polarities of "not wanting" or "wanting" touch and "inclusion" or "exclusion" may be encountered and worked with in Authentic Movement.

Free Writing: Giving the Unconscious Form

Here we focus on writing as a form of active imagination. Inspired by Natalie Goldberg's *Writing Down the Bones* (Goldberg, 1986), and Peter Elbow's *Writing Without Teachers* (Elbow, 1973), I designed an exercise to assist learners in (1) opening to the realm of spontaneity while suspending judgment; (2) discovering inner figures and images they have about themselves; and (3) bringing more consciousness to the dyad, where the original internalization of positive and negative self-concepts forms.

At AMI, I sometimes used this exercise before teaching witnessing skills, in part because it could unearth feelings and associations that learners brought to the act of "seeing" and "being seen." It also helped learners to listen sensitively and respond without judgment or projection, an important step in developing self-referencing language. Listening is a skill, which might not have been experienced satisfactorily in our family of origin, nor is it often taught in schools. For many participants "being heard" was a potent component in "feeling seen."

To illustrate, I would engage participants in a form of active imagination that began with a partner, paper, and pen. Each learner writes "seeing" at the top of one page and "being seen" on another page and then freely writes for five minutes under each heading. Before the exercise starts, I share Goldberg's writing guidelines with the group (Goldberg, 1986, p. 8). Generally, these involve encouraging learners to "keep their hand moving," to write freely and spontaneously, with vivid detail, and without judgment, evaluation, or attention to grammar or spelling. This allows the person to stay connected to the flow of feelings, associations, and psychic images without undue interference from the inner editor or critic. If the critic begins to talk, writing can be a vehicle for bringing more clarity to the critic's concerns, a vital step in becoming free.

After both pieces have been written, partners take turns reading what they are comfortable sharing. As one speaks, the listener witnesses the speaker, attending as she listens, noticing what resonates within her and about the process. When the speaker ends, the listener offers "re-call," a format I developed that involves repeating several words or phrases she heard the speaker say. The more specific the better, since each individual's images and metaphors are unique and meaningful. The listener is also encouraged to share bodily felt sensations or feelings that were awakened in her as she listened, using discernment and sensitive timing. Once both have had an opportunity to share, then the larger group reconvenes to discuss the experience, reflecting on such questions as (1) What was it like to bring voice to your experience? (2) To be heard without judgment? (3) To have your words reflected back? (4) What did it evoke in you to listen deeply?

Even though everyone enters the situation with unique patterns and psychic wounds, each shares the yearning to be seen clearly without danger to the self. This ambivalence between exposure and cover, visibility and invisibility is intensified in Authentic Movement through witnessing with clear attention, as illustrated in the analytic work with Sofia in Chapter 8.

What follows are excerpts from one learner's journal entry entitled "Seeing and Being Seen," which vividly portrays the writer's ambivalence.

Seeing

seeing seeing seen look see look pay attention see see what is there see what is present don't judge you just look at what is look carefully see details be with details what lies next to what what holds what what surrounds what what overpowers what what relinquishes what keep writing keep seeing no matter what see does that mean I'm not really seeing but feeling instead if you see something should there be a word to label it or describe it can I see feelings can feelings be seen I have few words for most of what I feel the things I see that I pay attention to have no words words define and confine and limit ...

Being Seen

I want to be seen but not judged being seen helps me be present being seen gives me a place being seen lets me know I exist being seen can be embarrassing being seen I feel angry and ashamed being seen brings me out of isolation brings me back to myself being seen frightens me and I leave myself I want to be seen as strong not weak deep not shallow of value not frivolous I am full of judgments about being seen and don't like discomfort of being whole being seen helps me find my wholeness

Movement Exploration: Patterns

After completing the writing exercise "Seeing and Being Seen," I would invite partners to witness one another moving. In one dyad a woman with long, thick, wavy hair moved, her hair covering her face, bending, arching, and curling up in such a way that she remained hidden from her witness. Here she described the movement that expressed itself that day, revealing a pattern that developed over months of moving with a witness in the studio:

> Sometimes I moved for fifteen to twenty minutes at a time with my back to the witness, though I was surprised to discover that this was the case. I hadn't consciously intended it and had been moving with my eyes closed. Over several months' time I began to trust that my witness was not going to interpret or judge my experience and began to emerge from behind my hair. Gradually, I allowed my face, neck, and chest to be seen. Fear emerged and subsided, then shame, then curiosity and excitement. My chest expanded, my breath deepened, and I began to move fluidly through the space, reaching out with my arms and hands. Finally, I began to contact other movers in an array of interactions—tenderly, assertively, playfully, sensually. This embodied experience brought my crippling sense of shame to the surface and allowed me to experience what had previously been hidden, enabling me to see myself and be with others more fully.

As this passage illustrates, over time movers may awaken to their specific patterns of movements and series of gestures, which are often repeated unconsciously. "Nothing is more revealing than movement," wrote Martha Graham (1984, p. 53). Through freewriting and reflective journaling learners bring awareness to their patterns (Stromsted, 1998, p. 7). In time these incomplete movements or statements can then be developed and brought to consciousness through this embodied practice (Schoop, 1974, pp. 153–158).

Moving the Work Forward

Authentic Movement practice includes identifying the bodily foundations of projection, emotional triggers, affect regulation, expression, containment, deepening empathy, and developing new behaviors. Movers and witnesses can recall and re-sense layers of experience, recognizing unconscious cognitions and biases. This awareness allows for exploration and the freedom to make more conscious choices.

For some, the mythic content of the work will lead to artistic creation or may evoke the divine. The social dimension may offer an opportunity to develop awareness within community. Patterns of relating and communication progress. Others may find satisfaction in theory and narrative research. For the clinician, it can mean an opportunity to explore the somatic underpinnings inherent in the therapeutic relationship.

Through moving, witnessing, drawing, and writing—identifying the unseen—what was invisible may become more visible. In practicing Authentic Movement developmentally, we move toward wholeness through direct psychic and somatic experience in relationship. Thus, the body's wisdom creates the possibility for a richer and deeper connection to one's daily life. Jung writes, "There is little use in teaching wisdom. At all events wisdom cannot be taught in words. It is only possible by personal contact and by immediate experience" (Jung, 1973, p. 447).

Epilogue

Following the passing of my dear friend and business partner, Neala, from cancer in 2004, the Authentic Movement Institute closed its doors after many rich years of personal and professional exploration. We did so with deep gratitude for the many contributions of the colleagues who had joined our faculty and the students and graduates who came to train.

In the years since, it's heartwarming to see the seeds of our shared explorations at AMI continue to flourish in various forms in the lives of our graduates. Many graduates carry this work forward, teaching new generations of practitioners across different continents and cultures. Some formats have been further developed with Janet Adler in her Circles of Four training before her passing in 2023. Others emerged through Joan Chodorow's seminars, international offerings and writings, in AMI's studio, in the beautiful work of colleagues in the US and abroad, in long-standing and developing peer groups, and increasingly through the inspiring explorations of new generations around the world. My ongoing international teaching, virtual seminars and consultation as a Jungian analyst and dance/somatic psychotherapist—along with my role as chair of the International Association of Analytical Psychology (IAAP) PreCongress Active Imagination in Movement teaching team—continue to bring a depth perspective to the practice. This work nourishes the healing process and supports our ongoing explorations in the development of embodied consciousness. We have also engaged with a wide range of applications, including explorations of the "collective body" (Adler, 1994/1999b, pp. 190–204), honoring the essential role of community in our divided world. And in moments of grace, the practice invites spontaneous ritual, a pathway to the divine within each of us.

The Authentic Movement Institute website serves as a historical record of the learning that developed there, including information about the curriculum, faculty, publications, further resources, and a video on the use of Authentic Movement in clinical practice, an ongoing offering: https://www.authenticmovementinstitute. com. As this depth-oriented, creative healing practice continues to spread to many parts of the globe, may it continue to support us in listening to our deeper callings, and witnessing what wants to rise and shine in one another.

Keeping Watch

In the morning
When I began to wake,
It happened again—

That feeling
That You, Beloved,
Had stood over me all night
Keeping watch,

That feeling
That as soon as I began to stir

You put Your lips on my forehead
And lit a Holy Lamp
Inside my heart.
                    Hafiz (2006), translated by Daniel Ladinsky

Neala Haze, MA, ADTR, REAT, Registered Dance/Movement Therapist and Registered Expressive Arts Therapist, cofounded and directed the Authentic Movement Institute (AMI) in Berkeley, California. With a master's degree in dance and counseling psychology, she studied Authentic Movement with Mary Starks Whitehouse and later trained with Janet Adler and Joan Chodorow. A dance/movement therapist for three decades, she integrated Eastern thought, humanistic psychology, and body-based and creative arts therapy approaches into her teaching and private practice. As the former co-coordinator and internship supervisor of the Graduate Program in Dance Movement Therapy at California State University Hayward, she produced two teaching videos based on Bonnie Bainbridge-Cohen's developmental theory. Her third video, *Authentic Movement and Performance: Imagining Brightly Colored Flowers I Rise*, documented bringing Authentic Movement into a performance setting. An adjunct faculty in the Expressive Arts Therapy Program at the California Institute of Integral Studies, Neala also had a private practice in somatic therapy. She passed away from cancer in June 2004.

References

Adler, J. (1999a). Who is the witness? In P. Pallaro (Ed.), *Authentic Movement: Essays by Mary Starks Whitehouse, Janet Adler, and Joan Chodorow* (pp. 141–159) Jessica Kingsley. (Original work published 1987.)

Adler, J. (1999b). The collective body. In P. Pallaro (Ed.), *Authentic Movement: Essays by Mary Starks Whitehouse, Janet Adler, and Joan Chodorow* (pp. 190–208). Jessica Kingsley. (Original work published 1994.)

Balint, M. (1986). *The British school of psychoanalysis: the independent tradition.* (Gregorio Kohon, Ed.). Free Association Books.

Bly, R. (1988). *A little book on the human shadow.* Harper & Row Publishers.

Chodorow, J. (1991). *Dance therapy & depth psychology: The moving imagination.* Routledge.

Chodorow, J. (1999). Dance therapy and the transcendent function. In P. Pallaro (Ed.), *Authentic Movement: Essays by Mary Starks Whitehouse, Janet Adler, and Joan Chodorow* (pp. 236–252). Jessica Kingsley. (Original work published 1977.)

Elbow, P. (1973). *Writing without teachers.* Oxford University Press.

Freud, S. (1961). Papers on techniques of psychotherapy. In J. Strachey (Ed. *and Trans.*), *The standard edition of the complete psychological works of Sigmund Freud* (Vol. 12). Hogarth Press. (Original work published 1915.)

Goldberg, N. (1986). *Writing down the bones.* Shambhala Publications, Inc.

Graham, M. (1984). *The dancer's notebook.* Running Press.

Hafiz. (2006). Keeping watch. In *I heard God laughing: Poems of hope* (D. Ladinsky, Trans.). Penguin.

Haze, N. (1994). Authentic Movement: Overview of origins, theory and practice. *Proceedings of the First International Clinical Conference in Berlin on Dance Movement Therapy* (pp. 102–105). Nervenlink.

Haze, N. & Stromsted, T. (1999). An interview with Janet Adler. In P. Pallaro (Ed.), *Authentic Movement: Essays by Mary Starks Whitehouse, Janet Adler, and Joan Chodorow* (pp. 107–120). Jessica Kingsley. (Original work published 1994.)

Henderson, J. (1984). *Cultural attitudes in psychological perspective.* Inner City Books.

Jung, C. G. (1916/1958). The transcendent function. In *The structure and dynamics of the psyche* (Vol. 8). Princeton University Press.

Jung, C. G. (1973). *C. G. Jung's letters, 1906–1950* (Vol. 1). (G. Adler, A. Jaffe, & R.F.C. Hull, Eds. & Trans.). Princeton University Press.

Jung, C. G. (1975). The psychology of the transference. In *The practice of psychotherapy* (Vol. 16) (pp. 163–323). Princeton University Press. (Original work published 1946.)

Lewis, P. (1993). *Creative transformation: The healing power of the arts.* Chiron Publications.

Mindell, A. (1985). *Working with the dreaming body.* Routledge & Kegan Paul.

Pallaro, P. (1994). *Somatic countertransference: The therapist in relationship* [Paper presentation]. "ECARTE," Third European Arts Therapies Conference, September 14–17, Ferrara, Italy.

Porges, S. (2011). *The polyvagal theory: Neurophysiological foundations of emotions, attachment, communication, self-regulation.* W. W. Norton & Company.

Porges, S. (2017). *The pocket guide to Polyvagal theory: The transformative power of feeling safe.* W.W. Norton & Company Ltd.

Reich, W. (1948). *The discovery of the orgone: The function of the orgasm* (Vol. 1). Orgone Institute Press.

Reich, W. (1961). *Character analysis.* Pocket Book.

Schoop, T. with Mitchell, P. (1974). *Won't you join the dance?* National Press Books.

Schwartz-Salant, N. (1982). *Narcissism and character transformation.* Inner City Books.

Stewart, L. H. (1986). Affect and archetype: A contribution to a comprehensive theory of the structure of the psyche. In N. Schwartz-Salant & M. Stein (Eds.), *The body in analysis* (pp. 183–204). Chiron Publications.

Stewart, L. H. (1987). Affect and archetype in analysis. In N. Schwartz-Salant and M. Stein (Eds.), *Archetypal processes in psychotherapy* (pp. 131–162). Chiron Publications.

Stromsted, T. (1994/95). Re-inhabiting the female body. *Somatics: Magazine-Journal of the Mind/Body Arts and Sciences, X* (1, Fall/Winter), 18–27.

Stromsted, T. (Spring, 1998). Re-inhabiting the female body. *A Moving Journal, 5*(1), 3–7, 10–11.

Stromsted, T. (2001). Re-inhabiting the female body: Authentic Movement as a gateway to transformation. *The Arts in Psychotherapy: An International Journal, 28*(1), 39–55.

Stromsted, T. (2007). The dancing body in psychotherapy: Reflections on Somatic Psychotherapy and Authentic Movement. In P. Pallaro (Ed.), *Authentic Movement: Moving the body, moving the self, being moved* (pp. 202–220). Jessica Kingsley. (Original work published 1998.)

Whitehouse, M. S. (1999a). The Tao of the body. In P. Pallaro (Ed.), *Authentic Movement: essays by Mary Starks Whitehouse, Janet Adler, and Joan Chodorow* (pp. 41–50). Jessica Kingsley. (Original work published 1958.)

Whitehouse, M. S. (1999b). C. G. Jung and dance therapy: Two major principles. In P. Pallaro (Ed.), *Authentic Movement: Essays by Mary Starks Whitehouse, Janet Adler, and Joan Chodorow* (pp. 74–101). Jessica Kingsley. (Original work published 1979.)

Woodman, M. (1983). *Addiction to perfection: The still unravished bride.* Inner City Books.

Chapter 12

Working with Authentic Movement in Groups

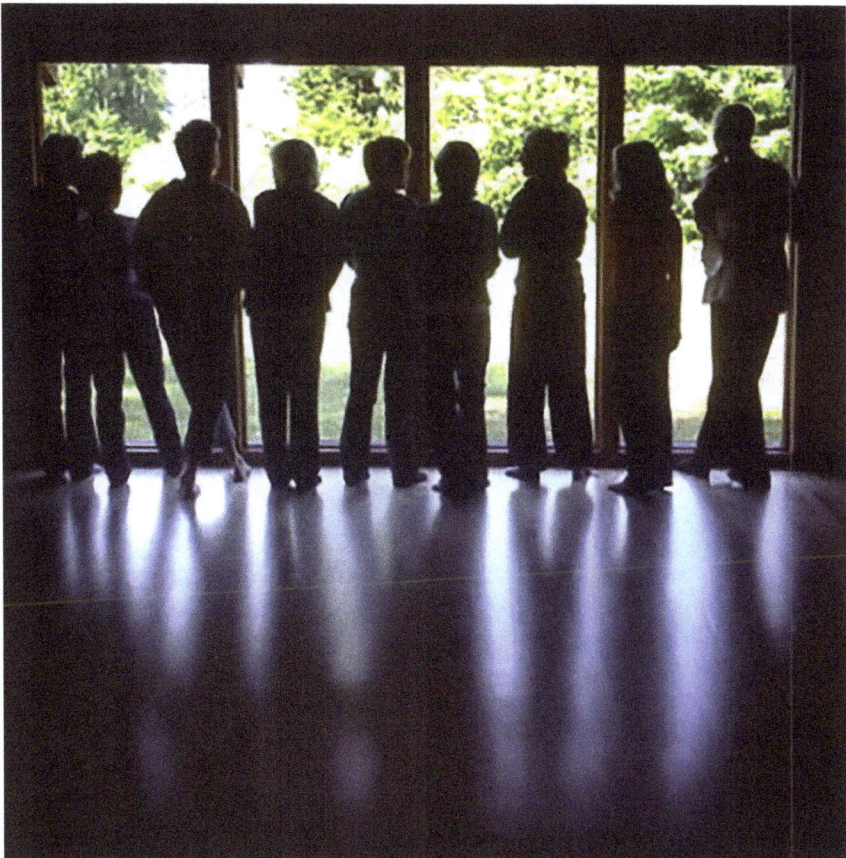

Figure 12.1 Author's Authentic Movement peer group, Whidbey Island, Washington, © Lizbeth Hamlin, 2009.

DOI: 10.4324/9781003538356-16

Authentic Movement can provide a profound resource for healing and growth both within the context of individual psychotherapy and in group settings. Here, I describe elements of group work, with a focus on the experience of a young man. Before assembling an Authentic Movement group, I screen group members to ensure that each member has sufficient ego strength to engage in this unstructured approach: each participant needs to be able to discern reality from fantasy and manage anxiety-provoking material. Screening includes asking applicants about their expectations of the work and how they have handled difficult feelings during challenging periods in their lives. I also ask about their history in therapy, including whether they are taking any medications or have ever been hospitalized in a psychiatric setting. What has been their experience with other forms of bodywork or movement, and what has been helpful for them?

It is also important to assess the congruency of their affect and how safe they might expect to feel working with their eyes closed. Though closing the eyes may seem like a subtle point, without sufficient object constancy, a person in contact with unconscious material can experience considerable anxiety when unable to track visually the presence of the witness/therapist and their responses. Orientation to time and space is also important, enabling them to maintain their bearings in the here and now as they connect with experiences from the past, remembered by the body. Though the work can contribute to deep healing and transformation, like any depth approach, there are cautions. Says Joan Chodorow,

> The major danger of the method involves being overwhelmed by the powerful affects, impulses, and images of the unconscious. It should be attempted only by psychologically mature individuals who are capable of withstanding a powerful confrontation with the unconscious. A well-developed ego standpoint is needed so that the conscious and unconscious may encounter each other as equals.
>
> (Chodorow, 1997, p. 12)

Jung also warned about the potential for the patient to get "caught in the sterile circle of his own complexes" or "remain stuck in an all-enveloping phantasmagoria" so that nothing is gained (Jung, 1916/1969, CW 8, p. 68). He emphasized how important it was to integrate what arose from the unconscious into the personality as a whole in order to receive the meaning and value of the experience.

If I am not sure that a person's ego strength is sufficient for engaging unconscious material and powerful affects directly at a body level, I may include a brief Authentic Movement experience in the interview process. If I sense that more preparation is needed, I may refer the applicant for individual Authentic Movement sessions to further prepare them for group work at a future time. Acknowledging each person's strengths and gifts and the resources they bring to the group can be a particularly rewarding part of the assessment process for participants and group leaders/therapists alike.

As an Authentic Movement group facilitator, I assume the simultaneous roles of witness and therapist. As a group therapist, I offer participants the essential elements and safety guidelines for moving and witnessing practice. These guidelines include encouraging group members to engage in deep inner listening with curiosity and respect for their own embodied experience, reminding them that there is no "right" or "wrong" way to move. I also counsel them to trust their "floodgates" as it is not necessarily wise to push themselves beyond their comfort level or sense of correct timing. To ensure everyone's safety, I ask that people open their eyes a little if they are going to make large or sudden movements.

Physical contact also sometimes occurs naturally between group members in Authentic Movement practice. When this occurs, I function as a therapist, encouraging movers to move away from any unwanted contact or to take the risk of engaging in respectful contact that feels genuine and consistent with their own process and development. Such experiences, when brought to consciousness, can be reparative, providing a sense of safety in their own skin while relating to another.

As the work unfolds, through my example as a witness, I demonstrate a containing sense of presence. The focus and concentration I bring and the group's quiet attention contribute to creating a safe and protected space for the movers. When I provide verbal responses at the end of a movement session, I am again a witness and a therapist as I look to guide the witnesses in giving responses that are as nonprojective, noninterpretative, and nonjudgmental as possible. I will, however, assume my therapist role if my clinical experience and judgment are required. I might intervene, for example, if I feel that projections are beginning to take over the process or if a group member is encountering a particularly difficult and prolonged impasse. Over time, participants also learn witnessing skills. Working with distinguishing their own material from someone else's and beginning to sense when to contain feedback and when to share it are important cornerstones of the work.

Authentic Movement groups can take on a wide range of formats. Though founder Mary Starks Whitehouse witnessed individuals in private sessions and participants in her groups, two of her students, Joan Chodorow and Janet Adler, began their own groups, taught their students witnessing skills, and influenced further generations as the practice continued to evolve. Several of Mary's other students also continued to explore the practice, integrating fundamental elements into their body-based and meditative approaches.

Ethical Guidelines

Ethical guidelines enhance the safety of the psychological space. Among these, it is essential that movers do not hurt themselves or others and that physical contact only occurs when both people consent to it. As the work can give rise to deep feelings, unmet needs, and initial projections, there is an agreement that sexual contact does not occur between group members. I share a precaution to observe sexual boundaries outside of the group space, given transference dynamics that can further complicate their relationship and the dynamics of the group. Mutual respect for diversity in gender, race, age, religion, physical abilities, and other elements is essential. A sense of dignity and autonomy for one's body is central to the practice, including respect for being the expert of one's own experience. Witnesses only speak if invited to give feedback, reflecting back what the mover has spoken of and their own embodied experience related to what they saw and heard, careful not to judge or interpret and mindful of owning their own projections. Confidentiality is essential for participants to feel free to explore elements from their unconscious; with the exception of confidential supervision, what is shared remains contained in the space. If group members need to further process their experience as a mover or witness with an outside analyst, therapist, or trusted loved one, they do so with a specific agreement. The focus remains on their *own* learning experience rather than identifying others.

Group Formats

Many of the major structural formats currently used in Authentic Movement practice were initially developed by Janet Adler with her students in our early trainings. She continued to elaborate on these over the years with an increasing emphasis on mystical practice. Joan Chodorow contributed explorations of the emotions and reflections on personal, cultural, and archetypal sources of movement from a Jungian and dance/movement therapy perspective in decades-long local clinical seminars and international professional conferences. Neala Haze and I developed training protocols at our Authentic Movement Institute (1993–2004). I continue to integrate current developments in neuroscience with psychological, somatic, spiritual, and artistic practices, weaving innovations into my analytic work, international teaching, and consultation. Wonderful colleagues and students in different parts of the world continue to bring their own areas of focus to the work, adjusting the practice to meet the needs of their patients and student populations. Group formats continue to develop in organic ways, enriched by the group leader's individual background, group focus, cultural context, and the spirit of the times.

Basics

Each movement session is decided on for a designated length of time—ranging from five minutes to over an hour, depending on the group, the context, and the format. Shorter times provide additional containment for newer movers, and the time gradually increases as group members gain more experience engaging with their unconscious through the body. Often, the witness uses Tibetan bells to begin and end each movement round—ringing once to start and three times for movers to begin to bring their movement exploration to a close.

Sometimes the group moves as a whole in a training or group therapy format, which consists of a group of movers and one teacher/witness or group leader/therapist. Once group members have more experience moving, they may become silent witnesses, learning sensitive, attuned observational and listening skills and awareness of what's arising in their own bodies in response to their mover's experience.

Over time, witnesses learn the verbal part of the practice of giving feedback, speaking in the present tense using "I statements" that are nonjudgmental and noninterpretive. For example, "When I see you rolling across the floor, I feel enlivened. As your arms curl in at your chest and your legs lengthen, I feel my whole body and remember rolling in the grass as a child."

The language component is an essential part of the practice. Distinct from the often-interpretive language of psychotherapy, it is more akin to psychologist Carl Rogers's reflective listening. Janet Adler adopted the "I statements" to name one's own experience used in "percept language" developed by John Weir (Eagle & Eagle, 2020) and others in the Humanistic Psychology movement. A vital part of Authentic Movement practice, this helps reduce projections and supports a sense of psychological and emotional safety for group members as they explore deep material. Verbal sharing occurs following individual or group movement sessions and is sometimes called a "talking circle."

The witness offers the mover eye contact before and after their movement experience, as seeing and being seen is a fundamental part of the practice. As noted in Chapter 5, the nature of eye contact can also differ somewhat from culture to culture, as I have learned while witnessing participants from diverse cultures in groups throughout the United States and other parts of the world. As I mentioned, in Japan, *direct* eye contact may seem intrusive in some instances; instead, *indirect* eye contact is more customary to demonstrate respect, particularly in deference to elders or authority figures. By contrast, in many parts of American culture, *direct* eye contact is often expected, indicating that one is *present*, paying attention, or signifying encouragement and importance. That said, as there are many cultures in the United States that draw on different traditions, this can vary widely.

The witness's visual engagement also varies during the movement practice. It can be direct when focusing on a single mover in the dyad or group session, or be softer and more indirect, engaging peripheral vision. Oscillating between a *direct* and *soft* gaze can serve to highlight the *individual* mover or allow the witness to "see" the mover within the wider landscape of the group—reflecting their possible place in the *collective* body. This softer, peripheral vision highlights the mover's role as a participant in the "group dance" within the circle in the studio or in nature. The type of gaze brings in other qualities as well. Says Chodorow, "The witness fluctuates between a solar, differentiated, objective, definitive way of seeing, and a lunar, merging, subjective, imaginative way of seeing. [Thus], the same movement event may be seen and described in many ways" (Chodorow, 1991, p. 50).

Groups can be formed of dyads and triads. A dyad consists of a mover and a witness, who then switch roles. In a triad, there may be a silent witness and a speaking witness, or, following the approach of Marion Woodman, a mirroring witness and a containing witness as described in the Dance of Three in Chapter 5. This dynamic can also reflect the relationships of mother and father (or other early caregivers) with their child, as well as the dynamics between client, therapist, and supervisor.

There are various types of group formats, each with specific guidelines. Below, I offer a brief summary of the major types and their descriptions.

Breathing Circles

Group members begin by sitting on the rim of the circle. Then, half of the participants become movers when the group leader (or in a peer-group setting, a group member designated for that round) rings the bell. At the conclusion of that movement round, movers exchange places with witnesses who become movers in the next round. A period of silent transition often follows the movement—for walking, resting, drawing, or writing—concluding with a talking circle after one or more rounds. Like the breath, this circle has cycles of inhalation and exhalation!

Long Circles

In this ritual format, everyone starts on the rim of the circle, taking time to witness and meditate on the empty space. Movers enter the circle when they feel drawn to move, responding to various sensations such as bodily discomfort, stiffness, or tiredness, or even the energy stirred by another mover's experience. Curiosity, or an inner urge to explore a specific emotion, image, or mood, can also inspire them to enter—whatever prompts them with the sense that "it's time to move!" Before beginning, the group determines how many witnesses will remain in the witness circle to enhance the sense of safety and containment. Unlike other Authentic Movement group formats, participants can freely alternate between moving and witnessing. They can choose to become a mover when they feel called to move or take on the role of a witness whenever their movement feels complete. It's even possible for them to enter, explore, and leave the circle multiple times in a single round.

The Long Circle typically lasts over an hour, sometimes extending into part of a day. During this process, participants physically leave their cushions in the witness circle. This action serves both as a literal and symbolic gesture, marking a place for their inner witness to remain present while they descend into their movement process. Some may also leave a sacred object beside their witness cushion or on the altar, symbolizing the larger spiritual witness that exists within and around them.

At the end of the Long Circle, as everyone returns to their original places, they collectively acknowledge the empty space. Although much has happened, the space is empty once again! This act serves as a reminder of the mystery at the core of our practice and our shared humanity. Focusing on this space—the fertile void from which all life emerges and ultimately returns—is fundamental to many meditation practices and vital for conscious embodiment.

Group members then extend their arms around the circle and make eye contact as the movement session comes to a close. Following a silent transition period for drawing, writing, walking, or resting, the group reconvenes for a talking circle, practicing verbal witnessing to reflect on their individual experiences. This may be followed by a "collective witnessing" session in which group members reflect on their movements as part of the larger "collective body" (Adler, 1994/1999, pp. 190–208). And perhaps by a Gesture Circle in which movement becomes the primary language for further reflection, creative expression, and integration.

Naming Circles

In a Naming Circle, a single mover moves for a specified number of minutes in the center of the circle. Once it is time to bring their movement experience to a close, their name is called along with the ringing of the bell, with an opportunity to share eye contact around the circle. Then the next person enters for their turn in the center of the circle.

Sprouting

Sprouting involves a witness extending their arms—like the branches of a deeply rooted tree—while making eye contact with other witnesses. This gesture can be initiated by any witness at any time, especially if they feel tired, unfocused, frightened, overwhelmed, upset, or vulnerable about what they are witnessing. Seeing other witnesses reaching out and making eye contact serves as a reminder that they are not alone—both they and the movers are being "held" by the larger circle—a caring and attentive consciousness that is co-created through everyone's intentional presence.

Gesture Circle

Participants start by standing in a circle, making eye contact, and observing the empty space. When the leader rings the bell, a mover steps in and repeats a gesture that was meaningful to them from the previous Long Circle. This could be a gesture they performed or one they saw another mover make. Precise replication isn't necessary, as everyone has unique bodies and movement styles. Instead, movers focus on capturing the feeling, shape, tempo, and qualities of the movement they remember. Others who resonate with this gesture can join in, creating a spontaneous tableau of reflective gestures that is vibrant with authenticity, aliveness, and depth—some of the best choreography I've seen! Once participants feel the gesture is complete, they return to the witness circle. The session concludes when the leader rings the bell three times.

Starting Points

Jung used starting points like moods, dream images, or life struggles as portals for Active Imagination. In my sessions with patients or groups, I often suggest a starting point based on an issue or theme they've shared, such as relationship tensions, current events, body discomfort, dream material, or important decisions. Alternatively, the session might begin with a kinesthetic focus, like exploring movements initiated by a specific body part or leading with the dominant or more receptive side of the body. I might also invite the mover to "drop their mind" into their heart, belly, pelvis, or feet, as Ann Skinner encouraged in BodySoul Rhythms.

Group themes often explore fundamental human emotions, such as being seen or unseen, feeling significant or peripheral, connected or abandoned, safe or in peril, understood or misinterpreted, overwhelmed or supported, alone or part of a transcendent whole. For more than three decades, I facilitated International Authentic Movement groups in Tuscany, Italy, with each year dedicated to a specific area of inquiry. These themes have included DreamDancing®, Embodied Alchemy®, and body symptoms. We explored the Motherline using family photographs and movement patterns, and integrative dances with Feminine/Yin and Masculine/Yang qualities. Our practice supported the reawakening of the healthy instinctual body. Participants charted their lifelines, mapping and reflecting on significant experiences and turning points. Myths and fairytales were often a vital part of our exploration. These gatherings served as soul retreats for deep inner work within community. They began gently, progressively deepening throughout the week, tracing the arc of descent and return that is essential for healing and transformation. This liminal space echoes elements of ancient Greek mystery schools and the spiritual journeys of many traditional cultures. During these retreats, participants step away from their daily lives and enter into sacred time. In clinical training groups, therapists and health practitioners alternate between personal experiences and professional seminars. In this setting, participants leave their professional roles behind, allowing them to explore their defenses at their own pace and discover hidden treasures. They return to their communities transformed, yet more authentically themselves, ready to share insights and make genuine contributions.

Art

Following the movement, group sessions often include artmaking, such as drawing, painting, sculpting, collaging, and writing. At other times, drawings can become prompts for movement; drawing a body symptom, dream image, emotional response to a relationship, life experience, or dilemma can be further explored through embodiment.

These art projects reflect the workshop's theme and can take various forms. For longer workshops, participants might create a mandala for the week, make a book and stitch a cover with pages for each day, or fill a Body Map with life experiences, dreams, poems, leaves, small stones, and twigs. They might also sculpt clay to represent their developing inner witness or write poetry, stories, or fairy tales. Artmaking helps integrate feelings and imagination, freeing them from inhibiting patterns caused by trauma, neglect, or shame. It often reflects new energies, joy, or even a sense of rebirth.

Closure

Each group experience—whether shorter or longer in duration—follows a natural progression, beginning with arrival, logistics, and introductions. Teaching themes are woven in as the practice deepens, develops, and draws to a close. The closure allows participants to acknowledge their experiences, celebrate their time together, and say goodbye before returning home to practice their learnings in daily life.

For example, at the end of the Tuscany retreat, we hold a sharing circle where each member reflects on their experience, something they intend to leave behind, and what they will take home. I offer guidance for transitioning back to the faster pace and responsibilities of daily life. On the final afternoon, we host an Art Gallery, displaying everyone's creations in the studio or a special outdoor spot they've connected with, like a tree, a hammock, or a place on the lawn. Participants witness the art in silence, and each artist briefly shares about their piece, with group members responding through gestures and a word or phrase written on a page nearby. This ritual concludes with a celebratory Italian dinner and a lively dance party, sometimes featuring live music, including the Italian host family!

Though a fuller description of group styles is beyond the scope of this chapter, for more information on locations, leaders, and types of groups, please see the Resources provided at the end of this book.

Group Example

Now, I will describe a specific group in which weekly movement sessions were an integrative part of training psychotherapists. The movement portion ranged from ten to forty-five minutes, building gradually throughout the course.

Our work was guided by group members' increasing capacity to attend to their embodied experience and to express and contain unconscious material. Participants engaged in individual psychotherapy concurrently outside the group to provide additional support for further exploration and integration of what emerged in the movement work. Confidentiality was also agreed upon so that group members could feel free to engage more fully.

The group met in a spacious, carpeted room with large windows. After a brief movement warm-up exploring the polarities of "open and closed," I invited participants to find a safe place in the room, close their eyes, and begin to attend to and be moved by their inner body-felt sensations, movement impulses, images, and feelings. Drawing and journal writing often followed the movement sessions, assisting in the transition to speaking. I sat to the side of the space where I could see everyone clearly. Over time, I taught group members witnessing skills as well. In the windows opposite, a large tree lost its leaves and then bloomed again during the months of our practice together.

Case Illustration—Daniel

Of medium height, lean, and agile, "Daniel" was a somewhat shy, though sometimes playful, man in his early thirties. He often felt that he was solely engaged in superficial conversations with his peers and said this exhausted him. Following his initial experience of moving in a group, he had *a dream in which he was sitting in a rowboat on a deep sea, terrified that if he "rocked the boat" and fell overboard, he would be eaten alive by a huge white whale.* He reported that his father was often absent or standoffish, and his mother had been intrusive and physically abusive. *In one dream, he had to stop her from looking at his nude body by using his elbows to push her away.* Daniel realized that for some time he had felt he could never escape her gaze; he had continued to see her in his mind's eye and attempted to read her facial expression to know how to act or what to make of what he was feeling. Over a few weeks, Daniel began to see how his mother had become a powerful internal reference point and, simultaneously, a source of painful and fragmented memories and low self-esteem.

As the other group members engaged in their movement explorations with eyes closed, Daniel spent a good deal of time curled up in a fetal position on the floor, sometimes still and frozen, sometimes rocking himself. Occasionally, he tried to stand but found himself returning again and again to these early movements, curling up in a ball on his knees with his head touching the ground and his arms either holding his belly or covering his head. Learning to stay with the sensations and feelings that he experienced, he began to realize that this position expressed the dilemma he felt so profoundly: on the one hand, he felt safe in it, but on the other, he felt unable to express the fear and the rage that he had never been able to show at home while growing up. He realized he was hiding from himself and others "out of a fear of being rejected" for who he was. He had an insight that this stemmed from not having had a safe place in his childhood to express his anger and fears.

Following this insight, two characters emerged in Daniel's imagination and his movements. The first was a huge, impish Hobgoblin who didn't care about anyone else and did what he wanted. Daniel felt both relief and repulsion. The second figure was a strong Stoic. At one point, he embodied the mischievous Hobgoblin and enjoyed feeling that he deserved whatever he wanted. He allowed himself to turn his back on all his witnesses in the group, embodying what it was that he wanted to hide from everyone and finding that it was a relief to be so "bad."

This movement was immediately followed by the appearance of the strong Stoic. Standing upright and tall, Daniel folded his arms over his chest in an authoritative pose. His head held high and pulled back, he occasionally shook his finger at an imaginary figure, grimacing and pulling his head in at the neck. "It was upsetting to go back to the Stoic. Do I have to?" he asked. "I feel like the child who was made to stop playing all too soon. In going back to the Hobgoblin, I am angry. I either want to be one or the other. There is not room enough for both. Anger wells up in my belly, and there is pressure on my heart. This responsibility that I feel I need to carry weighs on my heart. I feel myself caught between the hot belly of anger and the weight of the pain over my heart."

At this point in his process, I encouraged Daniel to stay with the tension between this pair of opposites, attending to his feelings and bodily sensations and allowing them to guide him in discovering a way through his dilemma. By following the heat he found in his belly while rolled up in the ball or "hiding" position, he began to pound on the floor with his fists. At first, the pounding was soft, but then it gradually grew louder and firmer with a definite rhythm. Discovering that he could not express himself fully in this position, Daniel sat up, experimenting until he found a position where he could feel safe and yet express his rage. With his legs curled under him in almost a lotus position, he leaned forward, placing his weight on his fists. From this position, Daniel could feel the weight of his emotions and his body behind the anger and banged his fists with renewed vigor. "I felt the anger," he said later. "I felt aggressive, yet I was able to honor my need to feel secure. I could honor the armor that I have created, even as I released my pain."

Following this movement session, another group member expressed her experience of needing to hide who she was. Daniel then shared what he had just written in his journal: "I am sick of hiding." Touched by her words, he began to sob, his body shaking for some time. Following this experience, he wrote, "It was amazing to be able to really express my feelings and not be judged by the witnesses. Now, I feel that a profound change has taken place within my psyche. Before, I was trying to fight this ghost of my mother who abused me from my distant past. I couldn't fight her. The catharsis brought my attention to the core issue behind my mother ... the degree to which I feel the need to hide things from her and everyone. Now, I am in a place where I feel like I can work on and learn from my issues as they unfold over time. I feel like my Imp and the Stoic are trying to find a common ground."

Daniel shared another entry from his journal: "Perhaps my movements are a dialogue between my mind and body ... I am desperately trying to find something valuable that I have lost. The mind is on top, looking down the tiny hole, trying to find what it has lost. And the body is a caged beast, trying to get out where there is no door. I feel like a lion; if I could get out, I'd kill something. I am trying to let loose, just trying to move away from the scrutiny of the mind. And maybe, just maybe, the mind is trying to find the key to unleash the beast." Robert Lewis Stevenson's famous tale of "Dr. Jekyll and Mr. Hyde" describes a similar dilemma. In the story an upright doctor struggles to cope with the tension between his primitive shadow aspects and his over-adapted, disciplined "good" persona. However, rather than using drugs to assist him in negotiating this impasse as Stevenson's character did, Daniel was engaging in the slow, careful work of bringing the shadow to consciousness, integrating these heretofore forbidden feelings and energies into a more empowered sense of self.

Following this breakthrough were several dreams in which Daniel found himself naked with an erection in public places with his girlfriend, feeling humiliated and needing to hide himself. In these dreams, his coat falls away, and he is mortified that everyone will see him—see his manliness. He pulls his coat around himself, feeling he must "harness" it. During the movement that followed these dreams, Daniel found himself alternately feeling strong and able to stand up, with his chest out, and then fearful. "I feel secure and not," he wrote about this dilemma. "I feel like I am just sitting there waiting for the blows to happen. I want to be more mobile, defensive, and active. I want to feel strong as well as safe, so it is important for me to find a new position."

In his next movement session, the image of a turtle came to him. While attending to this image, he began to close up like a turtle, bending over and covering his heart with his arms, cradling it like a baby. He returned to the rocking motion, having a sense of being both the infant being rocked and the one doing the rocking. He brought his knees in together, covering up his crotch and hips. He touched his torso down to his knees. He reported that at this point, he realized that he was not "weak" in this position, no less than when he was standing up, so he stood up again.

Daniel described this experience to the group: "I move back into the same position I was in before, only this time I feel the true nature of my stance. I am willing to show myself; I am willing to slowly come out of hiding … for myself and others, but I need to feel safe and protected," he says. "'How to do this?' I think. But then I remember Tina's voice encouraging me to listen to my body and trust that it will help me find a way. My arms have begun moving out in circles above my head and to my sides. I am taking and releasing a huge breath as I make each circle. Finally, my arms rest just over my belly, in what feels like a martial arts position. Not like 'Here I am, strong, taking on the world,' but rather, 'I am here, secure. I am prepared to defend myself if I need to, but … I would like to try to meet you.' I smile as I experience this new sensation, a zone of steadiness and comfort between my need to hide and my wish to be open and to release so much of what I feel I need to hide."

In the next movement session, Daniel had the image of being a scorpion, "twisting and turning close to the ground, [his] pinchers and tail raised to an unknown enemy." As one of his witnesses, I felt energized, alive, powerful, and mobile. Simultaneously, I had a sense of my own quiet stillness and felt a strong central axis moving down along my spine and into the floor. When he asked for my response, I shared my experience with him, adding that during his movement, I felt that I could be here with him in the presence of his power and fury, neither interfering with it nor abandoning him. His eyes welled up, and he heaved a huge sigh as a smile spread across his face.

As Daniel's work continued, he became more confident in himself. He spoke out more readily in the group, his voice deeper, enacting less of the jesting he had once employed so automatically in relating to others. He reported being better able to affirm his boundaries and later shared with me that by continuing to follow his dreams and bodily sensations, he was able to make a career choice that had previously been too difficult for him.

Through this movement work, Daniel became able to embrace his direct bodily experience. He also learned to develop a more discerning "inner witness," capable of stepping back and reflecting on his own life. As his feelings surfaced and found expression, he became more compassionate and discerning in his overall point of view. He no longer felt subjected to the moods that previously possessed him, blunting his awareness and his ability to make choices "until the storm had passed." As is so often the case in this work, the site of the wound had become the gateway to which he returned and moved through, as healing took place.

> Keep knocking, and the joy inside
> will eventually open a window
> and look out to see who's there.
> Rumi (Barks, 2005, p. 120)

References

Adler, J. (1999). The collective body. In P. Pallaro (Ed.), *Authentic movement: Essays by Mary Starks Whitehouse, Janet Adler, and Joan Chodorow* (pp. 190–208). Jessica Kingsley Publishers. (Original work published in 1994).

Barks, C. (Trans.). (2005). The sunrise ruby. In *Rumi, The book of love: Poem of ecstasy and longing*. HarperSanFrancisco.

Chodorow, J. (1997). *Jung on active imagination*. Routledge.

Chodorow, J. (1991). *Dance therapy and depth psychology: The moving imagination*. Routledge.

Eagle, J. & Eagle, H. (2020, August 22). *John Weir: Forgotten pioneer in the human potential movement*. https://beconsciousnow.com/2020/08/john-weir-forgotten-pioneer-in-the-human-potential-movement/

Jung, C.G. (1969). "The transcendent function." In *The structure and dynamics of the psyche* (Vol. 8). Princeton University Press. (Originally work published in 1916/1958.)

Part IV

Embracing the Body,
Healing the Soul

Chapter 13

Embodied Alchemy

A Pathway to the Sacred

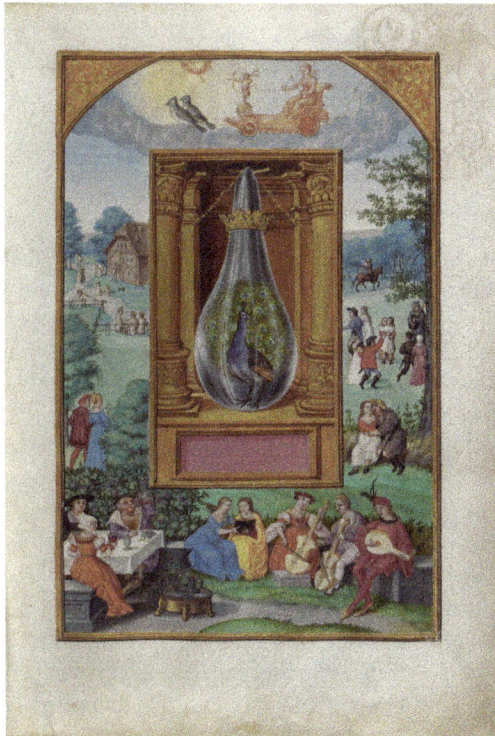

Figure 13.1 "The Peacock" in the alchemical flask whose appearance provided assurance of the color to emerge after a period of darkness and confusion. © The British Library Board, Harley 3469, f.28.

What can we learn from the ancient alchemists? And how might myths and legends guide the human soul on its journey? In today's Western world, cognitive therapeutic approaches often emphasize mental insight over embodied experience and the spiritual aspects of healing. Yet, true healing requires more than verbalization;

DOI: 10.4324/9781003538356-18

it involves *experiencing insight in the body* and integrating it within a conscious, empathic relationship to bring it into life and the community.

Both alchemy and psychotherapy transform the undervalued—the *prima materia* or base matter, the unconscious shadow—into something meaningful. Some analysts and body-oriented psychotherapists liken the body—with its unmetabolized emotions, implicit processes, and unknown interior landscapes—with the unconscious (Conger, 1988; Mindell, 1985; Stromsted, 2025; Wyman-McGinty, 1998). Understanding alchemy's stages can guide therapeutic work, especially in times of anxiety, dissolution, or impatience, ensuring clients persevere through natural phases of healing (Edinger, 1985).

Authentic Movement, which reconnects individuals to instinctual wisdom, mirrors alchemical principles by balancing embodied and spiritual dimensions, fostering development while grounding mystical states in life. Unlike institutions that separate spirit from nature, alchemy sought wisdom in nature's transformative powers. This chapter explores the interplay between alchemy, Jung's transcendent function, and Authentic Movement, revealing the process of embodied transformation.

Cultural Contexts

Long before the paternal God of Genesis, who created the world from "the Word," Mother Goddess cultures revered nature as the sacred ground from which all life emerged (Baring & Cashford, 1991; Gadon, 1989, p. 2). Nature and spirit were unified, with the sacred *immanent* in matter. However, a potent transition took place with the growth of patriarchal cultures and Christianity that moved toward a separation of body and spirit. Jungian analyst Anne Baring notes, "The belief that the body must be controlled, mortified, made to suffer for its desires and in general brought into a relationship of subjection to the mind is very deeply engrained in the Christian psyche" (Baring & Cashford, 1991, p. 529). In the West, and in some other patriarchal religious traditions, the feminine, the body, and a participatory connection to the sacred in nature have been devalued, suppressed, and exploited for personal gain (Stromsted, 1994/95, p. 19).

Today, the "Unholy Trinity"—the Body, the Feminine, and the Shadow (Chodorow, 1983; Jung, 1951)—remains undervalued in many contexts, except for the idealized, commercialized body. Movements like feminism, environmentalism, and practices such as yoga and mindfulness show a growing awareness of these elements. Still, industrialized culture prioritizes logic, efficiency, and profit over feelings, processes, and relationships, leaving the spirit "homeless."

Healing the body-spirit divide requires embracing the unconscious. In Western culture, embodied practices that emphasize conscious development are limited, and spiritual traditions become dogmatic when disconnected from the body. Similarly, bodily practices focused solely on aesthetics, like yoga for physical appearance, risk becoming mechanical. A balanced approach is essential to integrate body, brain, psyche, and spirit. In the Middle Ages, alchemists—mystics who aimed to create gold from base matter—sought to restore feminine consciousness by balancing it with the masculine traditions of the Bronze Age, symbolized by the sacred marriage of the king and queen, uniting spirit and matter in higher consciousness.

Alchemy: Early Beginnings

Various sources have pointed to alchemy having its origins in ancient Egypt, though it may actually belong to a lost tradition that goes back to the dawn of civilization (von Franz, 1980). Alchemy, the forerunner of modern chemistry, is most often understood as a primitive scientific attempt to create elemental gold, but in fact it had more to do with seeking "inner gold" through engaging the elemental makeup of matter—the wisdom of nature—in order to reveal her secrets and evoke spiritual experience. The physical aspect of alchemical practice involved heating materials in a hermetically sealed flask in order to "cook" them down to their most essential components. This brought about change not only in the physical materials in terms of color and consistency but also in the consciousness of the alchemist attending the process.

Jung's Transcendent Function

Having studied myth, religion, and fairy tales, Jung recognized that although these stories stemmed from individual unconscious experiences, they were shaped by tradition through countless retellings. Familiar elements were retained, while strange details were often discarded (von Franz, 1980). In contrast, Jung found alchemy rich with unconscious material, emerging without a fixed agenda, allowing for confrontation with the ego's rigidity. Emotional dysfunction, he believed, arises from psychological one-sidedness, where the conscious ego overvalues its viewpoint, creating tension with the unconscious (Chodorow, 1997).

Jung's transcendent function—holding the tension between opposites until a new "third" emerges—aimed to unite opposing forces within the psyche, "drawing polarized energies into a common channel" (Chodorow, 1997, p. 4; Jung, 1916/1969). Alchemy, too, involved the union of opposites, such as the Sun and Moon or masculine and feminine, transforming from an undifferentiated state to "gold."

The *coniunctio*, or sacred marriage, was the goal of the opus: the union of opposites into a more refined and conscious whole. This parallels Jung's transcendent function, where "either/or" becomes "both/and" (Jung, 1916/1969, CW 8). Jungian analyst Joan Chodorow describes a similar transformation in her work on containment:

For years I fostered cathartic release over suppression as if they were the only choices. But gradually, the image of containment became clear as a third option. To contain the affect is not to suppress or deny it, nor to purge it cathartically. To contain is to feel deeply, bear the discomfort, and express it symbolically. Symbolic expression holds the tension of the opposites ... the therapeutic relationship is both container and process ... the alchemical temenos.

(1991, p. 37)

Jung's work highlighted how alchemy is relevant to contemporary therapy: as a means of accessing the unconscious, a model for developing consciousness and individuation, and a process of healing and transformation. It contextualizes transformation within cultural myths and traditions, and emphasizes the harmonious marriage of opposites, offering a lens for addressing contemporary issues like rigid gender norms and the mind-body-spirit split.

Building a Conscious Container

In alchemy, the container or "cooking" vessel was essential for transformation. Kleopatra, an Alexandrian alchemist, compared it to an egg-shaped womb, whereas Maria Prophetissa described it as a Hermetic vessel, "completely round, in imitation of the spherical cosmos, so that the influence of the stars may contribute to the success of the operation" (Jung, 1968a/1953, CW 12, para. 338). These early alchemists saw the retort as a matrix or uterus from which the *filius philosophorum*, the miraculous stone, would emerge.

Warmth, presence, and focused attention were also vital. Throughout the alchemical phases—*calcinatio* (dismemberment through heating), *solutio* (liquefying), *coagulatio* (solidifying into the new form), *sublimatio* (raising consciousness), and *coniunctio* (the sacred marriage of opposites)—the alchemists regulated the flame's heat to achieve the right conditions for transformation.

Modern trauma theory uses "titration" to describe the regulation of emotional "heat" within a window of tolerance. This means managing emotional intensity and preventing *hyperarousal* (excessive stress activation) or *hypoarousal* (dissociation) (Carroll, 2005, p. 25). When this balance is lost, the therapeutic relationship falters because the client disconnects from their body. Freud noted that "the ego is first and foremost a bodily ego" (1961, p. 26), and James Hillman emphasized that "the body is the vessel in which the transformation process takes place" (1976, p. 146).

The body also needs time and the right conditions to support authentic feelings. Over time, it becomes its own conscious container within a warm and attuned healing relationship. Without this, the unconscious and the animating soul spark within it, remains repressed, unable to emerge and take root in the body. Marion Woodman said, "When there has been a radical split, a somatic container must be prepared to receive the psychic labor. There must be a greeting of the spirit, a chalice to receive the wine" (1982, p. 69).

Psychologically, the alchemical retort mirrors Winnicott's "holding environment," which softens the defensive "false self" constructed for survival in difficult environments (Winnicott, 1965). Alchemically, this is the descent, death, and rebirth central to depth analysis. Similarly, in Authentic Movement, without a safe "holding" presence from a witness who maintains awareness of the embodied self, the mover cannot relax her vigilance—her "inner self-care system" comprised of early object relations (Kalsched, 1996)—enough to open to her unconscious material. The witness holds and metabolizes affects and images the mover cannot process until the ego is strong enough to do so (a process described as the development of an *internal witness*) (Adler, 1987, p. 183). This process allows the mover to summon the *wounded healer* within, which in turn has a healing effect on the therapist/witness in a truly intersubjective relationship.

Dark Night of the Soul: Descent, Depression, and Dissolution in the Alchemical Process

In countless myths, we rediscover what early alchemists knew: that the transmutation of body and spirit requires enduring many ordeals in a death-and-rebirth process. The descent may be triggered by events such as divorce, death, or loss of home or job, or by physical impacts like illness, accidents, miscarriage, or menopause. The individual enters the *nigredo* phase, facing *mortificatio*—the dark, dismembering beginning—marked by confusion, disorientation, and the disintegration of the old self (Somers, 2004, p. 75). Sadly, depression is often stigmatized as weakness rather than seen as an opportunity to embrace internal darkness, the *Al-Khemia*, which can nourish the soul.

Surrender is key, as the ego's defenses soften, cook (*calcinatio*), and liquefy (*solutio*), humbling the identity once protected by familiar walls. This is genuine suffering, not neurotic pain. Helen Luke draws a crucial distinction between "neurotic depression," a passive collapse, and the piercing suffering that fuels individuation (Luke, 1995, p. 56). Neurotic suffering avoids real pain, while true suffering requires embracing the weight of consciousness. As Luke writes: "The only valid cure for any kind of depression lies in the acceptance of real suffering ... the roots of our neuroses lie in the conflict between longing for growth and refusing to pay the price in suffering" (p. 57).

Dissolution in this context is an active process—holding and deepening one's pain to facilitate growth. A *temenos*, or safe container, is needed to support this process. With compassionate help for the arising feelings and images, new life grows in darkness, transforming unbearable bodily sensations into meaningful imagery, enabling genuine mourning and healing (Bloch, 2010, p. 268). Over time, clients learn to do this for themselves, gaining empathy for others' darkness—a resonance that can be consciously held.

This capacity for compassion is vital to civilization. Compassion, meaning "suffering with," involves sharing in the carrying of human suffering. As Luke writes, each time we exchange neurotic depression for real suffering, we partake, however small, in bearing the world's darkness, leading to a greater sense of meaning (Luke, 1995, p. 59).

In this process, authentic feeling replaces neurotic guilt or distress from unresolved, unsymbolized somatic pain. A vivid example of descent and return is found in the ancient Sumerian myth of Inanna. Inanna descends to the underworld to attend her brother-in-law's funeral and comfort her sister, Ereshkigal. Inanna is killed by her sister's dark gaze and hung on a meat hook. Her maidservant, Ninshubar, seeks help from Enki—the god of wisdom and creation—who sends helpers to rescue Inanna and return her to the upper world, where she is revived (Perera, 1981).

This myth offers a blueprint for individuation: the soul's journey through death and rebirth, heartbreak and healing—necessary transformations for a conscious life.

As Inanna descends, she is stopped at seven gates, where Ereshkigal's servants demand she shed her jewels, fine clothes, and crown. Psychologically, this symbolizes opening to the unconscious, shedding outward signs of status and identity. Inanna descends further, becoming increasingly vulnerable, until she is naked, falling toward the dark, creative void from which all life returns and emerges (Ashton, 2007; Stromsted, 1994/1995, p. 26). Through witnessing Ereshkigal's anguish, Enkil's spirit helpers are able to secure Inanna's freedom (Perera, 1981).

Like Inanna, we often begin this journey due to external crisis, but our rational minds fail to grasp that we must undergo a kind of death to reconnect with our "dark sister"—or for men, the wounded hero in myths like the Holy Grail or the Egyptian myth of Osiris. This "sibling" represents our shadow side, and without embracing it, we cannot be fully human or compassionate toward others. What we have forgotten—and need to relearn—is how to surrender to this descent, trusting that something transformative can emerge (Stromsted, 1994/1995, pp. 24 and 26).

This journey is somatic, involving a descent into the body's primal regions to access memories, instincts, and "gut wisdom." It shifts us from an ego-driven existence to one guided by the deeper wisdom of the Self. Inanna's journey humbles and enriches her, allowing her to return as queen, integrating light and dark, spirit and body (Meador, 2000).

In Authentic Movement, safety and awareness foster *discovery of light in dense matter*, revealing consciousness in a body that may feel stiff, defended, or lacking vitality due to psychological constraints. As Janet Adler writes:

> The evolutionary process that we are each living, as clients, therapists, artists, seekers, is about the transformative power of suffering ... Much of the work in authentic movement is difficult, painful, redundant and frustrating. It involves hiding, risking, premature insight and paralysis, as well as reward. When it works, as when a piece of art works, the clarity and simplicity—the gift of wholeness—is stunning.
>
> (Adler, 1987, p. 158)

Natural movement, rooted in the instinctual brain, engages the neocortical brain in a more robust dialogue, fostering integration between hemispheres. Insight does not rely solely on cognition, making the descent process crucial. Authentic Movement practitioners follow bodily cues to access wisdom, reflecting the alchemical process of differentiating and integrating opposites.

In the alchemical opus, the King, representing the old patriarchal ruling principle—"the deficient values and belief systems that currently rule our culture" (Baring, 2003)—struggles to relate to the dragon, which personifies the reptilian and mammalian brain, the repository of our most ancient instincts. Anne Baring (1995, 2013) warns against trying to conquer the dragon, as the solar hero has failed to do for millennia. Progress occurs not through striving for higher planes, but by confronting and collaborating with the dragon—embracing death, illness, and descent rather than repressing or dissociating from them.

Through this journey, the King assimilates and transforms the mighty powers of the instincts, thereby gaining the "treasure" that enables wisdom and healing (Baring, 1995, 2013). Similarly, we descend, our egoic identities shattered, yet we reconnect with deeper wisdom as we emerge transformed. By mastering our own pain, we become "wounded healers," able to empathize with and tend to others' suffering. Baring's (2003) retelling of the myth highlights love's healing role: the King's compassion for the dragon awakens his own heart, healing them both and the kingdom—symbolizing the integration of the shadow and the consciousness that comes through transformation.

Alchemy and Contemporary Therapeutic Practice

Women's experiences with the cycles of menstruation and birth mirror the cycles of nature. This section explores why many women are drawn to this healing approach, illustrated through two examples. Some women feel a strong need for movement, sensing imbalance in their lives. Others seek healing for issues such as eating disorders, disconnection from instincts or sexuality, or feelings of being unmothered by women who did not have access to their own deep feminine natures. Symptoms may include distorted body image, low self-esteem, depression, physical injuries, autoimmune disorders, chronic infections, or cancer—signals from the ravaged body to be honored and understood anew.

Ironically, in today's culture, ancient and indigenous wisdom can enrich needed healing. Women with a "negative mother or father" complex—especially those with a harsh inner critic—may seek nourishment in the "archetypal mother," the fertile cycles of nature. By reconnecting with the flow of life in her body and the natural world, she accesses resources for healing. Jung noted, "The symbols of the self arise in the depths of the body" (Jung, 1940/1968b, CW 9i, para. 291).

Awareness of interpersonal relationships is also crucial in this process, as a lack of maternal nurturing can hinder embodiment. Mothers, and women before them, have often struggled for equality in ways that distanced them from their bodies, leaving few role models to pass on healthy embodiment to their daughters. The alchemical process can symbolically replace flawed parenting: "cooking" in a compassionate, conscious container becomes a form of nurturing.

Pamela Sorensen's description of the mother/infant dyad offers insight into the witness/mover dynamic, especially when working with preverbal material. Her three essential elements—observation, clarification, and emotional resonance—are foundational for the containing process. Sorensen writes: "When mother is uninterested or unobservant, we are worried … keen observation is necessary not only to keep the baby alive but also to form a loving relationship" (1995, p. 3).

Contemporary research in pre- and perinatal psychology, interpersonal neuroscience, and attachment theory supports the idea that a mother's or caretaker's responsive presence is vital for a developing infant's sense of self and embodied consciousness (Cozolino, 2006; Schore & Schore, 2012; Siegel & Hartzell, 2004; Wilkinson, 2010).

Containment and Rebirth: Cassie's Journey

"Cassie," a psychotherapist who studied at the Authentic Movement Institute (Berkeley, California, 1993–2004), longed for deeper intimacy with herself and others. In a safe witness circle, she risked allowing a vulnerable, mute part of herself to emerge, which she called her "stone child." As her defenses softened, a generative process unfolded. In her writing about the movement and subsequent drawing experience, she describes the emergence of this painful, hidden part of herself:

My stone child is here again. She is so terrified. I am so ashamed. I don't want anyone else to see her. I try to keep her hidden. She wraps herself around my heart turning it stone cold. She darts forward when I least want to see her. I feel her pain. I mark her presence in this circle again. She steps forward into the light. The ice around my heart begins to melt. A new person is here. Will she see my stone child with compassion, or will she be repulsed? This pain is almost unbearable. I cannot look. I am terrified. I do not want to see the rejection I imagine is there.

This moment embodies the alchemical metaphor of the *prima materia* in the *nigredo* (dark, initial, painful) phase. Cassie fears her underdeveloped, shamed shadow parts, that were unseen in childhood and relegated to the unconscious, will be rejected as they emerge. Yet, as she stays with her genuine feelings, a *solutio* (moistening/washing) begins:

Cold tears spill out of my eyes. My throat tightens and breath becomes shallow. I struggle to stay beside her ... I draw my feelings—the color and shape of a stone appears on the paper, empty inside. I am not empty, but my feelings are a tangled, matted mess. I cannot name them. I choose a color and make a mark inside the stone shape. It looks like a yolk sac. Another color and different gesture and a tiny fluke-like worm appears, attaching itself to the yolk sac. Out of the yolk sac a snake appears, uncoils, and strikes out.

Her tears give rise to new life in the yolk sack egg—*coagulatio*—signaling the alchemical transformation. Cassie's experience highlights the need to bear excruciating feelings within the container of Authentic Movement, and the healing power of being seen by a compassionate witness. She writes:

Compassion explodes into the empty place, dances throughout this stone container that has become uterus. There is a quickening. My stone child waits. Will she be welcomed? Will she find a place in the circle this time? There are other eggs waiting outside to be fertilized. What will become of them? She is placed in the circle. She will be seen by many eyes, by how many hearts?

Cassie's journey shifted from damaged, absent parenting toward a more primal, archetypal experience reflected in themes of incubation and birth. In the circle of empathic witnesses, she found a loving ground from which to draw resources for healthy growth. This process, similar to the *solutio* phase, is reflected in myths, fairy tales, creation stories, and dreams, which offer wisdom from a deeper source than the superego's "shoulds" and "rights and wrongs" (Jung, 1947/1969, CW 8, paras. 403–404) that the child navigated in the world of his or her parents, the infant's first gods.

Gail: Recovering the Ravaged Body

Illness often forces attention to neglected or undervalued aspects of the self. This story of a woman recovering from breast cancer illustrates how trauma can reshape the relationship with one's body. It also highlights a key aspect of transformation for women: cultivating a healthy relationship with the inner masculine, or *animus*, as Jung called it—developing discernment and cutting through overwhelming feelings (Hill, 1992).

"Gail" participated in a research project on Authentic Movement in recovery (Dibbell-Hope, 1989, 1992). Although the women in the group, all mastectomy survivors, were volunteers, many initially resisted, expressing profound disappointment in their bodies: "Why should I go back into my body? It betrayed me!" (personal communication, 1989). Over time, as trust in the group and process grew, each woman began listening to her body. Many recalled being "out of their bodies" during surgery, yet the group's supportive witnessing allowed them to consciously re-enter these experiences.

As each woman worked through her trauma by moving and being witnessed, she stayed in her experience while consciously feeling it, and many reconnected with earlier memories of sensuality and zest for life, surprising themselves by discovering that "blocking the difficult feelings blocked the positive ones too" (personal communication, 1989). A kind of renewal came about as each began to "reinhabit" her body, gaining a more accurate and accepting post-surgery body image, and pleasure in life. Gail, a slim, athletic woman in her thirties, shared:

> *I curl up from the ground and stand tall in the circle, my right hand over where my right breast used to be, my left arm raised to the heavens, then extended toward my witness. I have felt ashamed of my "flat, deformed side." But in the movement, I experienced my right side as masculine and my left as feminine, realizing how both have served me and how integrated I now feel.*
>
> (personal communication, 1989)

Gail had discovered the lump in her breast while breastfeeding and was terrified to learn it was not benign. Within the group's supportive space, its *temenos*, she grieved the loss of her breast, reconnected with her love for her children, and transformed passivity and grief into strength and appreciation for life. She experienced the *coniunctio*—a palpable sense of her masculine and feminine energies came together within her embodied awareness.

For all participants, movers and witnesses alike, grief became collectively palpable. Through the spontaneous enactment that Authentic Movement fosters, fear, alienation, and shame were replaced by a sense of empowerment, respect, care, and a new appreciation for the attuned relating and body wisdom that led them through these changes (Stromsted, 2007, pp. 139–140; Stromsted, 2009, p. 203).

The Future of Alchemy and Authentic Movement

The therapeutic field increasingly integrates neuroscience, attachment theory, trauma work, and other disciplines to address healthy development and interpersonal trauma. Yet only recently has the embodied dimension of experience gained recognition in traditional verbal psychotherapeutic models. Contemporary neuroscience reveals that early trauma is stored in the preverbal right brain and body, making these areas essential for effective healing (Schore & Schore, 2012; Wilkinson, 2010).

Nevertheless, there is still considerable work to be done in integrating the mind-body basis for trauma into psychotherapy (Stromsted, 2025). Body/somatic psychotherapy approaches sometimes focus solely on the literal body ("matter"), whereas verbally oriented approaches privilege words ("psyche"). If the latter work with dreams and images, they often do not heed the cries of the body, failing to decipher its meaning, and are at a loss for how to work with it. In fragmenting the body-psyche-spirit connection, hidden forces in nature, essential to healing, go untapped.

Alchemy offers a vital metaphor for this work, emphasizing the balance and integration of body, mind, and spirit. Healing arises not from language or the body alone, but through the interplay of symbols, sensations, emotions, and natural movement, unfolding in an organic, transformative process.

Intersubjective psychotherapy emphasizes relational healing through the co-created, co-transference energetic field, addressing early wounds for both patient and therapist. As Jung says, "The unrelated human being lacks wholeness, for he can achieve wholeness only through the soul, and the soul cannot exist without its other side, which is always found in a 'You'" (Jung, 1946, CW 16, para. 454). Yet a solely verbal approach can neglect the body, with its direct access to sensations, emotions, and the creative, self-healing energies of our inner wellsprings. Jung described alchemy as a process of individuation, moving from unconsciousness to a broader awareness of the Self, integrating body, brain, psyche, and spirit. Authentic Movement provides a pathway for this transformation. Jung recognized the need for embodied practices, stating, "The self has its roots in the body, indeed in the body's chemical elements" (Jung, 1948/1967, CW 13, para. 242).

Jung also warned, "The fate of the world hangs by a thin thread, and that thread is the psyche of man" (1971, p. 14). Personal and global transformation are linked: unresolved complexes (splinter psyches and their attendant, bundled affects) stored

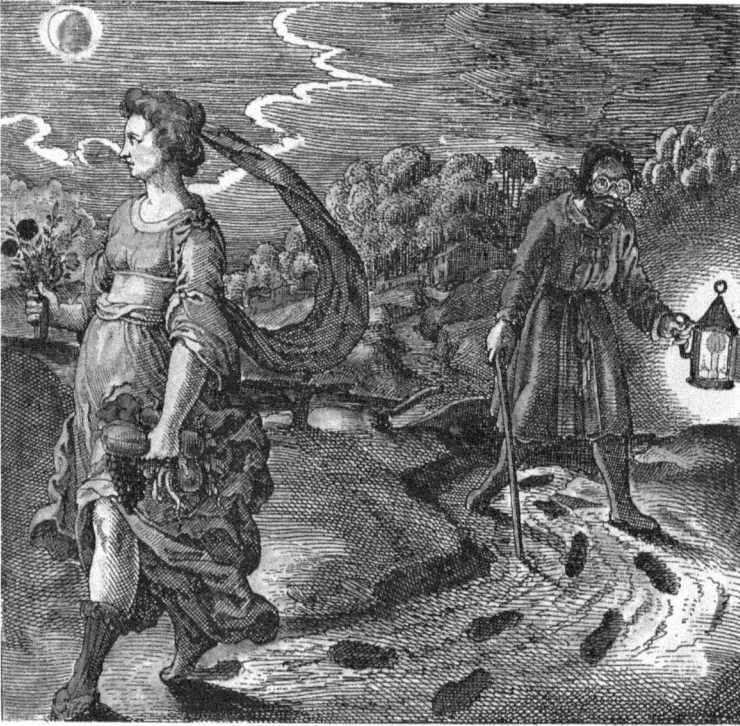

Figure 13.2 Dame Nature, whose clear footprints the alchemist
seeks to follow. Atalanta Fugiens, Emblem 42, Michael Maier, 1617.

in the body are projected outward, distorting perceptions and actions. By contrast,
a person attuned to their inner life develops more nuanced relationships with others
and the environment, fostering interconnection on interpersonal, political, spiritual,
and ecological levels.

The body plays a central role in this evolution. With a deeper awareness of embodied experience, individuals resonate with the life force animating all beings.
Rather than fleeing to spirit to escape discomfort, perpetuating trauma across generations, they can find a spiritual home in the body. Embodied consciousness is
vital for personal growth, therapeutic evolution, and the world's health. In the body
lies the gold, suspended in a dark matrix, waiting to be witnessed and cherished;
only then can its fragments coalesce into a vibrant wholeness.

> Some nights stay up till dawn,
> as the moon sometimes does for the sun.
> Be a full bucket pulled up the dark way
> of a well, then lifted out into light.
> Rumi (Barks, 2005, p. 129)

References

Adler, J. (1987). "Who is the witness?" A description of Authentic Movement. In P. Pallaro (ed.), *Authentic Movement: Essays by Mary Starks Whitehouse, Janet Adler, and Joan Chodorow* (pp. 141–159). Jessica Kingsley Publishers.

Ashton, P. (2007). *From the brink: Experiences of the void from a depth psychology perspective.* Karnac Books Ltd.

Baring, A. (1995, May 12–14). *The sacred marriage: Alchemy at the edge of history* [Presentation]. California Institute of Integral Studies, San Francisco, California.

Baring, A. (2003). *Seminar 11: The great work of alchemy—base metal into gold: The process of the soul's transformation.* https://www.annebaring.com/the-great-work-of-alchemy/

Baring, A. (2013). *The dream of the cosmos: A quest for the soul: Who are we and why are we here.* Archive Publishing.

Baring, A. & Cashford, J. (1991). *The myth of the goddess: Evolution of an image.* Penguin Books Ltd.

Barks, C. (Trans.) (2005). Die before you die. In *Rumi the book of love: Poems of ecstasy and longing.* HarperSanFrancisco. https://archive.org/details/colemanbarksrumithebook oflovepoemsofecstasyandlongingharperone2005

Bloch, S. (2010). Mercy: The unbearable in Eigen's writings and John Tavener's *Prayer of the heart.* In P. Ashton & S. Bloch (Eds.), *Music and psyche: Contemporary psychoanalytic explorations* (pp. 261–282). Spring Journal Books.

Carroll, R. (2005). Neuroscience and the "law of the self": The autonomic nervous system updated, re-mapped and in relationship. In N. Totton (Ed.), *New dimensions in body psychotherapy* (pp. 13–29). Open University Press.

Chodorow, J. (1983, October 21–24). *Dance therapy and the unholy trinity: Feminine, body, shadow* [Keynote]. 18th Annual Conference of the American Dance Therapy Association: The Healing Power of Dance Therapy, Asilomar Conference Center, Pacific Grove, California.

Chodorow, J. (1991). *Dance therapy and depth psychology: The moving imagination.* Routledge.

Chodorow, J. (Ed.) (1997). *Jung on active imagination.* Routledge.

Chodorow, J. (1999). Dance therapy and the transcendent function. In P. Pallaro (Ed.), *Authentic Movement: Essays by Mary Starks Whitehouse, Janet Adler, & Joan Chodorow* (pp. 236–52). Jessica Kingsley Publishers. (Original work published 1978)

Conger, J. (1988). *Jung and Reich: The body as shadow.* North Atlantic Books.

Cozolino, L. (2006). *The neuroscience of human relationships: Attachment and the developing social brain.* W. W. Norton & Company Ltd.

Dibbell-Hope, S. (1989). *Moving toward health: A study of the use of dance-movement therapy in the psychological adaptation to breast cancer, research jointly sponsored by the American Dance Therapy Association and the American Cancer Foundation* [Unpublished doctoral dissertation]. The California School of Professional Psychology.

Dibbell-Hope, S. [Director]. (1992). *Moving toward health* [video]. Available from sandydh@sonic.net.

Edinger, E. (1985). *Anatomy of the psyche: Alchemical symbolism in psychotherapy.* Open Court Publishing Company.

Freud, S. (1961). The ego and the id. In J. Strachey (Ed.), *The standard edition of the complete psychological works of Sigmund Freud* (pp. 3–66). Hogarth Press.

Gadon, E. W. (1989). *The once & future goddess.* Harper & Row Publishers.

Hill, G. (1992). *Masculine and feminine: The natural flow of opposites in the psyche.* Shambhala.

Hillman, J. (1976). *Suicide and the soul.* Spring Publications.

Jung, C. G. (1946). Psychology of the transference. In *The practice of psychotherapy* (Vol. 16). Princeton University Press.

Jung, C. G. (1948/1967). The spirit Mercurius. In *Alchemical studies* (Vol. 13). Princeton University Press.

Jung, C. G. (1951). Background to the psychology of Christian alchemical symbolism. In *Aion* (Vol. 9ii) (pp. 173–183). Pantheon Books.

Jung, C. G. (1968a). *The collected works of C. G. Jung: Vol. 12. Psychology and alchemy.* Pantheon Books. (Original work published 1953.)

Jung, C. G. (1968b). The psychology of the child archetype. In *The archetypes and the collective unconscious* (Vol. 9i) (pp. 151–181). Princeton University Press. (Original work published 1940.)

Jung, C. G. (1969). The transcendent function. In *The structure and dynamics of the psyche* (Vol. 8) (pp. 67–91). Princeton University Press. (Original work published 1916.)

Jung, C. G. (1969). On the nature of the psyche. In *The structure and dynamics of the psyche* (Vol. 8) (pp. 159–234). Princeton University Press. (Original work published 1947.)

Jung, C. G. (1971). *Psychological reflections.* Routledge & Kegan Paul.

Kalsched, D. (1996). *The inner world of trauma: Archetypal defenses of the personal spirit.* Routledge.

Luke, H. (1995). *The way of women: Awakening the perennial feminine.* Doubleday.

Meador, B. d. S. (2000). *Inanna: Lady of largest heart.* University of Texas Press.

Mindell, A. (1985). *Working with the dreaming body.* Routledge & Kegan Paul.

Perera, S. B. (1981). *Descent to the goddess: A way of initiation for women.* Inner City Books.

Schore, A. N. & Schore, J. R. (2012). Modern attachment theory: The central role of affect regulation in development and treatment. In A. N. Schore (Ed.), *The science of the art of psychotherapy* (pp. 27–51). W. W. Norton & Company.

Siegel, D. & Hartzell, M. (2004). *Parenting from the inside out.* Jeremy P. Tarcher/Penguin.

Somers, B. (2004). *The fires of alchemy: A transpersonal viewpoint.* Archive Publishing.

Sorensen, P. (1995). Thoughts on the containing process from the perspective of infant/mother relations. *Melanie Klein and Object Relations, 13*(2), 1–15.

Stromsted, T. (1994/1995). Re-inhabiting the female body. *Somatics: Journal of the Bodily Arts & Sciences, X*(1), 18–27.

Stromsted, T. (2007). Embodied imagination: Form grows from emptiness. In P. Ashton (Ed.), *Evocations of absence: Interdisciplinary encounters with void states.* Spring Journal Books.

Stromsted, T. (2009). Authentic Movement: A dance with the divine. *Body, Movement and Dance in Psychotherapy, 4*(3), 201–13.

Stromsted, T. (2025). Psyche's body: A brief history of engaging the body in analysis and psychotherapy. *IAAP News Bulletin* (36), January 2025.

Von Franz, M. L. (1980). *Alchemy: An introduction to the symbolism and the psychology.* Inner City Books.

Wilkinson, M. (2010). *Changing minds in therapy: Emotion, attachment, trauma, and neurobiology.* W. W. Norton & Company, Inc.

Winnicott, D. W. (1965). *The maturational process and the facilitating environment: Studies in the theory of emotional development.* International UP Inc.

Woodman, M. (1982). *Addiction to perfection: The still unravished bride.* Inner City Books.

Wyman-McGinty, W. (1998). The body in analysis: Authentic Movement and witnessing in analytic practice. *Journal of Analytical Psychology, 43*(2), 239–260.

Chapter 14

BodySoul Rhythms®

Marion Woodman and the Sacred Feminine

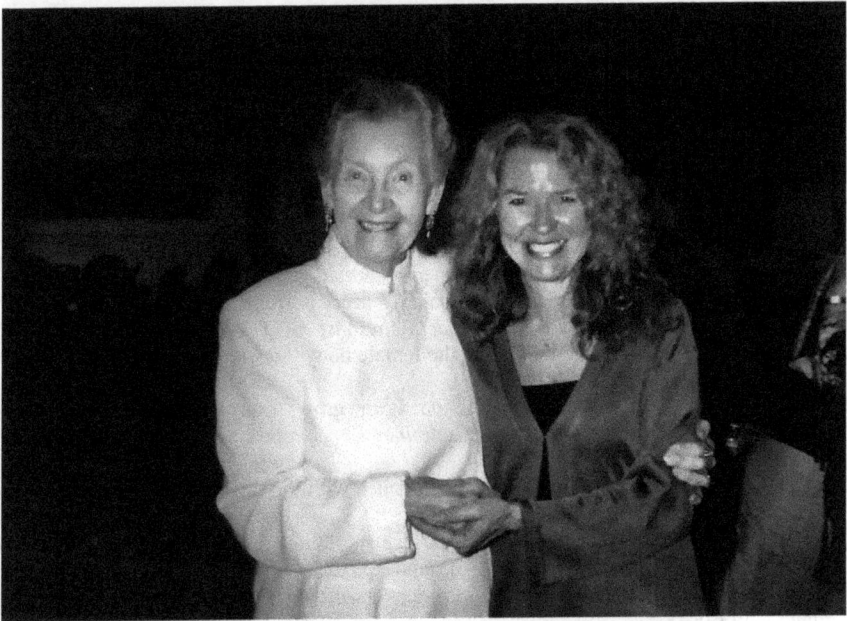

Figure 14.1 Marion Woodman & Tina Stromsted, Soul's Body Conference, San Francisco 2005. Photo courtesy of Baruch Gould.

My first contact with Marion Woodman's work was in 1981, when I read *The Owl Was a Baker's Daughter: Obesity, Anorexia Nervosa, and the Repressed Feminine,* which, like a good deal of Marion's writing, draws its title from classical literature. Eight years later, I met Marion in person at a workshop she was leading through the San Francisco C. G. Jung Institute. Following our meeting, I studied with her as often as possible, participating in the BodySoul Rhythms® intensive retreats she led for women. This chapter grew out of my dissertation

DOI: 10.4324/9781003538356-19

research, in which I interviewed Marion and other leaders in the field about their personal experiences and work with women in transformative movement practices.

Marion's early writings were followed by many other books, tracing the development of her work and ideas, including *Addiction to Perfection: The Still Unravished Bride* (1982); *The Ravaged Bridegroom: Masculinity in Women* (1990); and *Bone: Dying into Life* (2000); and five coauthored and edited books, including *Leaving My Father's House: A Journey to Conscious Femininity* (1992); and *Coming Home to Myself: Reflections for Nurturing a Woman's Body and Soul* (2001), coauthored with Jill Mellick. The Marion Woodman Foundation, a nonprofit organization, was founded to ensure that the work initiated through BodySoul Rhythms® intensives continues and flourishes (https://www.mwfbodysoulrhythms.org/).

At the heart of Marion's work was the development of "conscious femininity." When I first met Marion I was struck by her sense of presence, and her casual elegance. Tall, with thick, rich, wavy, graying brown hair, and sparkling blue eyes, she was energetic, vibrant, and articulate, packed a surprisingly wry sense of humor, and loved to dance. Marion's tone was informative, dramatic, and warm, taking care to engage the audience—even in enormous lecture halls—in something experiential that would support them in connecting with their bodies, and then drawing them out in relationship to the material she was presenting. Though the majority of her writing and teaching addresses women's experiences, she was also sensitive to the wounded inner feminine in men. A true crone—experienced, unsentimental, forgiving, and conscious of life's many paradoxes (Woodman et al., 1992, p. 202)—she embodied androgynous qualities, weaving rigorous theoretical material with experiential work that awakened deep feeling, body awareness, and creativity. She spoke passionately about the sacredness of matter and the sacredness of soul in Sophia (the feminine face of God), the relationship between the feminine individuation journey and bodily experience, and the value of dreams and intuition in guiding one's life from the depths of one's being.

Personal Background

Marion grew up in a small town in southwestern Ontario, Canada, the only girl in the family, with two younger brothers. Her father and mother met when he was giving his ordination sermon and she was a soloist in the choir. Both placed a high value on their Christian beliefs and on a life of service. An important element in the transformative movement work is the concept of being able to contact the unconscious and move freely, bringing feelings, images, bodily sensations, and memories to consciousness in a safe container, in the presence of a nonjudgmental "witness."

The daughter of a minister, Marion sought her soul through dance. "So how did the minister's daughter find dance?" I asked. Smiling, she told me that when she returned from England with Scottish dancing records, she was surprised to learn from her father's sister that she had probably inherited her Scottish Highland dance ability from her father. He had never revealed to her that he had won a number of gold medals before giving up his dancing to join the ministry! True enough, the steps had been easy for her to learn, and she had been in "heaven" on the dance floor.

When I asked her about her mother as her first "witness," wondering how her influence may have informed Marion's life and work, she replied:

"She was a suffragette who was very much ahead of her time in conservative London. She drove her own car. She had very lovely clothes. She had a job, and she had her hair bobbed before anybody else in 1926. That was big in her life because she had magnificent hair, and she decided to have it bobbed. That was more than her family could deal with. I've still got her magnificent braid that was cut off. But she was not in her body. She was very proud of her body, and she was a very good-looking woman, but she had no sense of herself as a woman, in terms of loving her menstrual cycle, or loving being a woman. She didn't like being a woman. Life would have been much easier for her in a man's body. I think that was one of the biggest things she had to deal with all her life: how to get along in a woman's body.

"In her day, she definitely suffered from being a woman. She was a very bright businesswoman—extremely clever. But because she was a woman, she had to fight her way. Then she married my father and moved to a village church. You can imagine a businesswoman marrying a minister. She was really put into a cage. The people of the church could not deal with this kind of person, especially since my father was the beloved of every girl in the congregation! And he went to the city and married a city girl and that did not sit well. By the time my mother arrived they were already against her. And so it was into that atmosphere that I was born."

Marion's independent-spirited mother felt sorry for Marion being a girl. In addition, these were Depression years, and she was aware of the added limitations that Marion would face. The family depended on farmers to bring them food. Her mother tried to provide for people who were coming in off the road hungry, and she couldn't afford to buy Marion even the simplest pretty clothes.

Then, when Marion was three years old, her mother became seriously ill and was, for the most part, bedridden for several years. While pregnant with her last child, she contracted tuberculosis of the glands through contaminated milk from the town dairy. With no one to look after her at home, Marion had to accompany her father on his ministerial rounds. Relegated to the parlors of parishioners while her father performed his duties, Marion made blankets out of doilies, playing in the world of her imagination and "pretty things." "My mother was the organizer in our household, and my father was my witness," Marion reflected. Marion spent very little time with her mother during her mother's illness and "didn't see much joy in the female body" during that time. "My mother hadn't been all that happy in her [female] body, and the illness took away what joy there was," she said sadly.

Marion's own body "shut down" during those years as she took on adult responsibilities that her mother wasn't able to fulfill. "All the spontaneous playfulness of a child was curbed by my feeling that I had to be quiet. I had to take responsibility beyond my years," she recalled. And this, she says, was a potent force behind her later putting on a great deal of weight, regardless of the number of calories she actually consumed. "The inner archetypal image was of the maternal body carrying the responsibilities," she said, and "matter follows image."

At the same time, Marion experienced her father as a friend. He would often say, "Leave the child to me," when she got into difficulties with other adults. Once they were in private, he would hear her out and empathize with her experience of the event. Reflecting on her development, Marion said, "I'm cut equally from the cloth of both parents." True enough, her mother's down-to-earth Irish-Canadian pragmatism and humor are reflected in Marion's sense of irony, which moves easily from speaking of matters of the spirit to the direct and practical experience of the body. Her father's dedication and sense of ministry have always been important to her, as has his profound connection with nature. Having grown up in the "bush," on land cleared by his Scottish parents, he was a natural gardener and a lover of animals. He took Marion fishing and hay-baling with him. The inner feminine was more accessible to him than it was to Marion's mother, who strove to overcome being a woman and all that womanhood meant in her day. As a man and minister, Marion's father was sensitive to the feelings of the people in his parish and concerned for the welfare of the Indigenous peoples on the nearby reservation, who were always ready to offer him a chair at their table whenever he came around.

Marion's father began teaching her to read at a young age. By the time she was six, she was looking forward to going to school, expecting to be able to immerse herself further in books. Instead, "public school was a horror for me," she said. The teacher had the children continually making "windmills," an activity Marion hated, and she told the teacher so. The teacher developed a "negative thing" for Marion, told her father she was rude, and hit her fingers with the pointer. Marion survived through the power of her will, deciding to sit at the back of the classroom, as far away from the teacher as possible, or perched atop a ladder, cleaning the blinds, in the home economics class. "I was out of my body by the age of six because of my anguish at school, though paradoxically I was never more aware of my body," she said. The life of the body was cut off again when she went to university, where she spent hour after hour looking into a microscope. "Again a paradox," she said, "as I was mesmerized in the biology lab."

Books and their authors were her constant companions during those difficult school years, as they continued to be throughout her life: Emily Dickinson, Shakespeare, the Bible, C. G. Jung, T. S. Eliot, William Blake, Marie-Louise von Franz, Rilke, Nikolai Berdyaev, and others. Her brothers, too, offered support. As "the preacher's kids" they didn't fit into any of the social cliques but were in a different category, with other children cleaning up their language around them.

As a little girl, Marion talked to God continually. She also carried a picture of the courageous young Joan of Arc in her apron pocket as a source of companionship—not the soldier Joan, but the girl in a simple mauve dress with bare feet, surrounded by the angel choir to whom she talked. "Wherever I went, I would put this picture down, put two stones on it, and she would take care of me. As long as she was there, I was safe," Marion recalled.

Marion, too, saw angels as a child. "Because my father was a minister I was with death all the time, and tried to tell my mother about the angels that I was watching when my father would be at a funeral and I was waiting for the soul to take off through the sky. I would sit at the window and explain to her what I was seeing, and she would come over and say, 'Marion, I tell you there are no angels!'"

Though her mother encouraged her to be more down-to-earth and practical, Marion's belief in angels was fine with her father. But it was her faith in God that ultimately made it possible for her to carry on. "I would not say that it was faith in myself," she reflected. "I thought that God gave me the angels, and God told me to follow the images in my dreams." Here, God functioned as her ultimate, larger witness, and her father as her personal witness. Marion's mother possessed a no-nonsense, practical style, a tough love that came from a "huge heart that refused to be sentimental." She was concerned that Marion did not have a strong enough hold on reality and gave her a grounding in this world, for which Marion now feels grateful, though it was difficult at the time. Not only was her mother a good businesswoman, but she was a wonderful cook as well. Marion remembers how, as a small girl, she would put on an apron and join her mother in the kitchen, standing on a chair to roll cookies on the counter. At the same time, her mother clearly conveyed the message, "I'm not raising a crybaby." Marion soon learned to hide her tears under her blankets when she encountered a heart-breaking experience, such as hearing the story of "The Little Match Girl." Though her mother was capable of projecting a public persona of practicality and strength in a crisis—wrapping the gangrenous legs of poor parishioners in newspaper, for example—she could experience feelings of vulnerability only in private.

At twenty-two, Marion became anorexic, believing that she "had to be thin to *live*," as dictated by the images of women at that time. She remembers feeling "beautiful and extremely feminine" during her years of anorexia. Being able to "touch my hip bones gave me a sense of security"; their presence "assured me that I was the 'right size.'" She had always been admired for her scholarship, yet nobody had ever said she was beautiful or attractive. Suddenly she found herself in a situation where "nobody cared a hoot about what was in my head." How "high" she felt dancing and how "out of prison," allowing herself to enter into "a paradisal state" as she "disappeared into the music"! Riveting energy accompanied her then, so much so that on one occasion, at the end of a polka, the man she was dancing with asked her politely, "Marion, would you mind putting me down?"

"There was a huge creativity in that space," she noted as she pointed out the discrepancy in her life then: she felt happy staying up much of the night dancing—waltzes, polkas, and ethnic dances with the Croatians, Finns, and Swedes in Northern Ontario—and then, though exhausted, turning around and doing a good job teaching at 9 o'clock the next morning. Determined to be thin and closer to spirit, she starved her body. "But I was on a straight rampage and I was being driven by forces that were killing my femininity. I had to change," she said. There came a day when she could no longer keep both worlds going: she collapsed on the floor while teaching. Unable to sustain her hectic lifestyle, she left for London, England, her "spiritual home," where she felt "free of the old images of responsibility for being a 'good upstanding citizen' in a 'good conservative town.'" There she danced "wonderful nights of intricate Scottish toe dancing!"

When the time came to head back home to her teaching job, Marion found that "the old heavy images of responsibility and perfection were still waiting" for her. This time she stayed, however, and married Ross Woodman. After recovering from a near-fatal car accident ten years later, she traveled to India in 1968. It was there that surrender began to play a significant role in her life, something that later profoundly informed her practice and teaching of inner-sourced movement. A severe case of dysentery led her to an out-of-body experience. Summing up her experiences, Marion said, "That was the thing that broke my relationship with the school. I did go back to the school, but I knew after I came back from India that there was a new life ahead somewhere." It was also in India that Marion discovered Sophia, the feminine face of God. She had gone there fed up with being a good "father's daughter" (a woman whose sense of identity is more closely affiliated with the father than with the mother), needing to "find out who I was when all my support systems were taken away." She describes walking home alone through the snow in Canada one night, lacking the courage, without her husband, to summon up the strength to stretch out her arm and hail a cab. It was at that moment that her inner rumblings grew into a volcano.

I knew I would buy a ticket to India, and I hoped I might encounter God in an ashram in Pondicherry. Six months later I arrived in New Delhi. God was with me all right, but His ideas were somewhat different from mine. 'He' turned out to be 'She' in India, a She that I never imagined existed in the narrow confines of my Protestant Christian tradition, a She that reached out to me not in the protective walls of an ashram, but in the streets seething with poverty, disease and love.

(Woodman, 1985, p. 176)

There, Marion underwent a number of transformative experiences that changed her life.

Personal Transformative Experiences: India

During her severe bout with dysentery in India, Marion had an experience that turned her life around. Too weak to stand, she fell on the tile floor of her bathroom.

How long I was there I do not know. I came to consciousness on the ceiling, my spirit looking down at my body caked in dry vomit and excrement. I saw it lying there helpless, still, and then I saw it take in a breath. 'Poor dummy,' I thought. 'Don't you know you're dead?' And mentally gave it a kick. Suddenly I remembered my little Cairn terrier. 'I wouldn't treat Gyronne that way,' I thought. 'I wonder what will become of it if I leave it here? Will they burn it? Will they send it home?'

(Woodman, 1985, p. 178)

She wondered why her body wouldn't stop breathing, why her spirit was not taking advantage of this opportunity to finally free itself: "I've been wanting to get out all my life. And here I'm out. All I have to do is take off," she thought.

Paralyzed by the immensity of my decision—either to leave my body there or go back into it—I saw it take another breath. I was overcome with compassion for this dear creature lying on the floor faithfully waiting for me to return, faithfully taking in one breath after another, confident that I would not forsake it, more faithful to me than I to it.

Now it was my choice—either to move into my body and live my life as a human being, or to move out into what I imagined would be freedom. I also thought of what a blow it would be to Ross, not to know what had happened to me, and did not want my body to be burned on the ghats in India. A profound shift took place: an overwhelming sweetness and love came into me for this poor thing on the floor. I saw it take another breath and there was something so infinitely innocent and trusting, so exquisitely familiar, in that movement that I chose to come down from the ceiling and move in. Together we dragged ourselves to the little bed.

(Woodman, 1985, p. 178)

Through this experience Marion was able to see her body as "separate" but not as a thing to be controlled. She forged a new awareness of her body-psyche connection, and, for the first time, was filled with good feelings and love toward her body. "She seemed so sweet," she said, recollecting the image of her body on the floor, "and like my beloved dog who was so loyal and dependent on me, I felt a loyalty in this creature. And I felt I didn't really know her at all, but I wanted to get to know her." Two weeks later she was still too weak to leave her hotel and negotiate the chaos of the streets of India. Providentially, another guest at the hotel sensed her weakened state and sent his wife to help her.

I was sitting at the end of the couch, writing my letter, frightened to death, because I had to go back out on the street again. Then I realized that I was terrified because now I wanted to live. Before I was able to go around because I did not care as much. But this woman came and pushed her way right up against me. And she had this fat arm, soft, black, black. And she pushed right up against me so I couldn't really read or write. Every time I moved, she moved. She knew her purpose, and we eventually got down to the other end of the couch. She knew no English at all and just kept smiling at me. But she was warm and I can remember relaxing *into* her a little. And that went on for a whole week.

And one day her husband came and said, 'You're all right now.' 'What do you mean?' I asked, startled at his intimacy. 'You were dying,' he said. 'You had the aloneness of the dying. I sent my wife to sit with you. I knew the warmth of her body would bring you back to life. She won't need to come again.' I thanked him. I thanked her. They disappeared through the door—two total strangers who intuitively heard my soul when I was unable to reach out my arms. Their love brought me back into the world. Having claimed my body and at the same time having surrendered myself to my destiny, I was undergoing both the joy and the pain of experiencing life in the flesh. ... I was no longer the victim, however. I no longer felt physically raped or in danger of death. I was participating in life with an open heart, ravished by the sights and sounds and smells of that extraordinarily paradoxical world. ... I knew something was being burned away that had to be burned away if I was going to live my life. I knew the pain was my pain. I had no idea what it meant, but I knew it had to be. I knew I was living my destiny.

(Woodman, 1985, pp. 178–181)

Upon returning to Canada, Marion taught at the university for two years and then took a sabbatical in England with her husband. There she began working on her dreams with Dr. Bennet, a wise old Irishman and Jungian analyst, whose compassion and directness helped her to get started on the task of identifying her true feelings and setting a direction for life. Eventually, Marion developed a severe kidney disorder. After twenty-four years of teaching English literature and directing theater productions in high school, her body once again forced her to reexamine her life. Since there were no Jungian analysts in Canada at the time, and Dr. Bennet was getting very old, he advised her to go to Zürich to work with an analyst there. Her conscious work in integrating imagery and movement with Mary Hamilton and the students, following on the heels of her dreamwork with Dr. Bennet, prepared her for the deep transformative work that she would later undergo on her own.

Partnering: Body and Analysis

Hoping to find healing, Marion moved to Zürich. Now she wanted to live, but *not* on a dialysis machine for the rest of her life. She studied depth psychology and dreams at the C. G. Jung Institute in Zurich and eventually became an analyst.

"When I arrived, there was nobody doing body work at the time. But my dream told me to take the images from my dreams and put them in my body, saying, 'Don't ask any questions, because it won't make any sense!' So many weekends I spent, maybe ten hours Saturday and Sunday, lying on the floor on a woolen blanket with another woolen blanket over me. I was in a womb, and I worked with the imagery from the dream and allowed the energy of the dream to go into my body. Over the period of four years, a very severe kidney condition was healed.

"I was in analysis, but my analyst was outraged at the thought of body movement. So he didn't want to know anything about what was going on. His attitude was, 'If you can't transform through your dreams there's something wrong with the way you're handling your dreams.' I knew that I could have a wonderful time with my dreams because I had been through two years of that, but it didn't change my body. In fact, I got higher and higher into spirit, so my body became more and more exhausted.

"[But] there was a great pact between me and God doing this work. It's like the container in analysis. ... If it's held absolutely sealed, it's much stronger than if there's a leak. So ... I had no leaks because I didn't have anyone to talk to. I didn't have anybody that was remotely interested in what I was doing. But my relationship with Sophia and God was sufficiently deep that I didn't have any fear. I trusted the dreams and I believed that the dreams were given by God. And I simply did what the dreams told me to do. And, of course, I was studying, so I was able to work with my studies, further amplifying and integrating my experience."

When I reflected back to Marion how amazed I felt at her ability to persevere under the circumstances, without a human witness and with so little support, she responded, "It was fear, Tina. I had to heal that kidney! I didn't go to Zürich to be an analyst. I went to Zürich to try to get this terrible problem healed. So I was profoundly faithful, simply because I wanted to live." Thus, her healing commenced through a profoundly integrative and transformative process, which was eventually to become her life's work.

The Development of Marion's Work

Marion had to contend with several life-and-death struggles through the course of her life: with her anorexia, her illness and out-of-body experience in India, her severe kidney condition in Zürich, and her healing from a cancer diagnosis and treatment she received. Marion described the importance of a lot of "good mothering" in the transformative process and the paradox inherent in the inner-sourced movement and analytic work: in the process one must build up the strength and flexibility of the body ego, while simultaneously dismantling the defenses.

"The work is to let the ego go and *become* the music. So that you are *being* danced. Many people can't sustain that kind of surrender. Their ego becomes inflated with the archetype; they begin to identify with the archetypal energy. The result is an inflated ego, functioning out of willpower. Instead of surrendering their ego to the Self, they cling to their willpower in their own ego. It's a failed spiritual journey. We can do all we want to try to change something with our will, but Jung says it's the archetypal energy that heals, and anything else is Band-Aid. In my experience that is true. It is the essence of the feminine experience. It's the secret of great lovemaking."

Body Integrity and Surrender

For Marion, each important experience of being touched by spirit, or "broken open" was accompanied by some kind of trauma to her body that profoundly changed her relationship with it.

Marion always acknowledged the importance of strength and the integrity of the woman's body structure as a ground for opening to consciousness, agreeing that some background in dance or other body disciplines can be of help with this. In fact, she felt that if it had not been for her "Scotch-peasant body" her story would have ended in tragedy. "It kept me walking on the ground, humble, and compassionate," she said. Marion realized in her own early crisis that the path to healing lay in surrender to what she "had no will power over"—in this case, her body weight. Paradoxically, this surrender was exactly what she needed in order to grow. At that point she had lost all faith in God and her will to live. "It was in the breaking of my health that the transcendent came through from the other side," she said. "And because of the anguish in my own soul I have been totally in communication with the anguish in others." She pointed out that this was where the love came in: "Until your heart breaks open, you don't know what love is about." Marion reminded me that it was the archetypal energy that healed. Since the turning point with the car accident and the brush with death in India, her life path had been one of "deeper and deeper surrender."

As Marion spoke with me during our interviews, paradox was ever present in many of her life's transformative experiences. For example, during her anorexic years she felt, on the one hand, that she was living life "with the intensity, and the joy, and the rapture" that she had never had before, while at the same time, "there was a death wish at the center of it" that she had not yet brought to consciousness. "I didn't care if I lived or died, so long as I was 'happy,'" she remarked with irony.

Loved Body: Living Body

Given the negative, distorted, limiting images that have been passed down in the projections of the patriarchy through the mother and father lines, learning to love our bodies played an important role in Marion's work. Body image is a mysterious phenomenon about which we still have much to learn. However, in listening to Marion, I began to have a sense that body parts that are loved and valued in early life often continue to carry their aliveness into adulthood. For example, although Marion's mother felt sorry for Marion for being a girl, she was nevertheless able to "witness" her daughter's hair, skin, and hands, parts of Marion's body that were vibrant and expressive throughout her life. Marion's mother was adept with her hands. "The consciousness that I have developed in my hands came through from a very early age," said Marion. Since those were Depression days, in the 1930s, when Marion's mother could not afford to buy her daughter even the most basic skirts and sweaters, she "didn't know what to do."

"But she knew how to fix my hair. ... As far as she was concerned, I had a head and hands. And if you know how I teach, and you do, I have a head and hands. I know when the kids used to parody me in high school, whoever was playing me would put on a long gown, which simply covered the body, and this extremely beautiful dance would go on with the head and the hands."

Creating the Container

Marion passed this "good mothering" and body witnessing down to her workshop participants in an evening partner exercise (modeled with Mary Hamilton) in which mother (Marion) cradled and rocked her daughter (Mary), singing and telling her stories as she brushed her hair. In this way the daughter felt held, nurtured, and accepted in the cells of her feminine body, and was able to release any excess bodily tension to this containing feminine presence. Marion also guided participants in giving each other hand and foot massages, loving the skin and easing the muscular constrictions that accompanied a "lifetime of holding oneself up, holding oneself together." Marion felt strongly that even women who had never had that loving touch or sense of being contained—"and many have not"—could "experience in their body the loving arms around them, which, in turn, gradually helps them to experience their own female body as a loving container for the soul." Working in pairs also helped women experience inner "self-holding" and relaxation, in contrast to the "drivenness" that characterized most "father's daughters." This facilitated an opening up to the vulnerability of the wounded inner child, in place of the compensatory stance that many women adopt with the use of various guises—tough Amazon, helpless little girl, seductress—or with the anesthetizing effect of various addictions, strategies that further alienated them from the source of their pain and thus from the potential for healing (Leonard, 1982, 1989; Woodman, 1980, 1982, 1985, 1990, 1993a, 1993b; Woodman & Bly, 1998; Woodman & Dickson, 1996). In the process, women began to learn to soften their defenses, trusting that their bodies, inner life, and the firm container created within the workshop could hold them.

Marion worked to create the container not only at a physical and interpersonal level, but also at an archetypal level as well, using ritual elements throughout her workshops. "I build a container at the altar so that Sophia is present. That's very important. And in analysis I always say, if you have to [telephone me in-between sessions], do so, so they know that the container has to hold. And they've got to take responsibility for holding it because, in my experience, the transcendent will come of its own accord when the container is strong enough. So I'm trying to build it with them so that when the transcendent does arrive, they'll be ready."

Marion began each day of her workshops with a prayer at the altar. This often took the form of asking for Sophia's guidance in assisting the group in working through specific emotional issues, as well as acknowledging important related events that were going on in the world at that time, linking inner and outer realities. From the altar, the group moved to experiential work, in which a group member volunteered to lead a warm-up or guided meditation to open the participants' bodies, in preparation for the day's work.

A Student's Transformative Story

An example of one of Marion's workshops illustrated the importance of the container provided by the feeling of the other group members. Their concentration played an essential role in the healing that occurred.

I've been in workshops where the tears run down my face, because I can see pain in somebody's body. The pain starts to come out in a shriek and I can see how the body is writhing. I'm describing a mask workshop that I was working in. All the members of the workshop were working with their clay to make the masks; they had their eyes shut. I was working with one woman who had broken on the floor. The other women just kept going with their masks. They all knew she had to go through it. Not one of them opened their eyes. They sent their love over to us in the corner—I could feel their love pouring in. And that little body writhed, and pulled, and pushed, and did its best to get born. And did. In that situation love is born in the whole group. There's a positive mother in the group. Nothing else will go through that wall [of the embodied negative mother] but that kind of love. If you confront the wall you come against it, but love melts it. And when you come through the wounding to the suffering, you see what the matter [the body] has endured. (Woodman, 1993b, tape 5)

Marion's work emphasized the importance of acknowledging and experiencing the energies of the shadow. For this reason, Marion felt it was crucial to keep a creative outlet open in the analytic process. Making faces, conscious breathwork, odd sounds, awkward or funny dances, masks that can be gorgeous, terrifying, ugly, or sympathetic—all helped to break down the stereotypical body image of perfect beauty that patriarchal culture set for women.

For me, body work is soul work, and the imagination is the key to connecting both. Most of us keep our breath as shallow as possible because the eruption of feeling is too intense if we inhale deeply. Breathing is very important because it is a matter of receiving, and that is the feminine principle incarnate. [Fear of rejection is related to our breathing.] If, for example, a person has an intense negative mother complex, this often manifests in a plugged throat, plugged nose, sinus trouble, asthma, and all kinds of difficulties.

Sometimes in body work, the mucus starts to pour out—it oozes out in ropes, out of the eyes, the nose and the mouth—when the complex is releasing! This often signals the end of asthma and related diseases. Such people often cannot give you their chest if you offer to hold them. They will arch. But when they start to trust, their body will begin to free itself and they will be capable of a full embrace.

However, as you solve these problems, you often encounter new ones. The whole vaginal area is related to the throat and the breath. So if you release something here, you also release energy at the other end. Then you're dealing with a problem that is sexual.

(Woodman, 1993a, pp. 16–17)

Finding Authentic Voice

Opening to one's voice was another essential part of Marion's BodySoul intensive, facilitated by vocal coach Ann Skinner. Marion pointed out that often a woman's voice was pushed up into the higher range by her negative animus, which squeezed her throat with inner criticisms, such as "You're worthless. You don't have any-thing to say. You don't expect anyone to take you seriously, do you? Who gave you permission to take up space? Anything you have to say has been said much better by somebody else!" Developing the capacity to stand up for her beliefs was another element of this work. Marion told the story about holding her ground with a man who wanted to borrow money. The tension between them grew so strong that the glass in a picture frame snapped spontaneously. "Better that, than your body!" I remarked, marveling at how she was able to develop a body that was strong enough to contain a remarkably high level of energy without snapping or becoming ill (UCSC Intensive, February 1995).

In the BodySoul workshops, movement and vocal exercises were often followed by drawing or painting a "body map," in which women traced each other's bod-ies and then filled in the tracings of their own bodies with colors or other media in response to how they perceived their bodies, and how they were experiencing themselves at the physical, emotional, and energetic levels at that time.

Once the participants' bodies were attuned and alive, Marion guided them in using their dreams to facilitate healing by placing positive dream images in "dark" parts of the body, much as she did to cure her own kidney condition. She allowed the image to move and transform as it wished. She also used inner-sourced and structured, directive movement work guided by Mary Hamilton, and often referred analysands in her private practice for sensitive and professional touch/bodywork when appropriate. These methods helped the body open, released the grip of the complexes, attended to the woman's wounded child, and helped the traumatized body catch up with the ego, which otherwise often tried to move ahead too swiftly in the analysis (Woodman, 1985, p. 55). Working with the unconscious through the use of dreams, active imagination, imagery, dance, art, music, voice, mask-making, and improvisational theater, Marion's work assisted women in building stronger, more flexible and feelingful bodies—vessels for feminine consciousness.

Addictions

In working with addictions, Marion attended to the metaphor in the behaviors, holding a larger frame of reference in helping the addict understand the meaning of the patterns that accompanied the illness. "I always try to grasp the metaphor at the root of an addiction. That varies. With food, it can be mother; with alcohol, spirit; with cocaine, light; with sex, union. Mother, spirit, light, union—these can be archetypal images of the soul's search for what it needs. If we fail to understand the soul's yearning, then we concretize and become compulsively driven toward an object that cannot satisfy the soul's longing" (Woodman, 1993a, p. 124).

Marion felt that it was through contacting this deep soul longing and bringing it to consciousness, rather than simply treating the external symptoms, that our culture might be healed of the addictions that still exist on such a massive scale. Her style in working with people was honest, direct, forceful, respectful, humor-ous, sometimes confrontational, and deeply supportive. Though Marion's mother "had no sense of loving being a woman," and Marion felt sad because she herself had no children, the mother archetype was generously expressed through her work with thousands of students, workshop participants, and analysands—"un-mothered women" and father's daughters who benefited a great deal from the healing her work provided them. Her own struggle with the death wish in anorexia was a testament to the work, which she modeled for women who wished to recognize and value their feminine being. Marion also illustrated a feminine mode of leadership, working collaboratively with Mary Hamilton and Ann Skinner, sometimes accompanied by psychologist Paula Reeves who assisted with witnessing the group. Their styles wove together naturally, as each took turns leading elements of the work as well as supporting one another in the process, seeming like mother and daughters in one moment, while at other times like sister muses as they integrated their gifts.

Cellular Resonance

Marion described an "overwhelming sense of sweetness and love" that came over her, sometimes accompanied by the scent of orange blossoms, in moments when Sophia was present. She also spoke of the change in the metabolism of the cells that came about through metaphor—how when she read Shakespeare, "the person that starts reading and the person that ends an hour later are two different people in the cells of the body." A "shimmer" came in, a higher metabolism, something that she likened to the old feeling she had when she was anorexic, only now she had a ground for it, a "body that [was] strong enough to take the intensity of what's coming through. And when the metabolism, the shimmer, gets to a certain stage, the transcendent comes in."

When I shared with Marion my longing to let go of some of my current work responsibilities and how, at times when my schedule would get too busy, my body sometimes felt as if it would burst in the presence of beauty or poetic metaphor (tearful with gratitude and resonating with energy that felt big enough to burst the tension in my tissues), she urged me to pay attention. "It's the edge, Tina. The very edge. The bursting is to be touched by God," she said, "and to deny that is to block energy. Repressed energy can kill. The experience needs to be brought to consciousness, through writing, making a poem." Here she reflected again on how the bodies had changed in the high school students whom she had invited to read and embody poetry. "It's the metaphorical body we're building. It's that place between spirit and matter."

Marion's questions brought her full circle to her early days as a teacher as she pursued research in psychoneuroimmunology to discover what it was that took place at the biological level—how *did* poetry change cell structure? Having sensed something of this in my own experiences in inner-sourced movement, I asked Marion to elaborate further.

"When I read a poem aloud and let it resonate through my body, if I love the poem, if I am really resonating with it, I get a 'shimmering' sensation. The resonators are open. They are really working. So that by the end of the poem I feel a real difference—you know, emotion, imagination, intellect, all come together—and it's as if psyche and body are whole. The only way I could describe that would be as an inner marriage where body and psyche are one."

"And does your subjective experience of yourself and your world change?" I wondered.

"Well," she responded, "if I don't read poetry every day and don't listen to music, I tend to get mired in mud. I fall into body and feel slow. I put on weight. My eating patterns don't change, but there's a slowness in the metabolism and everything is 'matter.' Whereas, when I read poetry aloud, when I listen to music, especially if I dance to it, my body is alive. Every cell is full of spirit."

"You're also really speaking about this as a 'living,' daily practice, as a way of life," I noted. "As, for example, differentiated from other images of 'enlightenment,' where people assume an 'endpoint' or something that you achieve—images that seem to be more characteristic of the masculine perspective."

"That's right," said Marion. "I don't see an endpoint to that, except death. And I've had a pretty good look at that one with cancer because with that in the wings you don't fool around."

In 1993, Marion was diagnosed with cancer at the base of her spine. With a healing process combining Western medical, homeopathic, and movement and dreamwork practices, she outlived all of her doctor's predictions. Her book *Bone: Dying into Life* (2000) articulated her experience living with and recovering from cancer. Integrating findings from quantum physics and information from current psychoneurological research, she remained passionate in deepening her understanding of the relationship between spirit and matter.

Personal Practices: Integration into Daily Life

Marion once reflected that it took her sixteen years "to understand why I went to India" and to integrate the transformative experiences that she had there. When I pointed out that I had rarely heard about the integrative aspects of the transformative process—because people usually focus on the "peak experiences" (Maslow, 1968, 1971)—Marion underscored how essential this was, and how "useless it [was] if you [left the transformative experience] alone."

"How do you integrate these experiences into your daily life?" I asked, to which she responded, "It's challenging to live in the body, and all of the things I do now—dancing, drawing, holding people, writing—are all part of my effort to continue to integrate and live this."

Though she became much more receptive to her body sensations and allowed "intuition to flow through her body," she stated that she still had to discipline her body. "Periodically it's like a wild racehorse. There's still a teenager in me. That energy is still in me periodically, but now my body and I are friends," she said. One of her daily personal practices was to put on music and "lie on the floor and spend half an hour letting my body do anything it wants to do." In this safe and free space, she often would speak as she moved, tape recording the movement patterns and images that emerged, or journaling following her movement experience to understand better what was going on "because I believe that you have to bring [the material] to consciousness." Over years of this practice, Marion developed a sensitive and refined "inner witness," capable of maintaining a conscious awareness as she allowed herself to be moved by unconscious material.

After moving, she often drew the images that came to her, working with them in the same way that she would analyze a dream, tracking the sequence of images "to see where the energy wants to go," as the imagery "has the transformation right in it." During this integrative phase of the work she first brought her own personal associations to the images and then used a dictionary of imagery and symbols and other relevant texts to amplify them further, historically and mythologically.

Marion also took daily hour-long walks to the river in London, Ontario, kept a daily journal, carried on research for her books, listened to music, and shared long conversations with Ross. The two worked on their dreams together as well. "I lost my daily six hours of imagery when I retired from my teaching job because I didn't sit down and read Shakespeare every day!" When she realized how deep her need for poetry was—"it's food for the soul"—she and Ross read poetry aloud to each other. "The older you get, the more you understand it," she said, again describing the "shimmer" that ran through her when she read Shakespeare, a shimmer that found a pathway through her work with inner-directed movement.

When Marion danced, her body came alive. "Every cell fills with spirit, so that I no longer feel weighted down and mired in the mud of matter." Having come to know the sacredness in matter, Marion always took time to "tune her body/instrument, as if preparing for Mozart." Her senses were considerably more heightened and intensified, and she experienced the same electric "shimmer" when she saw beauty in nature, such as the red tulips that created a "little epiphany" that stayed with her. After decades of work with the body, Marion found that her intuition grew keener as she picked up things going on with other people at greater distances. "When you've got more ground, the intuition can fly higher or more broadly," she said, referring to her psychic experiences. Marion's teaching combined a practical, grounded, sensation-specific use of language with profoundly metaphoric, symbolic, and spiritual images, grounding the latter with the former in daily life. The effect was often surprising, humorous, and powerfully integrative.

Sophia's Perfume

As our conversations came to a close, Marion reflected on another transformative experience she had had, which, like the others, engaged her directly at a body level. In this instance, she had been driven nearly crazy by the tinnitus that had been ringing loudly in her ear ever since her car accident, "to the point where I nearly didn't care if I lived or died," she said.

"But the tinnitus in my ear was the opening to Sophia, because I had a dream, filled with the scent of an orange blossom bush, in which I heard a clear voice ask, 'How does it feel on the eve of becoming everything you've fought against all your life?' And I thought, 'For heaven's sake, what does that mean?' Well, I found out, in a vision that immediately followed. I'd fought the feminine all my life, but I didn't know it. And, again, it was the love that healed me … this overwhelming sense of love, and the perfume … I could feel it, just cell by cell by cell. [Marion vibrated her fingers to demonstrate the shimmering sensation that grew from the ground up, traveling up her legs and through her whole body.] My body became limp with the beauty of the perfume. And I'd never known this kind of love before—pure, transcendent—feminine transcendence from below."

"How did you identify it as 'feminine' energy?" I asked.

"Remember the song you sang at the end of that workshop, Tina, with the words that were given to you from your dream? How did that go?"

Recalling the lyrics, still fresh in me, I sang to the tune of "Motherless Child":

> *I used to feel like a*
> *mother-less child,*
> *Now I know that I'm*
> *really wild,*
> *Right now I'm finding my*
> *personal style,*
> *Deep, down*
> *in my bones.*

> *Last night I dreamed of*
> *dance and perfume,*
> *Crazies and red wine filled the*
> *upstairs rooms.*
> *Downstairs the choir sang,*
> *"Sophia blooms!"*
> *Deep, down*
> *in my bones.*

> *There, I'm not alone.*
> *She gives us our Home.*

"What a beautiful expression of feminine energy, Tina!" Marion responded. "And I want to connect this with your story. The love I experienced was soft. It was warm … like the lady in India. I could relax into it like those little Japanese dolls … they can hardly hold their heads up. It was sinuous; it was flexible; it was total surrender. One hundred percent surrender. Yet I was totally immersed. And the healing would not have happened without that—I became totally concentrated on *being* the orange bush. The energy leapt beyond simile, 'like an orange bush'; it *became* the orange bush. That's metaphor.

"This is the secret of the transformation: when I see an orange bush in my meditation, I become the orange bush. I become the perfume. So the ego is not present, … there is union. My being is permeated; it is total intercourse with the Divine. And it feels like an orgasm, yes, it does. ... And there's nothing new about that."

Years of work with body and psyche, integrating dreams and inner-sourced movement, provided a tremendous healing and guide for Marion. She invited the women she worked with to find the discipline and surrender that could allow them to open to Sophia's gifts.

> The feminine
> has slower rhythms meanders,
> moves in spirals, turns back on herself,
> finds what is meaningful to her, and plays.
> This is your body, your greatest gift,
> pregnant with wisdom you do not hear,
> grief you thought was forgotten, and joy you have never known.
> (Woodman & Mellick, 1998, pp. 147–149)

Marion Woodman died in 2018 at the age of 89. After more than three decades of deep, embodied creative work with her—including soulful experiences, inspiring conversations, co-facilitating BodySoul Leadership Trainings, and her invitation to continue her legacy teaching her work, as well as my own, at Pacifica Graduate Institute—Marion will always have a special place in my heart. Her voice still guides me in analytic sessions, workshops, and life decisions whenever I seek inner wisdom. This quote captures the essence of Marion, her work, and the gifts she gave to us all:

> Love is the real power. It's the energy that cherishes. The more you work with that energy, the more you will see how people respond naturally to it, and the more you will want to use it. It brings out your creativity, and helps everyone around you flower. Your children, the people you work with—everyone blooms.
> Marion Woodman
> (as cited in Banitt, 2019, Chapter 10)

References

Banitt, S. P. (2019). *Wisdom, attachment, and love in trauma therapy: Beyond evidence-based practice*. Routledge.

Leonard, L. (1982). *The wounded woman: Healing the father-daughter relationship*. Swallow Press.

Leonard, L. (1989). *Witness to the fire: Creativity and the veil of addiction*. Shambhala Publications, Inc.

Maslow, A. (1968). *Toward a psychology of being*. D. Van Nostrand.

Maslow, A. (1971). *The Farther reaches of human nature*. Viking Press.

Woodman M. (1980). *The owl was a baker's daughter: Obesity, anorexia nervosa, and the repressed feminine*. Inner City Books.

Woodman M. (1982). *Addiction to perfection: The still unravished bride*. Inner City Books.

Woodman M. (1985). *The pregnant virgin: A process of psychological transformation*. Inner City Books.

Woodman M. (1990). *The ravaged bridegroom: Masculinity in women.* Inner City Books.

Woodman M. (1993a). *Conscious femininity: Interviews with Marion Woodman.* Inner City Books.

Woodman M. (1993b). "Conscious femininity, Part One." In C. S. Roth (Ed.), *Sitting by the well: Bringing the feminine to consciousness through language, dreams, and metaphor* [Cassette of presentation]. *Care of the Soul,* June 4–5. Sounds True Recording.

Woodman M. & Bly R. (1998). *The maiden king: The reunion of masculine and feminine.* Henry Holt & Company.

Woodman M., Dansen, K., Hamilton, M., & Greer Allen, R. (1992). *Leaving my father's house: A Journey to conscious femininity.* Shambhala Publications, Inc.

Woodman M. & Dickson, E. (1996). *Dancing in the flames: The dark goddess in the transformation of consciousness.* Shambhala Publications.

Woodman M. & Mellick, J. (1998). *Coming home to myself: Reflections for nurturing a woman's body and soul.* Conari Press.

Chapter 15

DreamDancing®

Embodied Consciousness

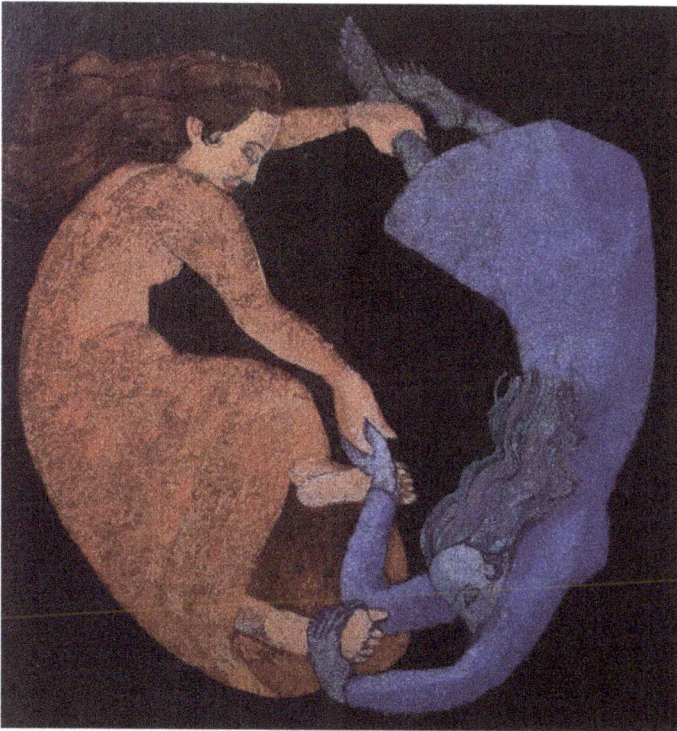

Figure 15.1 Peter Malone, Untitled, from *The Secret Language of Dreams* by David Fontana. (Illustrations copyright © 1994 by Duncan Baird Publishers. Watkins Media Limited. Reproduced with permission of the Licensor through PLSclear.)

We all move; we all dream. Dreams are reflections of the deep, formative processes that occur as we develop and grow. They help reduce stress, process emotions, and consolidate learning and memory. Dreams hold treasures that can enrich the meaning and depth of our life's journey. Reflecting our emotional state, our

DOI: 10.4324/9781003538356-20

spiritual condition, our feelings and struggles, they point to what matters most to us. Dreams can also reflect areas where we feel stuck and reveal ways to cultivate more freedom and wholeness in our lives. They invite us to engage with shadowy or disowned parts of ourselves, as well as new potentials—bringing fresh energy for healing, creativity, and personal development.

DreamDancing is an integrative approach I began developing in the 1980s. It was rooted in experiences with dancing dream figures in my childhood. When I was about eight years old, around the time of my parents' divorce, I had a repeating dream:

> *A young girl in a white dress lies in a field by the ocean. She is motionless and it's hard to tell if she is alive. Figures come toward her through the surrounding forests and from across the water. Each is dressed in a ritual costume, according to their tradition. One draws a mandala around the girl's body. Another dances, another plays the flute, still another drums a steady rhythm. One brings healing touch, as another sings a prayer over her bones until the girl revives.*

Later in life, I realized that "she" was me and that these dream healers were like shamans from many cultures conducting healing rituals that enabled my soul to return following frightening experiences in my childhood home. Though my father was warm and kind, he was often away traveling for work and lacked the strength to stand up to my erratic, reactive mother and, later, my punitive stepmother, fearing they would leave him. This triggered the sense of overwhelm he had felt at pivotal times growing up.

Dreams were always important to me as a child, opening me to the world within where I found resources lacking in my outer life. Often sitting at the base of a large oak tree, I would write them in my journal. Without adults to talk with about them, I often danced them to explore the feelings, actions, and stories in them as each character brought further dimension to the unfolding inner story, seeking awareness. Though I wasn't always sure what they meant, engaging them brought expression, meaning, and more balance to my life, often pointing to the path I needed as I found my way.

Later, when I read Jung's autobiography, *Memories, Dreams, Reflections*, I felt I had found a soul friend whose life was also guided by his dreams! Still later, following many years of dance and studies in psychology, anthropology, yoga, meditation, and other mind/body practices, I combined these worlds to become a dance/movement therapist and a Jungian analyst. Each of us has an origin story, revealing seeds that, with effort, courage, imagination, and adequate resources, can grow into a meaningful vocation and way of life that reflects who we really are.

A Brief History of Dreams

Although not everyone remembers their dreams upon waking, these experiences have provided important guidance throughout human history and are essential for our mental, emotional, and physical healing and growth. Early shamans and traditional communities from various cultures revered dreams as oracles and healing agents. For thousands of years, dreams were viewed as important inner navigational systems. They were "incubated" (invited) and interpreted as messages from the gods, a means of connecting with ancestor spirits for guidance, and even as opportunities to witness events in other realms. Ancient Egyptians, Hebrews, Greeks, Romans, Indigenous Peoples such as Native Americans, Māori, San Bushmen, African healers from the Xhosa and Zulu cultures, and many others around the world respected dreams, giving them an esteemed place alongside waking experiences.

For traditional Indigenous Australians dreaming has long served as a framework for making sense of the world, emphasizing the interconnectedness of all people and things. Dreaming is viewed as the "Spirit World," which exists alongside the physical realm, inhabited by Ancestors and Creator Spirits. Encompassing a continuum that links the past, present, and future, this view is transmitted through various traditions, including storytelling, music, dance, ceremonial body painting, and symbolic art.

The oldest known text on dreamwork is *The Book of Dreams* by the Duke of Zhou, around 1100 BCE in China. At that time the Zhou dynasty employed an official dream interpreter who reflected on the meaning and interpretation of dream images. Believing dreams could be predictive—implying auspicious and inauspicious things—the text included a wide range of symbols that were interpreted, with resonances even today (Pei & Zhang, 2000).

The ancient Greeks practiced dream incubation, traveling to a sacred place to sleep and receive a useful dream from a god. Up to four hundred temples were built in honor of Asklepios, the god of medicine and healing, and were in active use from the end of the sixth century BCE until the end of the fifth century CE (UNESCO). The Asklepion was the central healing sanctuary in the Hellenic and Roman worlds. Here, dreams were incubated to assist in the diagnosis and treatment of physical and soul illnesses (Meier, 1989). Our contemporary therapeutic use of dreams may well descend from these ancient practices. From what we understand, these early peoples were supported in their pilgrimages on every level of their culture. Dreams were believed to be direct messages from the gods. Asklepios often appeared in their dreams in a variety of forms—human and animal—touching the afflicted pilgrims, curing them, or advising them about what they needed to do in order to be healed, including what further offerings might be required (1989).

Modern Dreamwork

With the rise of secularism, rationalism, and materialism in the West, unfortunately, dreams have often become regarded as superfluous in the hustle and bustle of the daytime world in mainstream culture. However, when engaged with curiosity and respect, dreams can provide essential insights into daily life and restore a necessary balance.

Dreams have been extensively examined by Sigmund Freud, C. G. Jung, and other theorists. In the context of psychotherapy, dreamwork typically involves a verbal analysis of a patient's dreams to uncover unconscious wishes, impulses, feelings, motives, and memories. The aim is to help the dreamer gain a deeper understanding of themselves, develop a greater sense of agency and meaning in their life, and encourage new behaviors that align with their feelings and current life situation. Without this inner guidance, individuals may increasingly find themselves relying on external sources of guidance, such as unreliable news outlets or charismatic social media influencers. Alternately, they might fall into repeating unconscious patterns formed to cope with developmental traumas from childhood or feel stuck at a certain life stage, engaging in behaviors that have outlived their usefulness. The intimate connection between the psyche and the body is also significant. Arnold Mindell, an American Jungian analyst and quantum physicist, interpreted bodily symptoms as manifestations of dreams trying to express themselves physically—that is, body symptoms were dreams trying to happen in the body (Mindell, 1989).

Today many therapists specialize in verbal dream interpretation, gestalt enactments, or physiological work. DreamDancing engages the individual on all of these levels. In this approach, the image is seen as the inner representation of the person's unconscious, and the body as its outward expression or manifestation. Images, if not embodied, run the risk of becoming free-floating entities that can entertain, overwhelm, or be lost to the individual. Conversely, the body may be treated as an object to be fattened, dieted, exercised, directed, indulged, looked at, hidden, or ignored.

From my perspective, a deeper exploration and integration is facilitated when the unconscious images are given life and form. "The images give the movement meaning, while sensation and movement ground the image in emotional reality," says Joan Chodorow (Stromsted, 1984, p. ii). Through embodying the image, inner and outer expression and experience may become more unified and satisfying for the individual. Dance and movement therapy develops both the realms of image and body awareness, often experienced through subtle impulses to action.

In addition, the therapist's bodily and imaginal responses to the client's emotions, dreams, and movement qualities can be a valuable resource. This interaction brings attention to somatic transference and countertransference issues. Such work can be transformative for both parties, who suspend the limitations of their egoic "personalities" by engaging and giving shape to deeper levels of the psyche and bodily feeling.

Dreams & Neuroscience

Given the fundamental importance of sleep, contemporary medical science continues to explore the neurological basis of dreaming and its effect on our waking experiences (Mahr & Drake, 2023; Patel et al., 2019). Neuroscientists and researchers in sleep labs tell us that we dream four to six times each night, though we may not remember these dreams (Nichols, 2023; Siclari et al., 2017). Or when we do, we typically share and interpret them primarily through language. However, both early healers and contemporary neuroscience demonstrate that our bodies are home to our emotions, storing our memories and shaping our life experiences while helping us plan for the future (LeDoux, 2000; MacDuffie & Mashour, 2010). By embodying our dreams, we can better understand ourselves, integrate their insights into our everyday lives, and receive inner guidance as we navigate the uncertainties of our rapidly changing world.

From a neuroscience perspective, Jungian analyst Margaret Wilkinson (2010) and neuroscience researcher and psychologist Allan Schore (2003) speak about how the images in dreams form in the non-verbal midbrain area. Dream states, says Wilkinson, avoid overlearned portions of the brain, such as those responsible for rational thinking, reading, and writing. Instead, dreaming engages the visual-spatial brain regions that create metaphors, helping us see the larger picture to make meaning of our experience.

Dreaming often occurs during REM sleep. Psychoanalyst and dream researcher Mark Solms (1999) describes REM sleep as paradoxical, as one is active while resting—according to brain activity measured during REM cycles—as much as in waking. The eyes, too, move around in cyclic fashion, studying the images the brain is generating. We are paralyzed, to some degree, losing all muscle tone below the neck, yet amazingly able to fly, jump across canyons or from building to building, and perform otherwise impossible feats!

Stanley Keleman, one of the early pioneers of Somatic Psychology, worked with the interface between the body, psyche, spirit, and relationship. Keleman's development of Formative Psychology was based on the evolutionary process in which life continually forms the next series of shapes—from birth, through maturity, to old age. Keleman's "bodying practice" is a methodology with steps that can be experienced, repeated, and rehearsed in daily life. Drawing from anatomy, biology, embryology, physics, sports medicine, spirituality, relationship dynamics, and creativity in integrative healing, he described what he identified as the three phases of change:

1 *Endings*, when the current condition needs to come to an end.
2 *Middle ground*, a liminal time, when one can feel betwixt and between, a potentially confusing state of ups and downs when one form comes to an end before a new form is visible.
3 *New Beginnings*, marks the emergence of new form and behavior, the foundation of a growing sense of identity that requires practice to embody as a foundation for new life.

With parallels to the alchemical process, old forms are coming to an end while the seeds of new life are developing beneath the threshold of awareness, before taking new form—a new beginning. In this way, dreams are preparations for action; the body practices the necessary steps for further embodiment. This is a rich, natural process that goes on beneath the level of the ego within the dreaming, sleeping states.

Keleman understood the importance of dreams as "formative processes seeking embodiment in living one's life" (Keleman, in Stromsted, 1984). Having studied with Stanley since my early twenties, this was one of the most compelling parts of his work, given my early explorations with embodying dream figures.

Approaches to DreamDancing

There are many approaches to embodied dreamwork. In both educational and therapeutic groups as well as analytical settings, I facilitate explorations that incorporate several elements. These include embodying dream figures, exploring emotional states and qualities of energy, engaging in action sequences that promote new behaviors, and utilizing creative methods like movement, drawing, writing, or vocalization. Embodying elements from our dreams helps us access deeper instincts and emotions and provides avenues for healing and growth, beyond verbal dream interpretation alone.

During a thirteen-year period, I offered an annual DreamDancing group series for women that met monthly in a lovely dance studio in San Francisco. Guests who specialized in breathwork, storytelling, group improvisation, and voice sometimes joined us, including my colleague, Rhiannon. A noted jazz singer and teacher of Circle Singing and Vocal River, our co-facilitation supported group movement and vocal improvisations, which further expanded our ongoing DreamDancing practice.

During DreamDancing, the dreamer sometimes moves with eyes closed, attuning to their inner body-felt experience and imagery. Initially guided by me as the analyst or group leader in bringing the dream's landscape, characters, and action to mind, I soon step aside to hold space and presence as they deepen their engagement through Authentic Movement.

One approach involves embodying the significant shapes, gestures, and actions that form the core of each resonant dream scene, arranged in the order in which they appeared in the dream. These gestures are strung together to create a movement phrase, like a strand of pearls. This unique movement phrase becomes the "starting point" to enter an active imagination experience in which the mover can "dream the dream onward." As new postures and gestures begin to emerge spontaneously, the dreamer gradually releases their structured movement phrase to follow the life energy that can now guide their movement from a deeper place.

As they do so, as in Authentic Movement, the dreamer's witness sits quietly to the side of the space, watching the mover's experience as it unfolds. At the same time, the witness pays attention to how the dreamer's movement resonates in their own body, including any feelings, imagery, or memories that may arise—their somatic countertransference. The witness's comfort level with their own body and emotions is key, as it is the attitude of the witness that invites the body of the mover into the space. This connection allows the potentials contained in the dream to engage and awaken both participants. As Jung says: "In the deepest sense, we all dream not of ourselves, but of what lies between us and the other" (Jung, 1973, p. 173).

Intercultural Dances: Ancestor as Witness

There are many other possible formats for working with dreams in embodied ways that I've shared with individuals in analysis and with groups in a wide variety of communities and countries. In each setting the experience is shaped and enriched by the belief systems, traditions, attitudes toward the body, gender, sensuality and sexuality, movement patterns, and a variety of other cultural elements. Sharing and exploring dreams in embodied ways in these settings often brings further enrichment and insight into these vibrant cultural contexts, each with their ancient origins. It also provides a better understanding and appreciation for the shared needs, goals, and longings common to humanity, as well as the differences that arise from our diverse cultures.

During the height of the COVID-19 pandemic, when much of the world was in lockdown, I was invited to share a keynote presentation for the American Dance Therapy Association with participants from across the US and abroad. In the program announcement, I invited them ahead of time to bring a dream that felt meaningful for them—one they wanted to learn more about that they felt could provide some guidance or healing during that anxious, isolating time.

I recommended that it be a dream that felt life-enhancing in some way, not the worst nightmare they'd ever had, given the educational setting we were in, and the amount of time available. Difficult dreams and nightmares require additional containment and can be worked with more effectively in individual sessions with one's analyst—an established, familiar relationship, where there is well-earned trust.

During our Zoom gathering, I facilitated a DreamDancing exploration that involved working with three figures from the participants' dreams: (1) a positive figure that embodies the qualities the dreamer wishes to develop, (2) a shadow figure that represents challenges, and (3) a compassionate witness figure. This witness could be an inspiring character from a dream, a helpful spirit, or a person from their waking life—such as a supportive teacher or someone who shows love and encouragement. This figure is meant to hold space for the dreamer's movement exploration and witness them with compassion. Or it might be a guiding ancestor—real, historical, or imagined.

As movers explored the shape, feeling tone, and action of both the positive figure and the shadow character, I then encouraged them to transition back and forth between the two. This combined movement phrase—already a new third experience, with elements of the transcendent function—became their starting point for reentering the dream at a place of their choosing and "dreaming the dream on." This was not a process of purposefully acting out the dream step by step, but of discovering where their active imagination in movement process might take them. I was moved to witness them deepening in their explorations—with a wide range of expressions and gestures ranging from anguished and hiding, to curious, tender, caring, and joyous, among others.

When I rang the bell to gently signal the end of the movement time, I invited them to remain with eyes closed and return to a meaningful gesture, repeating it several times supported by their breath, noticing what word, phrase, or message might be there. And then to share their new gesture and message in an imaginal exchange with their guiding ancestor or spirit figure—feeling received by this compassionate witness. The spirit figure then offered a gesture in return. Finally, they brought their experience to a close and returned to the online community space.

Several then shared their gestures, accompanied by a word or phrase expressing how they felt, revealing deep resonances and messages that offered guidance during those challenging, sequestered times. As group members witnessed the dreamer's gesture, they then mirrored it back to them—evoking smiles, surprise, delight, and some tender tears as the dreamer felt seen and received in their offering.

To close, I invited everyone to share their gestures at the same time—resulting in a living quilt of movement that had arisen from their dreams—a vibrant community DreamDance! I invited them to take time to further integrate their experience through journaling, drawing, walking in nature, dancing, working with clay, or sharing their experience with a trusted loved one or analyst who could hold their experience without judgment or interpretation. I also encouraged them to consider spending time with and practicing what they had learned, especially with their ancestor or wise guide, as they continued to integrate their DreamDancing experience in the days and perhaps weeks or more that followed. Learning from dreams can evolve over time, deepening insights, emotions, and new actions in our ongoing life experiences, especially when supported by our ancestral ground.

DreamDancing in Analytic Practice

Working with dreams in the body can augment and deepen analytic practice. I begin with supporting the patient in attuning to their sensory experience—such as being aware of their breath, areas of tension and flow, comfort and discomfort, their sense of being connected to the floor, and feeling the support of their bones.

Introduced gradually according to the readiness of the patient, some of my initial questions to the dreamer might include: "If this dream were living in your body where would it be? What body part resonates most with this image? What sensations are in that part of your body; what qualities of aliveness are there— warmth or coolness, stiffness or softness, solid or liquid sensations, pulsations, and more?" Once made more conscious, I invite the client to amplify the sensations—letting them grow to incorporate more of their full body—resulting in a gesture that expresses something core to the dreaming process. "What sensations are you aware of now? Is there an emotion, an image, a sound? What word or phrase comes up as you repeat the gesture a few times, coming to know it better?" Here is a rehearsal for new behavior, something genuine that's informed from the inside-out.

Alternate questions for the dreamer may include: "What dream scene is most alive for you? What emotions are you aware of, and how are they being expressed in the dream; can you sense any of them now? What is the setting of the dream; how does it feel in your body—the sunny beach, mulchy marshes, rising skyscraper, mountain peak, solid brick house, mysterious hallway, new rooms, the field of flowers? And what is the unfolding action?"

Dreams in analytic work may reflect aspects of the transference relationship, as well as the dreamer's unconscious at the time of the dream. This includes feelings, dilemmas, obstacles, resources, and possible solutions. DreamDancing combines verbal analysis with embodied methods to engage the energies, emotions, and actions present in the dream. This process helps bring the dream to consciousness and integrate it into daily life. New elements also emerge spontaneously through the dream images, gestures, and intuitions of both the client and the analyst.

I describe various approaches in advance, allowing clients to choose what they would like to explore and to assess their readiness. I often include mindfulness and sensory awareness exercises, such as body scans, to enhance their sense of comfort and preparedness for engaging with their unconscious. We play with natural stretches that feel good, directive movement warm-ups that activate more of the body, and explorations of the space around us. I encourage them to feel the internal support of their bones, the earth beneath their feet, and the sky above their heads, as well as my presence, which holds the safety of the space and the timing for the exploration as a witness.

Then I invite them to share their dream, describing the landscape, feelings, and action in sensory-grounded detail. As a witness, I may reflect their gestures back to them, capturing the emotional essence of each dream scene as they share it. Gestures amplify the feeling and action within the dream and can then be strung together like beads on a necklace. The dance of expression communicates directly from the nonverbal, emotional midbrain, in concert with the image-producing brain networks that map our interactions with the world and the embodied self (Damasio, 2010, p. 64).

What follows is an example from my practice from some years ago.

Case Example: Jeff—Finding the Golden Key

"Jeff," tall, slim, with dark brown hair, was a woodworker in his mid-twenties who sought analysis after a painful romantic breakup. He also had chronic asthma and had worked hard to give up his dependency on alcohol. Weeks into our work together, he shared a repeating dream:

> *The tools I need are in a chest I can't open. The chest is locked and was stored away years ago, and I can't find the key. One night, as I walk in my stocking feet along the wooden floor of my childhood home, I see a light under the door to my mother's bedroom. Pausing, I realize the key was stored in her jewelry box, which she kept safely in her chest of drawers. Frozen outside her door, I'm afraid to retrieve the key as there's no entry without waking her up. I wake up feeling helpless.*

Though Jeff's mother had died some years before, she remained an imposing presence in his psyche. While growing up, when he brought young women home to meet her, without fail, she said, "That girl is not good enough for you; you could do better." This left him crestfallen, and though he was made to feel "special" in his mother's eyes, he couldn't help but feel that he, too, was not "good enough." And yet, she needed him by her side. Now, in adulthood, each time a new relationship began to deepen, and his heart began to open, something in him shut down; he would break off the relationship prematurely, without explanation. Though this helped him remain "in control," his girlfriend had left him this time, frustrated by his lack of warmth and his emotional unavailability. His asthma had worsened, and it was hard to resist a drink.

As Jeff shared the dream with me, I noted that he put his head down, curled in his shoulders, collapsed in his chest, and looked crumpled in his chair. When I reflected this back to him gently and invited him to notice what he felt throughout his body, he said, "It's hard to breathe, and … my belly, pelvis, and legs feel like wet cement." I encouraged him to feel his sit bones and spine in contact with the chair, to breathe into the disks between his vertebrae, and to release the sound of how he felt on the longer exhales. Then, inviting him to stand, I suggested, "How about if you spread your toes and press your feet into the floor on your exhale? See if you can draw support from the ground up while feeling the verticality of your spine." In this way, we were working to build more of a backbone in the face of his sense of defeat and despair with his mother.

Then, I asked, "Please tell me your dream again, this time without words, choosing a significant gesture to represent each important dream scene."

Jeff looked surprised, though he recounted the dream, choosing a gesture for each dream scene.

1 He placed his hands on his chest and turned his torso back and forth as if trying to open it up, his face drawn.
2 He walked warily on tiptoe, in his stocking feet, down the long, dark hallway in his childhood home.
3 He stopped, frozen outside his mother's bedroom door, looking scared, his shoulders bunching up, and his chest collapsed. Concluding his gestures, he paused as if awakening from his dream, feeling lost and hopeless.

With Jeff's permission, I reflected the main body postures and gestures I had witnessed him make for each of the three dream scenes, inviting him to notice how he felt as he watched me mirror them. Before beginning, I said I would not be able to reproduce them precisely—as they were his unique gestures, and we had different bodies—but that I would reflect the *quality* of the gestures, including the *feeling tone* they conveyed as faithfully as I could. I first asked permission as mirroring was a way to enter his world a bit more while being careful not to mimic him. Mimicry can carry an edge of ridicule if not done sensitively, whereas mirroring helps bring the gesture's feeling and potential meaning to consciousness.

Jeff's eyes widened as he watched me. Then, I invited him to do the gestures with me, putting the three gestures together like a string of pearls.

We touched our hearts, tiptoed timidly down the hallway, and then came to a rigid standstill, creating a three-part movement phrase that linked the dream's shapes into a conscious action sequence. Then, using elements from dance—tempo, space, intensity, and so forth—we slowed down the sequence and then sped it up. Then we made it smaller and larger, creeping in small steps and then taking long strides, so he could feel the difference and gain more of a sense of freedom, range of movement, and emotional access. Jeff's face flushed, and more erectness and vitality came into his body. I then asked if he would like to explore the dream further, "dreaming the dream on" through active imagination in movement.

When he nodded, I invited him to close his eyes and attune to any sensations or feelings he noticed in his body; and then, when he was ready, to begin his movement exploration with the three-part movement phrase or "dream dance," he had developed. We agreed on a ten-minute movement time, with the option to bring the movement to a close earlier if he wished, or pause if he felt uncomfortable and then begin again. "Go ahead and release the structured sequence whenever your movement begins to take on its own direction," I encouraged.

As he closed his eyes and repeated the movement phrase, his legs began to shake; soon, the shaking visibly vibrated up through his pelvis, belly, and chest. Enlivened, he began to pace through the room, first sneaking around, then stomping and saying "No!," thrusting his fists forward. Then he slowly started taking long strides, eventually sliding along the wooden floor, laughing with delight! Coming to a halt, his mouth grew determined as he leaned against the door to my office. Pausing and listening, he took off his socks and pressed his bare feet firmly on the floor. Breathing deeply, he released a gasp on the exhale, opening his chest and throwing his arms wide.

After standing still for a time, he reached forward, turned the doorknob, and began to open and close the door repeatedly. A cloud of fear began to form on his face, which was replaced by a release in his forehead and a renewed firmness in his jaw as he repeated the gesture with increasing assurance and assertion. Leaving the door open, he wrapped his arms around his chest in a hug, his right hand over his heart with tears streaming down.

When I rang the bell and invited him to bring the movement to a close, he opened his eyes and patted his heart. "The key is here...," he said. My heart melted as I heard these words; I, too, was struck by his discovery.

"Would you like to draw before speaking together?" I asked. "Or move directly into talking about your experience?" Choosing a large piece of paper and a range of colors, he drew a mountain against a rose-colored sky with a deep blue lake at its base. When I encouraged him to give it a title if he wished, he wrote "Sunrise" across the top of the page. Sitting on the floor with his drawing nearby, Jeff reflected on the dream and his movement experience. "I was surprised by the power I felt in my legs and pelvis," he said, "and how it made its way into my chest and arms—the chest that's been locked up without a key! And I was stunned to find myself opening and closing the door to your office. It felt so natural; I had to do it!" he said, looking directly at me with a trickster smile. I nodded and smiled, inwardly marveling at the power of the transference risk he had taken in my office. With me as the mother stand-in, he had found a way to assert his independence. One might consider messing with the door against the rules of conduct, as it's not protocol to do something like that. And that's exactly what he needed to do to break the mother bond that had been strangling him.

When he said he would like some witnessing, I offered, "I, too, felt aliveness throughout my body and a sense of caution when you tiptoed around the room. And joy as you glided across the floor! Then, I felt curious and smiled as you opened and closed the door. It was thrilling to see you leave it open, and I was deeply moved when you wrapped your arms around your chest and made the discovery of the key you had been searching for. Now, as I see your drawing, I feel strength and comfort in my body in the presence of the power of the mountain, and the mystery in the watery depths. The sunrise gives me a sense of peace and hope for a new beginning."

In the weeks that followed, Jeff reflected on how his "inner mother" had been forbidding him from growing up and choosing his own partner. He also recognized his ambivalence about separating from her, expressed in the dream through his frozen posture outside her bedroom door as he sought to retrieve the key to his own heart. "My father ran off with his young secretary when I was a boy; then, after they moved in together, he suddenly died of a heart attack." Looking thoughtful, he added, "I guess Mom was frozen, too; she was all I had, and I guess I was all she had, too." The trauma had shut both mother and son down on a heart level, causing them to close off to their feelings—unable to grieve and feeling angry at the same time. "It hurt so much that time stood still, and we couldn't talk about it," he said. "And it brought fear into opening up to new intimate relationships. That felt dangerous," he added, shaking his head, "look what happened to Dad."

Months into the analysis, Jeff's posture was more upright, his head erect, and his eyes and face more expressive. He could also hold healthier boundaries by saying "no" when he needed to, including invitations to share drinks with the guys after work. "How about a trip to the ballgame instead?" he quipped. Soon, he befriended the contractor on his new job, an older man who saw promise in him and guided his work. Over time, while exploring other childhood memories and current life experiences, Jeff expressed compassion for his mother and himself. "I wish I could tell her," he said. I suggested he write her a letter that he would not send, letting his thoughts and feelings flow onto the page. Respectful of his spiritual beliefs, I said it could be a way of communicating with his "inner mother," and perhaps even with his mother in the spirit world, depending on what felt true for him. He read it aloud in the following session, looking up from the page with an expression of relief and peace. Then he wrote a letter to his father—a corporate salesman who had emphasized money and prestige, whose natural instincts had also been curbed while growing up with his religious, disciplinary father and fearful mother. Jeff recalled how sometimes his father had forced him to eat peas and other things he detested as a child and shamed him for roughhousing. He hadn't known how to comfort his son when he was frightened or upset nor offer guidance that suited the boy's nature.

This letter was liberating, reawakening his voice. He also noted that he was breathing more freely, and his asthma was in remission. Within weeks, Jeff contacted his girlfriend and initiated a heartfelt conversation with her while they walked in Golden Gate Park, where the rooted trees and flowering plants mirrored his newfound growth. A year later, Jeff called for a few "tune-up sessions" as they made plans to marry, with hopes for a child of their own. As I reflected on Jeff's dream and his courageous work, I lingered at the thought of the key and the opening of the gates to the arboretum in Golden Gate Park—a place he loved to walk and sometimes sing quietly. Here, among the old trees, new blossoms, waterfalls, ponds, and all manner of birds and critters, he always found solace. They enjoyed these walks together now, and he smiled as he spoke of the warmth he felt when he held her hand as they moved together.

Here, we see the alchemical gold of the marriage of masculine and feminine, yin and yang, sol and luna, spirit and body—between us, and within us, that brings new life. Jeff's experience reflects how crystallizing a sequence of movements that engaged more of the body allowed him to commit more fully to the action and emotion—for it is within the dialogue of gestures that the conflict, message, and potentials of the dream are embedded.

My childhood dream journals were soul friends—a temenos for my evolving inner truth. Dance tapped body wisdom and provided a pathway to the divine. Embodying our dreams opens us to the mysteries, and offers guidance in living a richer, soulful life. No experience in dance is necessary—only curiosity, respect and a bit of courage to open to the unknown. As Rainer Maria Rilke wrote in *Letters to a Young Poet* (Rilke, 1984):

> You must give birth to your images. They are the future waiting to be born. Fear not the strangeness you feel. The future must enter you long before it happens. Just wait for the birth, for the hour of the new clarity.

References

Damasio, A. (2010). *Self comes to mind: Constructing the conscious brain*. Pantheon Books.

Jung, C. G. (1973). *C.G. Jung letters, vol. 1: 1906–1950*. Princeton University Press.

LeDoux J. E. (2000). Emotion circuits in the brain. *Annual Review of Neuroscience, 23*, 155–184. https://doi.org/10.1146/annurev.neuro.23.1.155

MacDuffie K. & Mashour G. A. (2010). Dreams and the temporality of consciousness. *American Journal of Psychology, 123*(2): 189–197. https://doi.org/10.5406/amerjpsyc.123.2.0189

Mahr, G. & Drake, L. (2023). *The wisdom of dreams: Science, synchronicity and the language of the soul*. Routledge.

Meier, C. A. (1989). *Healing dream and ritual*. Daimon Verlag.

Mindell, A. (1989). *Working with the dreaming body*. Penguin Publishing Group.

Nichols, H. (2023). What does it mean when we dream? *Medical News Today*. https://www.medicalnewstoday.com/articles/284378

Patel, A. K., Reddy V., & Araujo J. F. (2019). *Physiology, sleep stages*. StatPearls. https://pubmed.ncbi.nlm.nih.gov/30252388/

Pei, F. Y. & Zhang, J. (2000). *The interpretation of dreams in Chinese culture*. Weatherhill.

Rilke, R. M. (1984). *Letters to a young poet* (S. Mitchell, Trans.). Random House.

Schore, A. (2003). *Affect regulation and the origin of the self & affect dysregulation and disorders of the self* (2 Vols.). W. W. Norton & Company.

Siclari, F., Baird, B., Perogamvros, L. et al. (2017). The neural correlates of dreaming. *Nature Neuroscience, 20*: 872–878. https://doi.org/10.1038/nn.4545

Solms, M. (1999, March). *The interpretation of dreams & the neurosciences*. Institute of Psychoanalysis, British Psychoanalytical Society. https://psychoanalysis.org.uk/articles/the-interpretation-of-dreams-and-the-neurosciences-mark-solms

Stromsted, T. (1984). *Dreamdancer: The use of dance/movement therapy in dreamwork* [Unpublished master's thesis]. John F. Kennedy University.

UNESCO World Heritage Convention. Retrieved September 14, 2024. https://whc.unesco.org/en/list/491/

Wilkinson, M. (2010). *Changing minds in therapy: Emotion, attachment, trauma, & neurobiology*. W.W. Norton & Company.

Chapter 16

Earth's Body

Resonating with the Pulse of Life

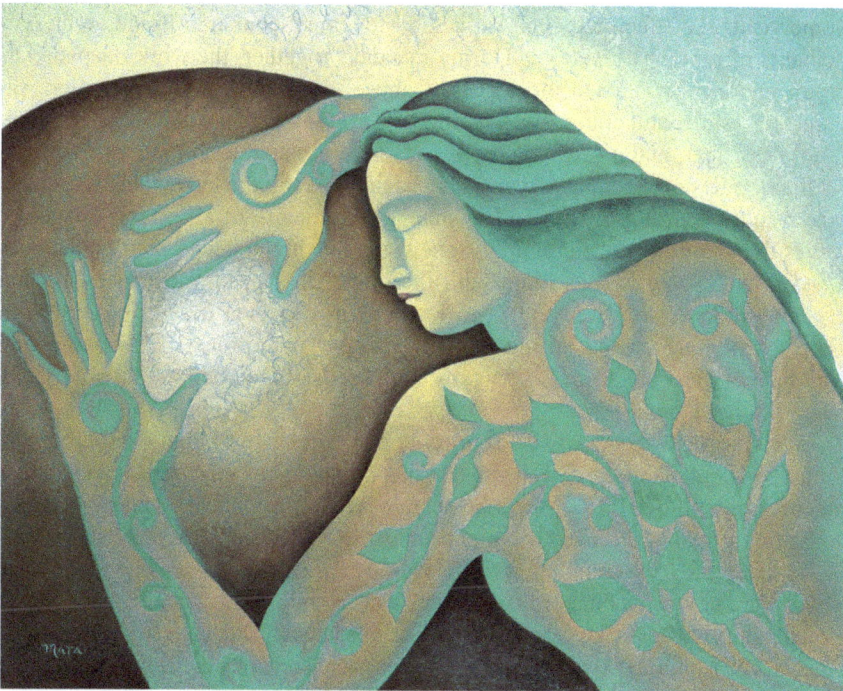

Figure 16.1 Gaia's Daughter © 1999, by Mara Berendt Friedman
@ www.newmoonvisions.com.

Our relationship with our bodies reflects how we connect with and treat the planet—a microcosm of the macrocosm. When we are not in tune with our senses and feelings we struggle to resonate with the Earth's body. Similarly, a lack of awareness of our unconscious emotions and attitudes often leads us to project them onto others and the environment. Any wounds or underdevelopment in our embodied sense of self are

DOI: 10.4324/9781003538356-21

reflected in the neglect and unconscious harm we inflict on the Earth. Just as disrespecting and manipulating our bodies is akin to misusing natural resources, both our bodies and the planet require awareness, compassion, and active engagement.

Authentic Movement practice can help us reconnect with our instinctual wisdom and foster a sense of responsible participation in the larger web of life. At times, Authentic Movement arises spontaneously in nature, and with the support of a developed "inner witness," it can be fully experienced. In these moments, we can access ancient images that reside within us, creating a feeling of connectedness that extends beyond our contemporary human community. This connection encompasses our embodied history as a species and our relationship with the Earth, our planetary body.

Earth Dance: Irish Tomb-Wombs

Some years ago I facilitated an Authentic Movement course in Ireland with participants of many nationalities. During our days together, the work deepened as group members contacted memories of abuse, drug and alcohol addiction, divorce, ancestors, and cultural and familial attitudes toward sexuality and religion. Emptiness, fear, and a sense of rootlessness were palpable in their expressions. As their bodies opened, participants also began to recall the land where they were raised and the strong hand it had in shaping their sense of aliveness. Images of waves thrashing the seashore, gray stone walls fencing in deep-green fields, huddles of small, cold houses filled with the thick scent of burning peat, bustling city sidewalks, sturdy tree trunks to lean against, Persian deserts layered with history—all were present in the room. Thus began the process of reconnecting with their earliest roots, alive, even now, in the cells of their bodies, but previously inaccessible to them.

Following the workshop, I visited my colleague Marian in Dublin; she told me that I must see *Lough Crew*, a sacred site that had not, until recently, attracted the attention of many visitors. Piling rubber boots, rain jackets, bag lunches, and candles into her station wagon, we drove the hour northwest to the ancient holy site. Not long after stopping to see the church in Kells, we turned onto a dirt road leading to the hills, which were now a national reserve. On top of each hill stood a small stone cave or mound: "tomb-wombs" of rebirth, according to ancient Celtic belief (Walker, 1983, pp. 298, 752), built 3,000 years ago, of tall stones covered with earth and grass. From a distance, they looked like nipples topping off the breast-like curves of the green hills. Approaching the opening of one, Marian unlocked the gate and invited me to enter first. Slipping between two tall stones, I stepped into darkness and felt the cool dampness on my skin. The deep quiet was broken only by the occasional howling of the wind as it sang its way through tiny cracks in the stones. I felt a spontaneous urge to pray and listen deeply to the earth and stone structures, sensing the potent presence of the past in them. Here is my journal entry following the experience:

Expecting to spend time in stillness and silence, I am surprised when, as I open my senses to the energies of this place, my body begins to dance. Pelvis, torso, arms, and neck trace shapes, curves, spirals, and circles. I feel as though I am being danced by the same soft yet powerful energy that pushed these hills up from the level ground—my body is an ancient song, clay for molding, responding to invisible forces. Following the energy current, I experience a deep sense of release, and surprisingly feel no fear in this darkened cave. Instead, I experience my unity with this timeless place. Stepping further into the center of the space, I plant my feet firmly in the dark earth. Snakes of warmth begin streaming up my legs, intertwining as they reach my pelvis, braiding themselves in the open bowl, gently rocked by the steady rhythm that is there. Soon they rise, warm and rippling, up my spinal column. As the snakes move up my lower and middle back, my belly releases in the front, electrified by their energy and surrendering to the support of the bones. As they continue to glide up my torso, the muscles around my ribs relax, creating more space for my expanding heart and breath. As the energy rises, warmth extends into my arms. Lifting over my head, they float on the currents that move through my body where I stand, firm yet electrified, on the ancient ground. Palms open, fingers spread into wings, lifting earth energy toward the curving dome of this ancient womb and out toward the sky beyond it. Breath opens me and my mouth releases a cry as I give myself to the sky. Still rooted in the earth, I experience myself as a tuning fork, a conduit, a channel uniting earth and sky. The snakes undulate. My torso swivels and circles, gaining momentum, liberated by the rootedness I feel in my pelvis and legs. With growing excitement and expansiveness, I sense that I am sprinkling seeds and water throughout the dark space. As I do so, I feel a certainty that "I am home" though I have never before been here. Earth and air mix in the dance as I hear the words Sacred Marriage *and sense the word made flesh.*

How many dances have gone on here, I wonder? How many births, how many deaths, how many prayers? Having completed their dance, the snakes gradually grow quiet, and my spine arches first back and then forward as my fingers extend to touch the cool earth. Blessing it with the heat in my hands, I feel simultaneously blessed by its vibrant, silent presence. Slowly, my spine rolls up, and I am myself again, a modern woman, though I feel enriched and am no longer a stranger to this place. In this moment I know in my bones that like our planet, our ravaged bodies and feminine and masculine psyches need to be understood in an entirely new way, which, paradoxically, has its roots in antiquity. Here on this land, I feel so poignantly the challenge of our times—to reintegrate mind, body, and spirit, both individually and collectively—and be made whole again through the dance. What happened spontaneously provided the vehicle for this ancient energy to enliven present life. Now Marian steps into the cave's opening. We light votive candles and place them on ledges in the cave. Their flickering light falls on stones the size of human bodies, some standing, others prone. Most are covered with carved spirals. Marian and I begin to chant—spontaneous sounds that glide, echo, lift off, and settle into the walls of this ancestral place of burial, ritual, and birth. Afterward, we climb to visit each mound, feeling its unique shape, size, and influence in our bodies. Before we leave, we pause to say blessings for our loved ones who are troubled or sick.

Later, tucked into the cross-shaped dugout just outside the last mound, we shared our experiences over sandwiches. As we talked, the memory of my encounter with the snakes came to life. I recalled how St. Patrick, believing snakes to be evil, was said to have banished them from the Irish Isle when he introduced Christianity—likely a metaphor for converting Celtic paganism. This thought sparked a stream of associations, leading me to the images of snakes found in yogic texts, where they represent kundalini energy. I also thought of the snakes coiled around the staff of Asclepius, the Greek god of medicine. Eventually, this image transformed into the two intertwining snakes that adorn Hermes's winged staff, which has been adopted as the symbol of the Western medical profession. In classical times, the snake's keen sight and ability to rejuvenate by shedding its skin were thought to symbolize a patient's capacity to overcome illness (Meier, 1989, pp. 20, 31, and 53).

The snake, with the spiral as its abstract derivative, was also associated with the Great Goddess, signifying the renewal of life in prehistoric times (Baring & Cashford, 1991, pp. 499–501; Gimbutas, 1989, p. 46). In fact, sacred vessels etched with intertwined double spirals, clearly resembling the pairs of double snakes with opposed heads, have often been found in her holy sites (Gimbutas, 1991, p. 53). Seated in this sacred Irish landscape, I felt a sense of gratitude as I was reminded that though the outer manifestation of this vital creature was "banished" here, the generative power of the snake was still as alive as ever as a spirited and creative inner force.

How could we have strayed so far from our bodies in our worship, I wondered, distancing ourselves from our natural, sensual relationship to ourselves, to each other, and to the earth in deference to a bodiless, transcendent God? In the earlier religions, all life was experienced as one, born out of the single body of Gaia, Mother Goddess of the Earth. And yet there was an inherent balance—sculptures of Goddess figurines with male characteristics were common. "Sacred marriage" was the phrase that had come from the dark earth with the rising energy of the snakes ... This pointed to a new paradigm, a deeply creative possibility, both within me and for our troubled world. I was reminded of Jung's words:

> When the great swing has taken an individual into the world of symbolic mysteries, nothing comes of it, nothing can come of it, unless it has been associated with the earth, unless it has happened when that individual was in the body ... And so individuation can only take place if you first return to the body, to your earth, only then does it become true.
>
> (Jung, 1976, p. 473)

On a personal level, the early loss of my mother through divorce and the subsequent lengthy business trips that took my father away from home throughout my childhood were potent contributors to the underlying sense of absence I had known. Here on this land, longing had given way to a profound experience of timeless, spaceless oneness. Absence had given way to presence.

A Memory of Wings

Distraught, a colleague—a dance educator—asked me this question: "If our world is really looking down the barrel of environmental catastrophe, how do I live my life right now?"

Sensing her anguish, and my own, we spoke for some time and then I wrote this response.

Years ago, during the winter solstice and holiday season I spent a few quiet days in a cabin in Bolinas, a small village overlooking the Pacific Ocean north of San Francisco, California. As the old year came to an end and the new year began, I turned on my computer and read news of the tsunami that had swept through Southeast Asia, claiming thousands of lives in a matter of minutes. I was shocked at the suddenness and magnitude of it and felt a longing to do what I could to help those who had survived. I had planned on a personal retreat in nature, a time for rest and hiking, away from the fast pace and noise of the city. And yet now I felt galvanized by souls I'd never met, who were leaving their bodies in electrified waves.

Under salmon-colored skies, I followed the sounds of the surf, a long walk that traced the edges of the Pacific—just "the other side of the pond" from Indonesia. Then, my feet took me back up through the fields on the high mesa, where I emerged from the trail to the sound of wings—dozens of startled quail who hopped about and then took flight. As my eyes followed them, I was amazed to see a Monterey Pine and a tall Eucalyptus tree filled with what looked like twinkling orange and gold Christmas lights. Once I got closer, I discovered they were covered with Monarch butterflies—a *dazzling* sight! Thousands of them rested, while others soared in bright, spiraling dances, waves of fluttering wings and lovemaking in midair, warmed by the rays of the sun.

On one side of the Pacific rim a deadly tidal wave, and here on the other, all this life. How to hold these two realities at the same time, and more importantly, how to direct our attention to reversing the steady deterioration and devastation of the delicately balanced ecology of our shimmering planet?

Tears streamed down my face as I sent a prayer to my neighbors across the Pacific. Then, I returned to commune with the butterflies, entering the new year with their fluttering songs at the peak of their long journeys. Remembering that the deaths of the crawling caterpillars preceded the growing of wings.

****

The sickness of our time is losing touch with our natural selves and sense of belonging as we try to fill the void with material goods, ravaging the Earth in the process. Our relationship with our body mirrors our relationship with the Earth; if we abuse our bodies—with overwork, addictions, and toxic experiences, we can exploit the planet without awareness or remorse.

Our fast-paced, increasingly technologically driven culture has lost much of its reverence for nature and our connection to the larger web of life. National parks, pristine forests, vital watersheds, and other untouched natural habitats that support essential biodiversity for plants, animals, insects, and other living beings are increasingly being overtaken by housing developments or exploited for oil. Vulnerable species lose their protections at the mercy of shifting political tides. Similarly, churches and temples that once held a sense of the sacred may no longer satisfy our longing for meaning or the direct *lived* experience of the sacred. However, if we can take the time to commune with nature, we can find restoration and renewal. We can once again experience ourselves as part of a larger whole—a deeper, broader "community" that connects us across time and space through our reverence for life. This connection encourages us to become more caring and conscious stewards of the Earth, as we appreciate, protect, and responsibly manage the gifts that Mother Nature provides to nourish all living beings.

This journey requires honoring our familial and tribal identities, then stepping *beyond* them, into a new level of consciousness. This requires working through and releasing the problems of the past to embrace a common purpose, becoming *global citizens*, recognizing that we who created the problem, must now address it if we are to save the beautiful, powerful, sensitive planet we call home.

As a Jungian analyst and dance/movement therapist, I focus on helping people reinhabit their bodies, nurture their souls, and rediscover what has been lost, both internally and externally. This journey is essential for living the life they were meant to lead—what Jung called the individuation process. By engaging the life within and around them, individuals can cultivate a deeper connection to their values, build meaningful communities, and experience the sacredness of nature. This connection is something that our industrialized and materialistic lifestyles have nearly stripped away from us.

Authentic Movement can assist in this transformative process. By moving from an inner source, the practice allows us to be touched and guided by a life force larger than anything our egos or brains can conceive—a pathway to fulfilling our destiny. I often begin teaching Authentic Movement workshops by inviting participants to recall a place in nature that they loved as a child. The room hushes as people reconnect with a place of safety, beauty, and freedom that still resonates deeply within them—a place that has had a strong hand in shaping who they have become. Gestures emerge from the part of the body where the life force in nature still resonates within them. Participants are visibly moved as they remember the naturalness they experienced then, the respite from fear and loneliness, and the felt sense of freedom and connection with all of life that comes alive again at that moment, still present in their cells, yet dormant—asleep but not dead.

For many, those beautiful places no longer exist, having been paved over to make way for apartment complexes, shopping malls, offices, parking lots, or repurposed as refuge camps, displacement facilities, or toxic waste disposal sites. Without this touchstone, we can easily become overwhelmed by despair at the plight of our planet, immobilized by a sense of hopeless and the question, "What can one person do?" How can I stop the relentless tide of unconscious destruction that we call *progress*? Paralysis sets in due to the sheer magnitude of the problem.

How can we thaw the "freeze" and address the grief, fear, and anxiety we feel in light of this grim trajectory?

The butterfly effect, from chaos theory in quantum physics, suggests that small changes in one part of a system can lead to significant, unpredictable effects elsewhere, highlighting the world's profound interconnectedness. This concept emphasizes that minor actions can have major impacts, though predicting which changes will instigate chaos is impossible (Dizikes, 2011).

First, we must access the vitality of the nature within us, thawing the frightened flesh and reawakening body wisdom. *Freezing* is not just a metaphor; it's a neurological reality linked to the vagus nerve—a protective response that helps conserve energy and disconnect from an inescapable or overwhelming situation. Like "playing possum," this is a last-ditch survival strategy when neither running away nor fighting can prevail. After this, grief sets in. Over time, we can begin to allow the deep Self within to rekindle our connection to our inherent vitality—our instincts and imagination—and with it, our connection to the wider web of life in the natural world. Only then does conscious action become possible—action informed by the heart, the mind, and a deeper resonant connection with the pulse and tides of the planet. Communion with others becomes possible and necessary as we realize that the overwhelm, outrage, and grief we feel are not ours to bear alone. Each of us has something valuable to contribute, fostering an awareness that together we *can* make a difference. Learning to sense the living body is an essential part of this process, reawakening a more natural experience of self and, along with it, our connection to the larger web of life.

Environmental Dances

How do we relearn to dance in Nature? After all, all of life began there, so in the scope of things, it's relatively recent that we've "moved indoors!" Now, it's a matter of attuning ourselves and re-membering our connection to the natural world.

I danced in the fields as a child (Chapter 1). These early dances were followed by many other experiences: formal classes in ballet, modern dance, African dance, Afro-jazz-Blues; theater; mime, improvisation; singing while moving with Rhiannon; tracing the flights of birds and listening for their songs; riding horseback; hiking; skiing, water skiing; running track; and playing basketball. I also spent time with the many animals in the fields and barn while growing up in the countryside in Massachusetts.

Skipping ahead to the mid-1970s, I vividly recall the environmental choreography dance classes I took with Susan Waltner, Professor Emerita of Dance at Smith College in Northampton, Massachusetts. Everything changed when we took our dances outside the studio and into nature!

Our bodies and psyches opened with the vastness of the sky above us. Our feet felt supported by the solid yet nuanced earth below. We danced up and down the steps in the garden, moved among the trees, and rolled in autumn's golden leaves. I remember a friend emerging from underwater in a nearby stream, clad in a wet suit with a mask and goggles—Nature gave way to a mythic dimension—an amphibian human discovering land for the first time!

Why Does a Walk in Nature Do Us So Much Good?

What happens when we walk in Nature? Why is it so beneficial? It's about finding a resonance between your body and the planetary body. It's an attunement, like tuning a violin, to the spirit of Nature. When I take forest baths in the woods, my breath becomes more attuned, my feet connect with the good earth, and my body aligns with the earth's body. I open myself to fuller oxygenation with the breath of the planet. This experience activates the cellular intelligence of my body and enhances my access to creative imagination, vitality, and the wisdom within the cells. That's when I start to create. This is the next step in Jung's "active imagination" approach—the creative process. I once heard that Marie-Louise von Franz said she had never known a problem that couldn't be solved by a walk. Personally, I have solved many a problem by spending time with trees and sitting among their roots.

From my earliest beginnings, Nature has been a source of healing and a numinous place of beauty and deep intelligence—the realm where the gods live. It also serves as a powerful metaphor for our relationship with our instinctual selves—our inner nature—a profound resource for potential renewal. The medical profession has long sought to better understand the intricate workings of our mind-brain-body-psyche-spirit connection to enhance healing. Despite major advances in medical science, the body's intelligence runs deeper than what we can fully comprehend.

When I teach in nature or in urban areas where people can access open spaces outside, I often invite participants to move, witness, and engage with nature—whether in their backyard, a park, near the ocean or a stream, or in a forest. Experiencing the containing and sustaining power of the natural environment, outside of the dance studio, classroom, conference hall, or Zoom meeting, can offer a refreshing sense of deep nourishment.

Moonlight Walk

During our weeklong International Authentic Movement Retreats in Tuscany, participants walk through olive orchards and among grapevines. They sleep in the grass, gently rock in the hammock, and raise a glass of local wine to the rolling hills that have been traversed by humans for thousands of years.

While walking with their eyes closed and guided by their partner/witness, a mover senses their environment, listens to the crickets, and hears the calls of the night birds. They feel the variations in the landscape beneath their feet as they walk softly, the witness providing a guiding and protective presence. Depending on the mover's preference, the witness may hold their hand or wrap an arm around their waist. This allows the witness to act as the mover's "eyes," looking out for any roots, rocks, potholes, or other obstacles on the path while adapting to the mover's pace. This arrangement frees the mover to fully engage with their sensory experience—attuning to the sounds, smells, and tactile contact with leaves and other natural elements their witness introduces them to. We conclude our moonlit walk in the vineyard, surrounded by grapevines illuminated by the soft glow of a full moon. After gazing at the starry sky and reflecting in silence for a few moments, we switch roles, allowing the witness to close their eyes and experience being the mover.

At our retreat house, partners share their experiences with one another, followed by sharing with the group as a whole over cups of tea before bed. On darker nights, when the moon is new, we dance among swirling fireflies (*lucciola* from the Latin *luceō*, meaning "to shine").

Dancing with Nature

As we return to group work in the Tuscany retreats (Chapter 12), our closing ritual on the final day invites everyone to move and witness in nature. After gathering in the studio, I briefly share these steps: "I invite you to revisit a 'Loved place in Nature'—a place where you have felt safe, inspired, and held in beauty—a place where you've walked, rested, or prayed." This exploration begins with an invitation and the following steps, which I share here with you, the reader. If you're not already dancing with nature—feel free to adapt this exploration for your own use.

1 Go out and visit a special place in nature, perhaps a place you've spent time before that holds meaning for you.

   a Alternately, simply follow your intuition and see where you feel drawn to spend some time.
   b See, hear, sense, and touch—be a witness to something in nature: a tree, a plant, an animal, or a bird (though birds may not linger long!).

2 Notice what resonates in your body, and use this as an opportunity to start saying goodbye to the landscape in Tuscany as well (or to another special place you are visiting or departing from).

   a Be a witness to something in nature, to nature's movement.
   b Be a mover and let nature hold and witness you.
   c Dance *together*: Move *with* this element, a *living being* in nature—taking on the roles of both mover and witness.
   d Gradually bring your dance to a close, returning to a gesture that held particular meaning for you. Repeat this gesture several times so you really get to know it—fully embody it.
   e Allow the movement to become smaller, subtler, until it's no longer visible from the outside, though the feelings and rhythms are still resonant within you.
   f When you hear the Tibetan Bells, please return to the studio in silence. (Or you can also set this timing for yourself.)

3 With paper and colors, draw your experience in nature.

4   Now we will have our last Long Circle (if you are in an Authentic Movement group setting, see Chapter 12) for this year's retreat. Please put your drawing in a safe place to the side, where you can see it if you choose to use it as a movement score. Then, take your place in the large Witness Circle in the studio to begin the Long Circle.

5   As movers, here's an invitation to let your "starting point" be your movement from one of three options, choosing what feels best for you at this time:

    a   Option #1: Let your drawing serve as a musical score to move to. The images and energies originated from your embodied experience in nature. Now try putting the image—its colors, shapes, and textures—back into your body, exploring it in movement. See what draws your attention: a color, a line, a shape, or a specific part of the drawing?

    b   Option #2: After creating your essence drawing of your experience in nature, begin your movement experience using the gesture from your Nature Dance.

    c   Option #3: Begin with what you currently feel in your body, what is *present* at this time.

And now we begin the Long Circle:

6   The whole group moves; Tina and Margareta Neuberger, my dear, gifted colleague and assistant for many years (or perhaps another assistant) will be the only witnesses on this last morning as you move together.

7   We devote 30 minutes to this movement round:

    a   When you feel that your movement has come to a natural completion, please take your place in the Witness Circle, becoming a witness until all movers have returned to the outer rim of the circle, or when the Tibetan bell rings three times—whichever occurs first.

    b   Afterward, take a silent transition in the dining room with tea and snacks (for 15 minutes, in silence).

    c   Witnessing Circle: Return to the studio for the Talking Circle to name your experience and share a gesture, receiving "recall" if you like.

These and countless other explorations are among the ways we can relearn to resonate and dance with Nature—the pulse of life. May your Nature Dance reflect the essence of Nancy Wood's poem.

> Because I spent the winter sleeping with a fish,
> there is a fin within me now.
> Because I spent the spring with an eagle in her nest,
> there is an egg within me now.
> Because I spent the summer with the buffalo,
> there is a bone within me now.
> Because I spent the autumn growing with one tall tree,
> there is a root within me now.
>
> Nancy Wood

References

Baring, A. & Cashford, J. (1991). *The myth of the goddess: Evolution of an image*. Penguin Books Ltd.

Dizikes, P. (2011, February 22). When the butterfly effect took flight. *MIT Technology Review*. https://www.technologyreview.com/011/02/22/196987/when-the-butterfly-effect-took-flight/

Gimbutas, M. (1989). *The goddesses and gods of old Europe*. Thames and Hudson.

Gimbutas, M. (1991). *The civilization of the goddess*. Harper & Row.

Jung, C. G. (1976). *Vision seminars* (Vol. 2). Spring Publications.

Meier, C. A. (1989). *Healing dream and ritual*. Daimon Verlag.

Walker, B. (1983). *Woman's encyclopedia of myths and secrets*. Harper Collins Publishers, Inc.

Chapter 17

Further Reflections and Looking Forward

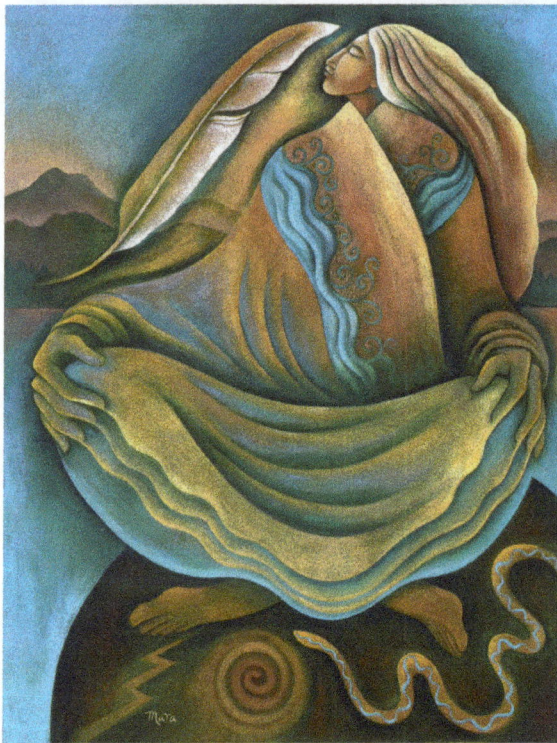

Figure 17.1 listen ... She will teach you Her ways © 1995, by Mara Berendt Friedman @ https://www.newmoonvisions.com/.

Our world is experiencing significant changes and challenges, and practices such as Authentic Movement offer valuable tools for navigating these turbulent times. The body and the unconscious mind are central to this process, which can be accessed through active imagination, movement, and somatic practices that foster

DOI: 10.4324/9781003538356-22

creativity and resilience. These approaches are particularly invaluable during chaotic periods, providing pathways for resilience and transformation.

Recent social challenges—including racial injustice, struggles with gender identity, sexism, a widening income gap, gun violence, political polarization, environmental crises, immigration and population displacement, authoritarianism, and warfare—underscore the importance of shifting from an egotistical mindset to one that embraces communal awareness. Individuation, often misunderstood as individualism, is a lifelong journey of psychological growth and self-awareness that does not culminate in isolation. As social beings, we thrive in relationships, communities, and natural environments.

Embodied practices, even in virtual settings, along with trauma-informed approaches, remain essential. Daily spiritual practices that promote balance and resilience, alongside healthy expressions of sensuality and sexuality, are critical to well-being in the digital age. The impact of social media further necessitates mindful navigation.

To address societal issues, we must create networks to encourage equality and connection. Embodied practices ground us, sustain our sense of gratitude, and support conscious activism. They help prevent burnout and strengthen community resilience. Looking to the future, I envision somatic practices becoming integral to various fields, such as education, psychotherapy, parenting, medicine, spirituality, and the arts. These practices cultivate emotional intelligence, empathy, and collaboration, equipping us to address today's challenges. Teaching children to embrace their bodies and emotions in safe, supportive environments will lay the foundation for a healthier society. This integrative approach enhances our understanding of both ourselves and our communities.

Expanding the West's individualistic tendencies to incorporate collectivist values can foster respect for diversity, reduce conflict, and build a future rooted in embodied presence and meaningful connections. In this chapter, I share several stories illustrating how Authentic Movement, dreams, and various forms of conscious embodiment can help address these challenges.

Movement as Medicine

Re-inhabiting the body and experiencing life through the senses foster a healthy imagination, which is distinct from unproductive thoughts and negative behaviors. In addition to Authentic Movement, many methods address challenges related to embodiment. These include Sensory Awareness, Focusing, Somatic Experiencing, dance/movement therapy, neurofeedback, Eye Movement Desensitization and Reprocessing (EMDR), alongside other somatic psychotherapies. Hands-on bodywork techniques, such as craniosacral therapy, acupressure, trauma-informed touch, massage, and self-touch techniques, also contribute to overall well-being. Recently, closely monitored psychedelic sessions have emerged as promising tools for engaging altered states of consciousness. When combined with psychotherapy, they show potential for addressing complex issues such as PTSD, severe anxiety, and treatment-resistant depression (Barber & Aaronson, 2022; Ellis et al., 2025; Reiff et al., 2020).

The COVID-19 pandemic has accelerated the growth of telehealth, which has been shown to be surprisingly effective. Although online therapy lacks the full embodied presence of shared physical space, a body-oriented approach can broaden the therapeutic environment. In this way both and client co-create a resonant field that fosters intimacy and accessibility, even in an online setting.

As discussed in Chapters 3 and 13, Authentic Movement has shown promise in addressing medical conditions that inhibit embodiment. Elyn Selu, a doctoral student in my courses at Pacifica Graduate Institute who had been diagnosed with multiple sclerosis (MS), explored these themes in her dissertation (Selu, 2020). Multiple sclerosis significantly impacts movement, cognition, and mood, creating a challenging disconnection between the body's desires for coordination and the reality of physical limitations. Individuals with MS often experience muscle spasticity, tremors, and fatigue, which, as her research reflects, leads to an identity shift as familiar movements become difficult. This sense of betrayal is not just physical; it necessitates a reevaluation of one's relationship with their body and environment (Selu, 2020).

While many manage their symptoms with conventional medications, the psychological impact of living with an unpredictable body is frequently overlooked. Mindfulness-based methods such as Authentic Movement, provide valuable opportunities for improving both mental and physical well-being. Elyn's research emphasizes the importance of enhancing body awareness among people with MS, revealing that greater self-care and control can be achieved through meditative practices. Additionally, her findings suggest that a lack of body awareness can exacerbate mental health issues, highlighting the need for culturally adapted awareness techniques for diverse groups (Selu, 2020).

Authentic Movement as Social Activism and Engaged Ecology: The Community Long Circle

Authentic Movement connects the conscious and unconscious aspects of ourselves as well as our relationships with others and the larger community. Jung emphasized that once something is made conscious, we have an ethical obligation to *live* it. This practice not only fosters awareness and growth on psychological, creative, and spiritual levels but also promotes social action as a means to build healthier communities. Through this practice, we learn to minimize harm to ourselves, others, and our animal cousins; to live in harmony with the Earth; and to honor the more-than-human world.

In May 1998, Neala Haze, our Authentic Movement students, and I hosted an ecological event at César Chávez Park in Berkeley, California. This land, once home to the Native American Ohlone people for thousands of years, had become a garbage dump and was eventually transformed into a public park named after labor activist César E. Chávez. Park designers honored the land's history by including wildlife sanctuaries, scenic trails, and open grassy spaces where dogs can play off-leash and people can fly kites.

To celebrate and bless the reclaimed land while fostering social and ecological awareness, we invited guest faculty Lisa Tsetse and Sox Sperry, who were exploring Authentic Movement as a form of nonviolent social activism, to lead a Community Long Circle practice (Tsetse, 2007; Tsetse & Sperry, 1998). Tsetse and Sperry's work honors Authentic Movement as a nonviolent practice with the potential to "create a bridge crucial to our planetary healing" (Tsetse, 2007, p. 407). Tsetse noted that, similar to my early dances in the fields, "the earth itself is our witness, and it asks the same of us" (p. 407). Drawing inspiration from the civil rights movement, Tsetse emphasizes nonviolence as a practice of presence, compassion, and steadfast action to build structures that treat everyone as equals. These principles resonate with listening practices, such as South Africa's Truth and Reconciliation Commission (https://www.justice.gov.za/trc/) and Braver Angels (https://braverangels.org/ten-better-angels-skills/) in the US, which seek meaningful dialogue and shared humanity. However, more work is needed to address global inequities rooted in racism, sexism, classism, gender identity, medical and mental health issues, and the challenges faced by people with disabilities and other challenges.

Authentic Movement aligns with these values by teaching empathy, resilience, and compassion—"to suffer with." Practitioners experience a deep connection as both witness and mover, engaging with both pain and resilience while returning to their "home base"—the body's breath, sensations, and grounded presence. This embodied awareness helps limit burnout and fosters sustained activism. While often practiced outdoors, where it intersects with public life, it can also take place indoors as part of a retreat process that bridges personal and collective growth.

Tsetse and Sperry envision the Community Long Circle as a public form of the practice, structured with three concentric circles. An inner circle of movers explores a shared question or intention, while a second circle witnesses both the movers and the world beyond. A third, outer rim of "Keepers" faces outward, holding space for dialogue with community members who observe and choose to engage (Tsetse, 2007, p. 412).

At César Chávez Park, we formed these three circles. To our surprise and delight, a spontaneous fourth circle emerged—off-leash dogs running joyfully around us! Drawn to our energy, these instinctual beings seemed to sense the depth of feeling generated by our movement practice and became an integral part of the experience. Movers and witnesses switched roles to explore the fullness of each perspective. By the end, local community members had gathered, curious about our activities. When they asked if we were meditating, praying, or clearing the land's energy, we replied "yes" to all. The event sparked meaningful conversations and deepened our connection to the land, the community, and one another.

It was a beautiful, unforgettable experience—a living example of how Authentic Movement bridges inner transformation with social and ecological awareness.

Transforming Suffering and Becoming Agents of Change

Many individuals in our communities are applying similar principles in their work. Joanna Macy, PhD, a scholar of Buddhism, systems theory, and deep ecology, is renowned for her contributions to peace and environmental justice. Over four decades, she developed *The Work That Reconnects*, a methodology to transform suffering into empowerment, helping individuals become agents of change. Her approach includes group activities such as conversation, meditation, singing, and body exercises, which deepen connection with others and the planet.

Macy began her journey as an anti-nuclear activist in the 1970s, organizing workshops worldwide to help people articulate their pain. One significant workshop took place in Russia in 1992, addressing the trauma experienced by those impacted by the Chernobyl disaster. I met her shortly thereafter when we both taught at the California Institute of Integral Studies in San Francisco. During her presentation and in subsequent conversations, she shared insights about how alarming messages regarding the health of the planet often caused people to shut down instead of taking action. In response, she refined her methodology to inspire creative, embodied solutions to sustainability challenges. Her book and free online course, *Active Hope: How to Face the Mess We're In with Unexpected Resilience and Creative Power* (Macy & Johnstone, 2012/2022), coauthored with Dr. Chris Johnstone, a resilience specialist based in Scotland, has reached more than sixty countries.

In another example of becoming an agent of change, my friend, artist Jen-Ann Kirchmeier, returned to Alaska to help clean oil-poisoned wildlife following the 1989 Exxon Valdez oil spill, which devastated Alaska's Prince William Sound and killed hundreds of thousands of animals. As a soulful painter, she gained the trust of a Native Alaskan tribe and offered to paint portraits of their elders. Later, when the tribe faced clear-cutting of their land, Jen-Ann protested with them, as they tied themselves to the tree trunks.

For the first time, she heard the trees' cries as the bulldozers tore through the forest, feeling the distress ripple through their vast network of roots. She had never been able to perceive this frequency of sound before, but sitting quietly with the other women allowed her to attune on a deeper level, forging a profound connection with nature that transformed her life. Although several of the tribe's elders have since passed, her paintings remain a sacred gift to both their families and the tribe.

Inner and Outer Nature

As we move forward, it's vital to take embodied healing practices further into the world, especially into nature. In Chapter 16, I discussed the value of walking in nature to enhance mental and physical health—a practice called "forest bathing" in Japan. During a walk to a mountain shrine in Kyoto, I encountered a magnificent noble tree that took my breath away. Standing tall with outstretched branches, it was adorned with ceremonial ropes and brightly colored sashes. This sacred site included a nearby hut where hikers, pilgrims, and meditators could sit, pray, and rest.

While speaking with someone on the path, I learned about the *shinboku*—a tree or forest regarded as a *shintai*, an object of worship at or near a Shinto shrine believed to house spirits, or *kami*. These trees, often encircled by a sacred rope called a *shimenawa*, hold deep cultural and spiritual significance. Locals consider them an integral part of shrine grounds and surrounding forests, cherishing them and protecting them from logging (Shinboku, 2022). As I witnessed these sacred trees during my walk, their profound presence and wide trunks wrapped in multi-colored scarves reminded me of the moving prayers shared by women at an international Authentic Movement retreat in Tuscany in 1992, which coincided with the outbreak of war in Bosnia.

As planes flew overhead toward Bosnia, some women's bodies began to tremble, their eyes drawn to the studio ceiling. Those with PTSD, from their own experiences or their parents' wartime trauma, quivered. One woman recalled her mother's stories of Nazi soldiers occupying their home in Holland—the sound of their boots pounding the streets still unsettled her.

Tension escalated as participants from Germany and Austria protested, saying they weren't alive during that time and weren't to blame for the actions of their ancestors. In contrast, those from Holland and other occupied countries felt painful memories resurfacing—of hunger, forced labor, reprisals, and the persecution of Jews. One Jewish woman expressed anxiety, asserting her right to feel fear, even though the trauma was from a generation ago. Despite their restraint, the group's tension intensified as people shared their feelings using "I feel" statements, acknowledging their experiences.

At lunch, group members ate mostly alone, with little of the usual socializing.

My assistant Margareta, who grew up in Germany, and I went for a walk. She asked, "What will you do?" I replied that I didn't know and spoke about how we all carry wounds—both individual and collective—and that along with the horrific atrocities some have faced, we all share some form of hardship, pain, and loss. I acknowledged the old tribal divisions that the warplanes above had stirred, and wondered about how we could create a space for safety and groundedness in our bodies, allowing us to explore these feelings together? After our walk, I meditated and rested, waking with a *dream of women wrapping each other in shawls.*

In the afternoon session, I acknowledged the devastating history we carried—the trauma of neighbors turning against each other. I reminded the group that our parents and grandparents often didn't have the opportunity to heal their wounds, and now it was our generation's turn to face and heal them. "Let's see how we can use our practice to work with what's here," I said, inviting them to return to their rooms for two items:

1 Something precious, like a favorite piece of jewelry or a flower, to place beside their witness cushion.
2 A scarf, sweater, or shawl to wrap around themselves.

The women eagerly returned with their items. I led a warm-up to open their bodies and ease their breathing. Then, I invited them to find a quiet space in the studio, close their eyes, and notice a place in their body that felt grounded and safe. After that, I invited them to identify a wounded area that needed protection and to wrap their scarf around this injured part. Then, they took their places on their cushions for the Long Circle, entering and leaving the space as they wished.

One by one, movers entered the circle, their wrapped bodies expressing a range of emotions—tears, rage, fear, tenderness—as the work deepened. Then, two women—"Silka" from Germany with a Christian background and "Ariel," a Jewish woman from New York—unexpectedly came together. Silka, who had lived on a Kibbutz to better understand Jewish culture, felt a deep connection to Ariel's background. With her eyes closed, Ariel crawled into Silka's lap, and Silka wrapped her in her skirt, singing a Hebrew lullaby as Ariel wept. The witnesses, many in tears themselves, looked on in awe.

When I rang the bell at the end of the movement session, Silka and Ariel opened their eyes, surprised to see each other. They shared a long, healing embrace. After this, the group's drawings transformed from stiff and constrained to fluid and colorful. During the talking circle, each person shared their experiences, marveling at the healing that had unfolded naturally. "You couldn't have planned that," one said. It was clear that something deeper, beyond personal histories, had worked its healing magic. Taking hands in the circle, we shared a moment of silence before leaving the studio to break bread together under the Tuscan sky.

The Dreaming Land

Marie-Louise von Franz, a protégé of Jung, taught that walking barefoot connects us to the spirit of the land, fostering dreams of ancestors, a practice known as *earthing*. Friends in their eighties have experienced this in their daily walks along the Northern California beaches. Similarly, Zulu healers (*Sangomas*) I met in South Africa emphasized that dreams extend beyond the individual psyche, offering messages for the community (Chodorow et al., 2009; Cumes, 1999; Stromsted, 2009; van Löben Sels, 2024). Such a dream message gave me guidance as I struggled with the decision about whether to accompany friends on an ocean journey to Greenland, given timing and expense. *In the dream a polar bear beckoned me to a fire on the ice, where I embraced her and began to see as if through her eyes. In that profound connection, I keenly perceived her reality: a beautiful world threatened by climate change.* I sensed that the bear was a conduit to my Norwegian grandmother, "Bestamor." This connection felt even more powerful when our ship paused in Newfoundland, the site of an eleventh-century Viking settlement she had written about in her book, *Ancient Pioneers: Early Connections between Scandinavia and the New World.* This journey intertwined our familial and ancestral legacies with the pressing issues of our time, echoing the calls of the land and its spirits.

Dreams often remind us of our deep connection to nature. Whether through the healing power of green spaces or the resonance of ancestral lands, the way we interact with the environment—both consciously and through our bodies—becomes a conduit for personal and collective healing.

Embodied Walking in the World

In these polarized times, C. G. Jung's insights into the psyche offer valuable guidance. As discussed earlier in Chapter 4, engaging with our shadow material reduces projections of unwanted traits onto others. Embodied practices, even in virtual settings during the pandemic and beyond, aid in trauma recovery and emotional expression, particularly for those who find it difficult to articulate their feelings or tend to intellectualize them.

It's also crucial for therapists, educators, parents, medical, and healthcare professionals to connect with their own embodiment in relation to others. We resonate body-to-body, often right-brain to right-brain, beneath the threshold of language. Our bodies can perceive the music of the other person—their tone of voice, the rhythm of their steps, the sound of their footfall, and their gestures—each as unique as fingerprints.

In uncertain times, engaging in simple spiritual practices can foster balance and resilience, while being attuned to our bodies helps us remain present and authentic. Somatic practices nourish equanimity, perseverance, and overall well-being, supporting both self-regulation and co-regulation in our relationships with one another and the greater life force.

As we navigate the present moment and look toward the future, many embodied practices, movement experiences, and mindfulness meditations can guide us. These include important work in diversity (Brewster, 2023; Caldwell & Leighton, 2018; Johnson, 2018; Johnson & Akomolafe, 2023; Kimbles, 2021; Menakem, 2018), ecology (Halprin & Kaplan, 2019; Kampe, McHugh, & Münker, 2021; Kiehl, 2016), and other essential areas for reflection and active engagement. A list of resources for conscious embodiment, particularly focusing on Authentic Movement and other forms of Dance/movement therapy, follows this chapter. Additionally, multiple sources of trauma-informed somatic work can be found online.

To conclude, I offer a mindful walking meditation that can be practiced daily or as needed. This version, shared by Valerie Brown—a Buddhist practitioner, lawyer, and activist—comes from her work with Thích Nhất Hạnh, a wise and compassionate Vietnamese monk and peace activist (Brown, 2024). In this tradition, walking is accompanied by a *gatha*—brief lines that focus the mind. The practice invites you to return to your true home—your body, breath, and surroundings—as you take each step along your path. As Valerie noted, "At Plum Village, there's a *gatha* for everything—brushing your teeth, turning on hot water, looking in the mirror" (Brown, 2024).

These reminders encourage gratitude for the present moment. For instance: *I have hot water. I have food brought by the Earth and others. I am surrounded by those who bring meaning to my life.* With moments like these to pause, we are reminded of gratitude for what life offers as we navigate uncertain times, and indeed all times. By repeating *gathas* like these, we relearn *I am here. I am reminded of the gift of life.*

As you walk—whether indoors or outdoors—feel your feet on the ground and take in your surroundings. Notice the path, particularly if it is uneven, and attune yourself to the nature and life around you. Walk slowly, matching your pace to your breath, for 10, 20 minutes, or longer. Here is the *gatha* Valerie shared, which you can adapt to suit your own sense of presence:

Listening, hearing, with each breath and step:

> I have arrived, I am home, in the here, in the now, I am solid, I am free. In the ultimate I dwell.
>
> Thích Nhất Hạnh, shared by Brown (2024)

As the poet Rumi opens the door to what's to come:

> The wind is pouring wine: Love
> Used to hide inside images. No more!
> The orchard hangs out its lanterns.
> The dead come stumbling by in shrouds.
> Nothing can stay bound or be imprisoned.
> You say, "End this poem here and
> Wait for what's next." I will. Poems
> Are rough notations for the music we are.
> Rumi (Barks, 2005, p. 27)

References

Barber, G. S. & Aaronson, S. T. (2022). The emerging field of psychedelic psychotherapy. *Current Psychiatry Reports*, *24*(10), 583–590. https://doi.org/10.1007/s11920-022-01363-y

Barks, C. (Trans.). (2005). The music we are. In *Rumi, The book of love: Poem of ecstasy and longing*. HarperSanFrancisco.

Brewster, F. (2023). *Race and the unconscious: An Africanist depth psychology perspective on dreaming*. Routledge.

Brown, V. (2024, November 15–17). Walking meditation. In Halifax, J., Solnit, R., Williams, T. T., Brown, V., & Figueres C. (Presenters), *Awakened action: Opening to all of life conference* (in person and online).

Caldwell, C. & Leighton, L. B. (2018). *Oppression and the body: Roots, resistance, and resolutions*. North Atlantic Books.

Cumes, D. (1999). *The spirit of healing: Venture into the wilderness to rediscover the healing force*. Llewellyn Publications.

Chodorow, J., Fay, C. G., Adorisio, A., Gerson, J., Mendez, M., & Stromsted, T. (2009, August 12). Moving journeys-embodied encounters: The living body in analysis [Presentation]. Pre-congress Day, XVIIth International Congress for Analytical Psychology, Capetown, South Africa.

Ellis, S., Bostian, C., Feng, W., Fischer, E., Schwartz, G., Eisen, K., Lean, M., Conlan, E., Ostacher, M., Aaronson, S., & Suppes, T. (2025). Single-dose psilocybin for U.S. military veterans with severe treatment-resistant depression: A first-in-kind open-label pilot study. *Journal of Affective Disorders*, *369*, 381–389. https://doi.org/10.1016/j.jad.2024.09.133

Halprin, A. & Kaplan, R. (2019). *Making dances that matter: Resources for community creativity*. Wesleyan University Press.

Johnson, D. H. (2018). *Diverse bodies, diverse practices: Toward an inclusive somatics*. North Atlantic Books.

Johnson, R. & Akomolafe, B. (2023). *Embodied activism: Engaging the body to cultivate liberation, justice, and authentic connection—A practical guide for transformative social change*. North Atlantic Books.

Kampe, T., McHugh, J., & Münker, K. (Eds.). (2021). Embodying eco-consciousness: Somatics, aesthetic practices and social action. *Journal of Dance & Somatic Practices*, *13*(1&2), Article 00063. https://doi.org/10.1386/jdsp_00063_2

Kiehl, T. (2016). *Facing climate change: An integrated path to the future*. Columbia University Press.

Kimbles, S. L. (2021). *Intergenerational complexes in analytical psychology*. Routledge.

Macy, J. & Johnstone, C. (2022). *Active hope: How to face the mess we're in with unexpected resilience and creative power* (Revised ed.). New World Library. (Original work published 2012.).

Menakem, R. (2018). *My grandmother's hands: Racialized trauma and the pathway to mending our hearts and bodies*. Central Recovery Press.

Reiff, C. M., Richman, E. E., Nemeroff, C. B., Carpenter, L. L., Widge, A. S., Rodriguez, C. I., Kalin, N. H., & McDonald, W. M. (2020). Psychedelics and psychedelic-assisted psychotherapy. *American Journal of Psychiatry*, *177*(5), 391–410. https://doi.org/10.1176/appi.ajp.2019.19010035

Selu, E. (2020). Authentic movement as a movement meditation practice: Support for immune mediated inflammatory disease. *International Body Psychotherapy Journal: The Art and Science of Somatic Praxis*, *19*(1), 55–63.

Shinboku. (2022, May). *Wikipedia*. Retrieved October 30, 2024, from https://en.wikipedia.org/wiki/Shinboku#:~:text=remove%20this%20message)-,(Learn%20how%20and%20when%20to%20remove%20this%20message),for%20the%20construction%20of%20shrines.

Stromsted, T. (2009) Healing soul's body: An introduction to Authentic Movement. In P. Bennett (Ed.), *Journeys & encounters: Clinical, communal, cultural, proceedings of the 17th International IAAP Congress for Analytical Psychology*. Daimon Verlag.

Tsetse, L. (2007). Moving the outer rim in: Authentic movement and nonviolence. In P. Pallaro (Ed.), *Authentic movement: Moving the body, moving the self, being moved: A collection of essays, volume two* (pp. 406–415). Jessica Kingsley Press.

Tsetse, L. & Sperry, W. (1998). The community long circle: Authentic movement as nonviolent community action. *Authentic Movement Journal*, *5*(3), 11–14.

van Löben Sels, R. (2024). *Dreamwork(ing): A primer*. Trout and Mountain Press.

Glossary

Active imagination A Jungian therapeutic method that involves engaging the unconscious through creative modalities such as art, writing, movement, music, or dialogue with inner figures or symbols. This process bridges the conscious and unconscious, facilitating the exploration and integration of hidden thoughts and emotions—fostering personal growth, creativity, and psychological wholeness.

Alchemy (a) A precursor to modern chemistry in which elemental substances were cooked at regulated temperatures to transform them. (b) A metaphorical process of inner transformation that involves confronting and working through unconscious material to refine consciousness—"turning lead to gold."

Affect The outward expression of a mood or emotional state, often observed through facial expressions, tone of voice, and body language.

Archetype A universal, innate symbol or pattern that represents fundamental human themes or experiences. Archetypes manifest in myths, dreams, and cultural narratives that shape behaviors and perceptions across individuals and societies.

Authentic Movement A subtle yet powerful therapeutic approach that bridges the conscious and unconscious through movement; a somatic practice involving a mover, a compassionate witness, and their relationship—used in psychotherapy, meditation, and creative expression.

Body armoring A protective physical response to emotional pain, trauma, or repressed feelings that involves the tightening or constricting of muscles and tissues.

BodySoul Rhythms® A somatic and expressive healing approach developed by Marion Woodman, Mary Hamilton, and Ann Skinner that integrates Jungian theory with dreamwork, movement, voice, mask-making, theater, and embodied wisdom to bridge the body, psyche, and soul.

Breathing Circles A group format in Authentic Movement where participants take turns with half the group moving and half witnessing, before switching roles at the sound of the bell—reflecting cycles of inhalation and exhalation, inner exploration and conscious attending.

Chthonic Unconscious, primal forces or energies that originate from deep within the psyche, often linked to repressed emotions, shadow aspects, or ancient, instinctual patterns.

Collective unconscious A universal layer of the unconscious mind made up of archetypes—primordial images, symbols, and psychic structures that are inherited from previous generations.

Complex A group of unconscious emotions, memories, or ideas that are organized around a specific theme or archetype, often influencing an individual's thoughts and behaviors.

Coniunctio The symbolic union of opposites that reflects the deep process of bringing together the conscious and unconscious aspects of the self, including reconciling polarities within the psyche, such as masculine and feminine energies, or the integration of the shadow.

Dissociative Identity Disorder (DID)   Typically a response to severe trauma, DID is a mental health disorder characterized by the presence of two or more distinct personality states or identities within a single individual.

DreamDancing®   An approach that integrates verbal dream sharing with embodied practices like movement, somatic awareness, art, voice, and writing to work with unconscious material.

Embodied Alchemy®   A therapeutic approach that integrates the body's unconscious material into the healing process, facilitating the transformation of uncomfortable, repressed experiences into meaningful experiences and embodied insight.

Formative psychology   A field within somatic psychotherapy developed by Stanley Keleman that explores how the body's structure and movement reflect emotional and psychological development.

Gestalt therapy   A humanistic approach to psychotherapy that focuses on unified patterns of thoughts, feelings, and behaviors (gestalts) and their relationship to the world, often using techniques like role-playing.

Individuation   The life-long self-realization process in which individuals integrate conscious and unconscious elements, leading to a more cohesive, authentic sense of self toward wholeness.

Long Circles   A ritual format in more experienced Authentic Movement groups in which movers enter and leave the circle in their own sense of time, with a designated number of witnesses to hold safe space.

Mirroring   A process of reflecting back the movements, feelings, or experiences of a person in an empathetic and nonjudgmental manner.

Naming Circles   A group format in Authentic Movement in which a single mover moves for a specified number of minutes in the center of the circle. When the bell rings they bring their movement to a close, and if they wish, make eye contact with group members who say their name before the next person enters for their turn in the center of the circle.

Organic Research Method   A qualitative approach that emphasizes in-depth exploration of individual cases, presented in a narrative form, with the goal of promoting transformation rather than offering generalizations or conclusions.

Percept language   A language practice fundamental to witnessing in Authentic Movement in which "I statements" are used to own one's own experience, reducing projections and fostering psychological and emotional safety for group members as they work with unconscious material.

prima materia   An alchemical term for the unconscious, unrefined aspects of the psyche, the "base matter" that has yet to be transformed.

Process-Oriented Psychology   A holistic therapy developed by Arnold Mindell, based on C.G. Jung's ideas and quantum physics. It focuses on exploring and integrating inner and outer experiences, such as dreams, body symptoms, altered states, synchronicities, relationships, group dynamics, shamanism, and nature.

Projection   The process of externalizing unwanted emotions and unconscious aspects of the self, such as the shadow, onto others or external situations.

re-call   A conscious listening practice in which witnesses reflect back words and phrases used by the mover, together with how the mover's expression moved the witness through body sensation, emotion, imagery, or memory.

self   The ego, or the part of the psyche that individuals are aware of and identify with.

Self   The central archetype symbolizing wholeness and the totality of the psyche, encompassing the conscious and unconscious aspects of an individual.

Somatic therapy   A therapeutic approach that focuses on the connection between the body and mind, exploring how emotions manifest in the body by using body awareness, movement, and physical touch.

Synchronicity   The seemingly coincidental yet meaningful alignment of an inner, psychic experience with an external, physical event.

Temenos   A sacred, contained space that symbolizes the wholeness of the psyche and its link to the collective unconscious, protecting the core of the personality from external forces during deep inner work.

Titration   The gradual, controlled exposure to intense emotions or experiences in order to safely process trauma, addressing one moment of an experience at a time to allow for deeper emotional processing without becoming flooded or retraumatized.

The shadow   The unconscious aspects of personality rejected by the ego—including both denied negatives and unacknowledged positives—that can influence behavior and perceptions until they are integrated into consciousness.

Transcendent function   The process through which opposites within the psyche, such as the conscious and unconscious, are integrated and reconciled.

Unconscious   The part of the psyche that contains thoughts, memories, emotions, and desires that are not currently within conscious awareness, yet influence behavior and experiences.

Unholy Trinity   Jung's Underworld Triad: The Shadow, the Body, and the Feminine, representing elements repressed by culture that emerge from deeper levels of the psyche in compensation for the masculine one-sidedness of the Holy Trinity.

Resources

Internet Resources

American Dance Therapy Association (ADTA)
https://www.adta.org/
Authentic Movement Facebook Resource Page (International offerings)
https://www.facebook.com/groups/48153313102/
Authentic Movement Institute Resource Archives
https://www.authenticmovementinstitute.com/authenticmovement
Center for Energetic Studies—Stanley Keleman's work
https://www.stanleykeleman.com/
European Association for Body Psychotherapy
https://eabp.org/
European Association Dance Movement Therapy (EADMT)
https://eadmt.com/
Integral Somatic Psychology Program
https://integralsomaticpsychology.com/isp-professional-training/
International Association for Analytical Psychology (IAAP)
https://iaap.org/
International Expressive Arts Therapy Association (IEATA)
https://www.ieata.org/
The International Somatic Movement Education and Therapy Association (ISMETA)
https://ismeta.org/
Jung Platform: Psychological & Spiritual Perspective Webinars
https://jungplatform.com/
The Marion Woodman Foundation & BodySoul Rhythms® Globally
https://www.mwfbodysoulrhythms.org/
https://www.mwfbodysoulrhythms.org/bodysoul-rhythms-globally
Somatic Experiencing International®
https://traumahealing.org/
Soul's Body® Center
https://authenticmovement-bodysoul.com/
United States Association for Body Psychotherapy
https://usabp.org/

Training Programs Internationally

Asociación Argentina de Psicología Analítica
https://www.apa.org.ar/

Art Therapy Italiana (Italy)
https://www.arttherapyit.org/

Authentic Movement Australasia (Oceania)
https://www.authenticmovementaustralasia.com/

Authentic Movement: Psychotherapeutic Modality Trainings (Russia)
https://irina-biryukova.tilda.ws/modalnost

Centro Internacional do Movimento Autêntico (International Center for Authentic Movement) (Brazil)
https://movimentoautentico.com/

Circles of Four: Discipline of Authentic Movement (International)
https://disciplineofauthenticmovement.com/

Contemplative Dance/Authentic Movement (USA)
https://www.contemplativedance.org/

Discipline of Authentic Movement (UK, International)
https://authenticmovementcirclesblog.wordpress.com/

Healing & Counseling Graduate School (South Korea)
https://hcg.ac.kr/bbs/content.php?co_id=030101

Inspirees Educational Group (China, International)
https://www.inspirees.com/trainers/
https://www.inspirees.com/authentic-movement/

Institute for Integrative Bodywork & Movement Therapy (UK, Lithuania, and Russia)
https://ibmt.co.uk/

Institute for Poetic Medicine
https://www.poeticmedicine.org/

International Dance/Movement Therapy Programs Listing
https://adta.memberclicks.net/international-programs

Korean Association of Expressive Arts Psychological Counseling (KAEPA)
http://www.keapa.or.kr

Korean Dance Therapy Association (KDTA)
http://www.kdmta.org/en/kdta/introduce01.php

Naropa Graduate School of Counseling (USA)
https://www.naropa.edu/academics/schools-centers/graduate-school-of-counseling/

Queen Margaret University, Edinburgh (Dance Movement Psychotherapy) (Scotland)
https://www.studyinuk.global/courses/msc-dance-movement-psychotherapy

Seoul Women's University, Dance/Movement Therapy Programs
https://www.swu.ac.kr/englishindex.do

Somatic Academy Berlin (Somatische Akademie Berlin) (Germany)
https://www.somatische-akademie.de/en/home

South African National Arts Therapies Association (South Africa)
https://sanata.org/
Studio for Movement Arts & Therapies (India)
https://smartmove.co.in/
Tamalpa Institute (Expressive Arts Therapy; US & International)
https://www.tamalpa.org/

Journals

American Journal of Dance Therapy
https://www.adta.org/american-journal-of-dance-therapy
The Arts in Psychotherapy Journal
https://www.sciencedirect.com/journal/the-arts-in-psychotherapy
Art Therapy: Journal of the American Art Therapy Association (AATA)
https://arttherapy.org/blog-art-therapy-journal-covid-19-resources/
Body, Movement and Dance in Psychotherapy: An International Journal for Theory, Research and Practice
https://www.tandfonline.com/journals/tbmd20
Creative Arts in Education and Therapy (CAET; Eastern, Western, & Global Perspectives)
https://www.iacaet.org/caet-journal/
Drama Therapy Review
https://www.nadta.org/drama-therapy-review--dtr-
International Body Psychotherapy Journal: The Art and Science of Somatic Praxis
https://www.ibpj.org/
Journal of Analytical Psychology
https://onlinelibrary.wiley.com/journal/14685922
Journal of Dance & Somatic Practices
https://intellectdiscover.com/content/journals/jdsp
Journal of Music Therapy (American Music Therapy Association)
https://www.musictherapy.org/research/pubs/
Journal of Music Therapy (Oxford Academic Research)
https://academic.oup.com/jmt
Journal of Poetry Therapy
https://poetrytherapy.org/Journal-of-Poetry-Therapy
Jung Journal: Culture & Psyche
https://www.tandfonline.com/journals/ujun20
Somatics Magazine—Journal of the Bodily Arts & Sciences
http://www.somaticsed.com/magJournal.html

Index

Note: – *Italicized* page references refer to figures.